Spasticity and Muscle Stiffness

Preeti Raghavan
Editor

Spasticity and Muscle Stiffness

Restoring Form and Function

Springer

Editor
Preeti Raghavan
Departments of Physical Medicine
and Rehabilitation and Neurology
The Johns Hopkins University School of Medicine
Baltimore, MD, USA

ISBN 978-3-030-96899-1 ISBN 978-3-030-96900-4 (eBook)
https://doi.org/10.1007/978-3-030-96900-4

This Springer imprint is published by the registered company Springer Nature Switzerland AG
The registered company address is: Gewerbestrasse 11, 6330 Cham, Switzerland

... Behold the outward moving frame,
Its living marbles jointed strong
With glistening band and silvery thong,
And linked to reason's guiding reins
By myriad rings in trembling chains,
Each graven with the threaded zone
Which claims it as the master's own.

—Oliver Wendell Holmes, The Living Temple

To Dr. Robert Stern, for his everlasting inspiration,
and to my family, for sharing in my joy of discovery.

Foreword

I had the privilege of being part of the gait and biomechanics laboratory of Dr. Justus F. Lehmann at the University of Washington in Seattle, where it became clear that there was a viscous and elastic component to spasticity which we sought to understand. With the help of mechanical engineers at the University of Washington, we developed a lower limb spasticity measurement system with which we could tease out the viscous stiffness from the elastic stiffness and thereby assess the effect of various interventions.[1] However, significant gaps remain in our understanding and treatments of the components of spasticity. This long-needed book seeks to address those gaps and will be of great value to those of us who participate in the management of patients with spasticity.

The first part of the book respectfully describes the historical definitions of spasticity as it proceeds to newer definitions that account for more of the developing data sets. The distinction between spasticity and spastic movement disorder takes the process to the next level. In spastic paresis, the neural and non-neural components are teased apart by a systematic assessment of upper and lower limbs as well as the various types of resistance during active and passive movement. The forms essential to this assessment are supplied for the convenience of the reader. A quantitative assessment of the resistance to passive joint motion in chronic stroke survivors shows how the neural and non-neural elements may be disrupted together, which may account for the variance in response after injections of botulinum toxin. The challenges of managing children with spastic cerebral palsy are pointed out; growth must be facilitated despite the structural changes that occur. These changes are, in several ways, different from those in adults.

The reader is prompted to read the important chapter on mechanisms of development of passive mechanical muscle stiffness by the introductory question: "spastic muscles are weaker, shorter, and stiffer…how do they get that way?" A description of the hyaluronan hypothesis of muscle stiffness alone would be worth careful reading of this chapter. All the preceding would be intellectually satisfying but perhaps not practical without knowledge of the symptomatic and functional effects of spastic paresis. The extensive descriptions and illustrations in this chapter on structural

[1] Lehmann JF, et al. Spasticity: quantitative measurements as a basis for assessing effectiveness of therapeutic intervention. *Arch Phys Med Rehabil.* 70 (1): 6–15, 1989.

effects are very helpful to the clinician. The order of intervention becomes apparent by studying these photos.

In the second part of the book, the framework for treatment logically follows the preceding chapters. Medical exacerbation of spasticity will have been observed by clinicians who specialize in management of spinal cord injury, for example. But it is important for all clinicians to be alert to these occurrences and manage them first, if possible. The remaining chapters on oral spasmolytics, intrathecal baclofen, botulinum toxin injections for focal muscle overactivity, and hyaluronidase injections for focal muscle stiffness would justify a book on their own; but I'm glad they are included in this book. Last but certainly not least, the chapter on emerging non-pharmacologic therapies, such as electrical stimulation, is a *tour de force* that describes the studies assessing these interventions in various conditions.

The reader will benefit by reading this superb book more than once. I will refer to it again and again.

Barbara J. deLateur
The Johns Hopkins University School of Medicine
Baltimore, MD, USA

Preface

Docendo discitur: by learning you will teach; by teaching you will learn.
—Latin Proverb

The word "movement" conjures up images of fluid motion, executed with grace, precision, and power. The human form is an engineering marvel and, as D'Arcy Thompson wrote in his treatise *On Growth and Form*, "living forms are diagrams of the forces that hold them together." In contrast, the word "spastic" suggests choppy, erratic, or uncontrolled movement, and "stiff" suggests rigid, inflexible movement, both of which lead to a breakdown in its form and function.

In my career of over 20 years, I have encountered individuals with "spasticity and/or muscle stiffness" almost daily either in clinical practice or in my research lab where we study motor recovery after neurologic injury. It is a vexing problem that causes significant disability and interferes with rehabilitation and recovery. In fact, "spasticity" is often used as a catch-all term whose definition continues to evolve.[1] Although "spasticity" is a hallmark of injury to the central nervous system (CNS), we now know that it encompasses both neural *and* non-neural changes in skeletal muscles that affect movement. How do these neural and non-neural components develop, evolve, and manifest into the movement disorder that affects posture, motor control, function, and recovery? Indeed, paraphrasing Winston Churchill, spasticity is a riddle, wrapped in a mystery, inside an enigma. Is there a key to solving this mysterious and vexing riddle?

During the winter of 2013–2014, my colleagues and I were writing a review article about the changes in muscle architecture in individuals with spasticity to try to understand this enigmatic problem.[2] Around the same time, my son was doing an experiment for an upcoming science fair. The experiment used Oobleck – a mixture of cornstarch and water. Oobleck is popular with kids because it can behave both like a liquid and a solid. You can drop things into it slowly, but when it is stirred quickly, it can act like a solid and things no longer fall through it. It has paradoxical properties – just like the changes in resistance I observed in my patients when moving their joints at different speeds! At first the connection between Oobleck and

---

[1] See Chap. 1.

[2] Stecco A, Stecco C, Raghavan P. Peripheral mechanisms of spasticity and treatment implications. *Curr Phys Med Rehabil Rep*, 2014. https://doi.org/10.1007/s40141-014-0052-3

spasticity was not obvious. But the more I learned about the architecture of muscle and the chemical and physical interactions that take place between the muscle fibers and their extracellular matrix, the more relevant the properties of Oobleck became. A clearer understanding of spasticity and muscle stiffness, and how they differ, began to emerge. Muscle function is beautifully illustrated by Alexander Tsiaras and described by Barry Werth in *The Architecture and Design of Man and Woman*: "Bundled into ropelike cables equipped with armlike cross-bridges that bend, detach, straighten, and then repeat the process, billions of muscle cells hauling in unison can raise a finger, or an arm." Now imagine what would happen if these ropelike cables were stuck to one another? Clearly, both the form and function of the muscles would be affected.

This book arose out of an attempt to reconcile what we already know about spasticity – directly from the experts who have studied its many facets – and new information we are gleaning about muscle stiffness. It is as much an attempt to learn as it is to teach and is guided by two objectives. The first is to explain the cascade of neural and non-neural changes that influence both the architecture of muscle, and its effects on muscle function and movement. The second is to help practitioners use this information and the new understanding of muscle spasticity and stiffness to develop a framework for treatment. The chapters cover many key aspects of pathophysiology, assessment, and treatment, but they are by no means exhaustive. Furthermore, movement therapies, such as physical and occupational therapy strategies, are not described in detail, nor are neurolytic treatments such as nerve blocks using anesthetics, alcohol and phenol, or surgical techniques for the treatment of spasticity and contracture. The choice and order of topics aim to create a logical progression of ideas.

Part I of the book deals with the pathophysiology and assessment of spasticity and muscle stiffness. The goal here is to trace our collective understanding from the earliest descriptions of the upper motor neuron syndrome by John Hughlings Jackson as consisting of a "duality of symptoms" to its neurological and neurophysiological underpinnings, functional consequences, clinical and quantitative assessment, and eventually to changes in structure of the muscle and its effects on posture, movement, and function. Chapter 1 outlines the neural basis of spasticity, how it is invariably accompanied by some degree of weakness or paresis among other symptoms (hence the term "spastic paresis"), and its consequences on the mono-synaptic stretch reflex. Chapter 2 discusses how the neural dysfunction also affects afferent and polysynaptic reflex pathways and leads to an inability to adapt muscle activity during movement. These neural changes in combination with secondary non-neural changes in muscles contribute to spastic movement disorder. Chapter 3 describes a five-step clinical assessment for the syndrome of spastic paresis which includes an assessment of function and the neural and non-neural resistance encountered during passive and active movements. Chapter 4 demonstrates the pitfalls in our perception of resistance when examined through a quantitative lens. Chapter 5 describes the structure of muscle, how muscle force generating capacity is intricately associated with muscle length, which in turn is associated with changes in extracellular matrix (ECM) content and passive mechanical stiffness of muscle fibers and bundles in contracture. Chapter 6 attempts to bridge the gaps between muscle paresis, spasticity, stiffness, and contracture. It explains the hyaluronan hypothesis – how both paresis and spasticity lead to the accumulation and aggregation of hyaluronan in muscle ECM which leads to stiffness and triggers a cascade of biochemical events which, if untreated, eventually lead to fibrosis and muscle contracture. Chapter 7 concludes Part I by detailing the symptomatic and functional after-effects of the neural and non-neural changes on both muscle form and function in the upper and lower limbs that necessitate treatment.

Part II of the book explains the rationale, framework, considerations, and evidence for various treatments for both spasticity and muscle stiffness, although it is not an exhaustive compilation of all available treatments. Chapter 8 provides a brief overview of a framework for the treatment of spasticity and muscle stiffness considering the new information presented in Part I. Chapter 9 explains the basis for the exacerbation of spasticity by illness, infection, and/or discomfort from various causes and how they can be addressed. Chapter 10 discusses the various oral medications used and studied in the treatment of spasticity as well as their mechanisms of action and side effects. Chapter 11 details the use of intrathecal baclofen therapy for individuals with poorly controlled spasticity, including the selection of patients, trialing of the treatment and indicators of success, considerations on dosing, and troubleshooting. Chapter 12 describes the use of botulinum toxin injections to treat focal muscle overactivity as well as their mechanisms of action and guidelines for use. Chapter 13 describes the use of hyaluronidase injections to treat focal muscle stiffness, their mechanisms of action, and the preliminary evidence on their efficacy. Chapter 14 concludes Part II by describing promising emerging non-pharmacologic treatments and the available evidence on their efficacy.

I am grateful to my many colleagues who have contributed to this book and have been patient and understanding while it took its present form. I want to thank them for their knowledge, wisdom, and the many discussions that have shaped the writing of this book. I also want to acknowledge the support of my colleagues at New York University and at Johns Hopkins University who provided clarity to several ideas presented here. I would like to especially remember Dr. Robert Stern, who described the role of hyaluronan in many diseases, and whose lab sequenced the gene for the human recombinant hyaluronidase commercially available today. I was fortunate to get to know him before he passed away in 2017. He took a personal interest in helping me understand the biology of hyaluronan and its possible role in muscle stiffness. I will never forget the wonderful dinner we had together with my family – his curiosity about everything he encounters is most memorable. Most importantly, I want to thank my family – my husband, for being a fountain of knowledge and my strongest support through all situations, and our two sons, who have each in their own way contributed to my understanding, whether through their science experiments or asking questions. I am also grateful to my sister and her family for their support, to my father-in-law who never tired of listening and providing encouragement, and to my mother, my constant inspiration and cheerleader.

Baltimore, MD, USA Preeti Raghavan

Contents

Contributors

Marjolaine Baude, MD BIOTN Research Unit, UPEC University, Créteil, France

Mary K. Cowman, PhD Tandon School of Engineering, Grossman School of Medicine, New York University, New York, NY, USA

Sudarshan Dayanidhi, PT, PhD Biologics Lab, Shirley Ryan AbilityLab, Chicago, IL, USA

Joanne Delgado, MD Department of Physical Medicine and Rehabilitation, Memorial Physician Group at Memorial Healthcare System, Hollywood, FL, USA

Volker Dietz, MD, FRCP Spinal Cord Injury Center, University Hospital Balgrist, Zürich, Switzerland

Alberto Esquenazi, MD Thomas Jefferson University, Philadelphia, PA, USA

Gait and Motion Analysis Laboratory, MossRehab, Elkins Park, PA, USA

Jourdan K. Ewoldt, MS Department of Mechanical Engineering, Boston University, Boston, MA, USA

Steven R. Flanagan, MD Department of Rehabilitation Medicine, NYU Grossman School of Medicine, New York, NY, USA

Gerard E. Francisco, MD McGovern Medical School, The University of Texas Health Science Center at Houston, Department of Physical Medicine and Rehabilitation, Houston, TX, USA

TIRR Memorial Hermann Hospital, Houston, TX, USA

Mouna Ghedira, PhD Service de Rééducation Neurolocomotrice, CHU Henri Mondor, Créteil, France

Alexandra Gordon, BS Albert Einstein College of Medicine, Bronx, NY, USA

Jean-Michel Gracies, MD, PhD Service de Rééducation Neurolocomotrice, CHU Henri Mondor, Créteil, France

Cynthia Hung, MD Department of Rehabilitation Medicine, NYU Grossman School of Medicine, New York, NY, USA

Isaac Hernandez Jimenez, MD Department of Physical Medicine and Rehabilitation, McGovern Medical School, The University of Texas Health Science Center at Houston, Houston, TX, USA

Yaowaree Leavell, MD Department of Neurology, Division of Neuromuscular Medicine, Oregon Health and Science University, New York, NY, USA

Sheng Li, MD, PhD McGovern Medical School, The University of Texas Health Science Center at Houston, Department of Physical Medicine and Rehabilitation, Houston, TX, USA

TIRR Memorial Hermann Hospital, Houston, TX, USA

Elaine Magat, MD Department of Physical Medicine and Rehabilitation, McGovern Medical School, The University of Texas Health Science Center at Houston, Houston, TX, USA

Manuel F. Mas, MD University of Puerto Rico, School of Medicine, Department of Physical Medicine, Rehabilitation and Sports Medicine, San Juan, PR, USA

McGovern Medical School, The University of Texas Health Science Center at Houston, Department of Physical Medicine and Rehabilitation, Houston, TX, USA

TIRR Memorial Hermann Hospital, Houston, TX, USA

Nathaniel H. Mayer, MD Lewis Katz School of Medicine at Temple University, Philadelphia, PA, USA

Motor Control Analysis Laboratory, MossRehab, Elkins Park, PA, USA

Rajiv Menon, PhD Bernard and Irene Schwartz Center for Biomedical Imaging, NYU Grossman School of Medicine, New York, NY, USA

Robert Petrucelli, MD Department of Rehabilitation Medicine, NYU Grossman School of Medicine, New York, NY, USA

Maud Pradines Service de Rééducation Neurolocomotrice, CHU Henri Mondor, Créteil, France

Preeti Raghavan, MBBS Departments of Physical Medicine and Rehabilitation and Neurology, The Johns Hopkins University School of Medicine, Baltimore, MD, USA

Mark Ragucci, DO Department of Rehabilitation Medicine, NYU Grossman School of Medicine, New York, NY, USA

Ravinder Regatte, PhD Bernard and Irene Schwartz Center for Biomedical Imaging, NYU Grossman School of Medicine, New York, NY, USA

Ryan Roemmich, PhD Department of Physical Medicine and Rehabilitation, Johns Hopkins University School of Medicine, Baltimore, MD, USA

Haresh Sampathkumar, MD PAM Health Rehabilitation Hospital of Dover, Dover, DE, USA

Michael Saulino, MD, PhD Cooper University Health Care, Camden, NJ, USA

Department of Physical Medicine and Rehabiliation, Cooper Medical School of Rowan University, Camden, NJ, USA

David M. Simpson, MD Department of Neurology, Icahn School of Medicine at Mount Sinai, New York, NY, USA

Antonio Stecco, MD, PhD Rusk Rehabilitation, NYU Grossman School of Medicine, New York, NY, USA

Nina L. Suresh, PhD Department of Physical Medicine and Rehabilitation, Shirley Ryan Ability Lab, Chicago, IL, USA

Elina Zakin, MD Department of Neurology, Division of Neuromuscular Medicine, NYU Grossman School of Medicine, New York, NY, USA

Part I

Pathophysiology and Assessment

Neural Basis of Spasticity

1

Preeti Raghavan

...dissolution is not only a "taking off" of the higher but is at the very same time a "letting go" of the lower.
– John Hughlings Jackson,
Croonian lectures, Royal College of Physicians, London, 1884.

- Spasticity arises after a neurological injury; hence it clearly has a neural basis. However, it has many definitions and manifestations, and the underlying mechanisms are still not clearly understood.
- This chapter reviews the definitions of spasticity, the time course of its development, and the types of neural injury that may cause it by disinhibiting inhibitory brainstem pathways as well as by facilitating excitatory brainstem pathways, that result in an excitatory-inhibitory imbalance in the spinal cord interneuronal network.
- The descending pathways modulate persistent inward currents via serotonin and norepinephrine, which provide a low-level depolarizing synaptic drive to the resting motoneuron pool resulting in increased afferent sensitivity and can account for hyperreflexia.
- However, the abnormal brainstem descending inputs and persistent inward currents cannot fully account for other spasticity-related motor impairments, such as muscle stiffness.

P. Raghavan (✉)
Departments of Physical Medicine and Rehabilitation and Neurology, The Johns Hopkins University School of Medicine, Baltimore, MD, USA
e-mail: praghavan@jhmi.edu

P. Raghavan (ed.), *Spasticity and Muscle Stiffness*,
https://doi.org/10.1007/978-3-030-96900-4_1

Definition of Spasticity

It is well-known that damage to the descending motor pathways anywhere from the cerebral cortex to the lower end of the spinal cord can give rise to a set of symptoms called the upper motor neuron syndrome. John Hughlings Jackson observed in the late nineteenth century that neural injury often leads to dual symptomatology. For example in hemiplegia, in addition to loss of movement (negative symptoms), excess activity also develops (positive symptoms) such as increased tendon reflexes and excess muscle tone, which he attributed to the "release" of the lower centers from control by the damaged higher centers that are "taken-off" [1]. The idea of "release" phenomena characterizing the upper motor neuron syndrome continues to inform our understanding of spasticity.

In fact, Lance and colleagues defined spasticity at a consensus symposium in 1980 [2] as:

> a motor disorder characterized by a velocity-dependent increase in tonic stretch reflexes with exaggerated tendon jerks, resulting from hyperexcitability of the stretch reflex as one component of the upper motor neuron syndrome.

Subsequently, Pandyan et al. [3] attempted to validate Lance's definition by reviewing the literature since, and concluded that spasticity is not a pure motor disorder and that it does not result exclusively from hyperexcitability of the stretch reflex. The changes in resistance to imposed passive movement were also not found to be uniquely related to increased muscle activity, and the phenomenon of velocity dependence was not exclusive to stretch reflex hyperexcitability. Hence spasticity was redefined as:

> disordered sensorimotor control, resulting from an upper motor neuron lesion, presenting as intermittent or sustained involuntary activation of muscles.

This definition suggests that spasticity is a disorder of sensorimotor control, rather than a motor disorder alone. Furthermore, it suggests that spasticity presents as muscle overactivity, rather than solely as stretch reflex hyperexcitability, which had major implications for treatment that was then directed to reducing muscle overactivity.

A more recent definition of spasticity proposed by Li et al. [4] is even broader, and specifies a neuroanatomical substrate for the hyperexcitability, rather than the release of control by the higher centers as alluded to by Hughlings Jackson. By this definition, spasticity is:

> manifested as velocity- and muscle length–dependent increase in resistance to externally imposed muscle stretch. It results from hyperexcitable descending excitatory brainstem pathways and from the resultant exaggerated stretch reflex responses. Other related motor impairments, including abnormal synergies, inappropriate muscle activation, and anomalous muscle coactivation, coexist with spasticity and share similar pathophysiological origins.

Abnormal excitability of the stretch reflex is still the central mechanism as per this latest definition of spasticity. However, it also attributes spasticity-related motor impairments to the excitatory brainstem pathways.

Time Course of the Development of Spasticity

Although hyperreflexia is central to defining spasticity, several studies have shown nonreflex-related resistance to movement in patients with "spasticity" [5–7]. Furthermore, although hyperreflexia is elicited relatively early after injury, the resistance to passive movement measured using the Modified Ashworth Scale (MAS), which is commonly used to assess spasticity clinically, tends to increase in prevalence over the ensuing weeks and months [8–10]. Even mild hyperreflexia early on is an important predictor of severe spasticity and increased resistance to passive movement later [11, 12], suggesting that hyperreflexia may trigger a cascade of events that lead to a build up of the resistance to movement. In a retrospective study of chronic stroke survivors with moderate-to-severe upper limb motor impairment, 97% of subjects demonstrated increased resistance to passive movement which was associated with impaired motor control [13]. Thus, it is important to understand the characteristics of the neurologic injury that lead to the development of spasticity and the ensuing resistance to movement to initiate measures for prevention and early treatment. Untreated, spasticity leads to fatigue, pain, sleep problems, and urinary dysfunction among others, affecting physical health [14], and restricting activities of daily living (ADL) and mobility that contribute to disability and increased health care costs [15, 16].

What Types of Neural Injury Lead to the Development of Spasticity?

Several recent studies have shown a positive correlation between spasticity and the overall degree of injury to the sensorimotor system – the greater the lesion volume and severity of injury, the greater the likelihood of developing spasticity [17]. However, small lesions involving specific regions of the brain such as the putamen, internal (posterior limb) and external capsule, thalamus, and insula, which are involved in sensorimotor processing, have also shown to be correlated with the degree of spasticity [18]. Note that in these studies, the resistance to passive movement on the MAS, which is not specific to the neural component, was used to measure spasticity (see Chaps. 3 and 4). More recently, the velocity-dependent neural component of hand spasticity was shown to be related to lesion load of the corticospinal tract (CST), after controlling for motor impairment and lesion volume [11].

To fully comprehend the effect of neural injury, especially given the strong correlation between motor impairment and spasticity reported recently [13], it is helpful to review the origin and termination of the CST, which modulates brain stem and spinal cord activity. The CST originates from a wide range of cortical areas having different functions, including the primary motor cortex (M1) which is involved in the execution of movement, the dorsal (PMd) and ventral (PMv) premotor areas involved in the sensory guidance of movement, the supplementary motor area (SMA) involved in planning and coordination of internally generated movement sequences, the cingulate motor areas involved in emotional aspects of voluntary movement, including changes in autonomic function [19], and corticospinal projections from the parietal lobe including the primary somatosensory cortex, posterior parietal cortex, and parietal operculum (SII) [20, 21].

The termination of the corticospinal projections within the spinal gray matter is also varied (Fig. 1.1) [22–24]. Projections from the somatosensory cortex terminate

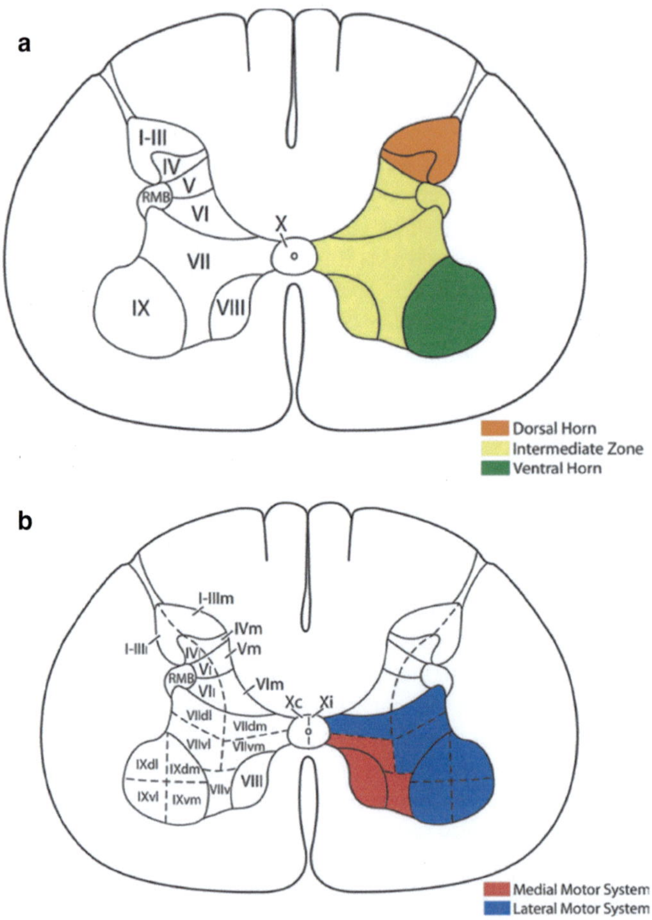

Fig. 1.1 Schematic diagram of the general anatomical organization of the spinal cord adapted from Kuypers [23]. (**a**) The ventral horn consists of lamina IX (green), the intermediate zone laminae V, VI, VII, VIII, and the reticulated marginal border (RMB) (yellow), and the dorsal horn laminae I–III and IV (orange). (**b**) The Rexed laminae are further subdivided into 20 subdivisions in each half of the spinal cord. The blue shaded regions of laminae VII and IX represent spinal components of Kuypers "lateral motor system" [24]. The red shaded region of lamina VII and lamina VIII constitute parts of his "medial motor system". (From Morecraft et al. [22], with permission)

mainly in the more dorsal parts of the spinal gray matter (Rexed laminae I–V) and are involved in the descending control of sensory afferent input. These projections are an important source of presynaptic inhibition of primary sensory afferent fibers [25, 26], and are responsible for sensory reafference or gating of inputs arising from one's own movement [27, 28]. Projections from M1 target most areas of the intermediate zone of the spinal cord gray matter (Rexed lamina VII). These are the indirect oligosynaptic projections that mediate corticospinal input to motor neurons via a premotoneuronal network [22]. Inputs to the premotoneuronal network originate in a variety of descending motor pathways, in ascending and descending propriospinal pathways, in local segmental interneurons, as well as in sensory afferent inputs from the periphery. Integration of information in this network is critical to achieve the precise timing and balance of activity in the motoneuron pool, contributing to highly flexible movement responses in the healthy state [29]. Recent evidence suggests that corticospinal projections from the dorsal and ventral premotor areas terminate in laminae VII and VIII, and govern proximal upper limb musculature involved in postural stabilization and control of the proximal limb during reaching and grasping through the indirect oligosynaptic neural networks [30]. These projections, as well as the corticospinal projections from the leg area of M1 to motoneurons of more proximal leg muscles, are bilateral [30, 31]. Injury to these pathways can account for increased spasticity when standing [32, 33].

In contrast, direct cortico-motoneuronal connections in the ventral horn (Rexed lamina IX) originate from both M1 and SMA, but the corticospinal projections from M1 to the hand muscle motor nuclei are denser than those from the SMA [34]. In humans, fast-conducting direct mono-synaptic cortico-motoneuronal connections have been found to be responsible for precision grasp, but not power grasp [35, 36]. Selective lesions of the CST may therefore only impede individuated finger movements as has been shown in monkeys [37].

Thus, injury to the CST at its origin, especially when it involves both sensory and motor areas [38, 39], along its path, or at the level of the spinal cord, regardless of etiology leads to widespread consequences depending on the corticospinal projections affected and their particular function. The function of the CST reflects its origins and terminations and includes: (1) descending control of afferent inputs, including nociception [25, 26]; (2) selection, gating, and gain control of spinal reflexes [40]; (3) direct and indirect excitation of motoneurons [41, 42]; (4) inhibition of motoneurons [43, 44]; (5) autonomic control [45]; (6) long-term plasticity of spinal cord circuits [46]; and (7) trophic functions during development [47, 48]. Individuals who present with spasticity invariably present with symptoms reflecting additional corticospinal dysfunction depending on the pathways affected.

How Does Injury to the Corticospinal Tract Lead to Spasticity?

In 1946, Magoun and Rhines found an area in the brainstem, the ventromedial medullary reticular formation, which when stimulated could inhibit any type of muscle activity, including stretch reflex activity. This region receives facilitatory influences from the premotor cortex [49]. Extensive lesions involving premotor and supplementary motor areas, and/or their projections were found to inhibit the medullary reticular formation, leading to release or disinhibition of stretch reflex activity, causing hyperreflexia [50]. The inhibitory influences from the medullary reticular formation are transmitted to the spinal cord by the dorsal reticulospinal tract (RST), which runs very close to the lateral corticospinal tract. Stimulation of the dorsal RST in decerebrate cats was also shown to inhibit excitability in the spinal interneurons [51, 52]. Section of the dorsal half of the lateral funiculus, which contains the dorsal RST in humans, to treat parkinsonism was also followed by spasticity [53]. This lent further support to the idea that the disruption of cortical inputs to the brainstem, specifically injury to cortico-reticulospinal fibers, and/or damage to the dorsal RST, releases the spinal neural network from inhibitory control causing an imbalance between excitatory and inhibitory inputs [54, 55].

While disinhibition can explain hyperreflexia that is seen soon after injury, the question of what leads to the development of increased resistance to passive movement, abnormal synergies, inappropriate muscle activation, and anomalous muscle coactivation remains. One possibility is that the imbalanced neural excitability becomes amplified through increased facilitatory influences involving alternative brainstem control pathways. Magoun and Rhines also found that stimulation of the reticular formation of the dorsal brain stem (pontine reticular formation) can facilitate or exaggerate any type of muscle activity, including the stretch reflexes [49]. The facilitatory influences from the pontine reticular formation are transmitted to the spinal cord by the medial RST, which along with the vestibulospinal tract (VST) provides excitatory input to the spinal neural network. The VST is thought to play a minor role, as section of the anterior funiculus of the cord to relieve hypertonia resulted in only transient reduction in spasticity [56]. In contrast, extensive unilateral or bilateral anterior cordotomy, which is likely to have destroyed both the VST and the medial RST, was followed by a dramatic reduction in spasticity [57].

Recent studies in monkeys demonstrate that the projections from nonprimary motor cortices (PM and SMA) are denser and end mainly ipsilaterally in the pontine reticular formation, whereas the projections from the primary motor cortex (M1) are less dense and end contralaterally [58]. The importance of the denser ipsilateral projections from the uninjured PM and SMA is that these projections are thought to compensate for injury to the contralateral CST and enable at least partial recovery of motor function in monkeys [59–62], and in humans with mild impairment [63–68]. However, severely impaired individuals also show increased activation of the ipsilesional premotor regions [69–71] associated with compensatory movement strategies [72–74]. Hence it is hypothesized that the motor overflow from the ipsilesional to the impaired side contributes to increased spasticity and disordered motor control [75]. Indirect support for this hypothesis was noted in an imaging study which showed strong correlation of synergistic arm movements with the functional reorganization in the reticulospinal pathways suggesting a contributory role in the development of compensatory motor strategies [76]. Hence it is suggested that spasticity and the related motor impairments are exacerbated by the ipsilateral excitatory contribution from the medial RST to the spinal neural network as shown by the dashed line in Fig. 1.2 [77].

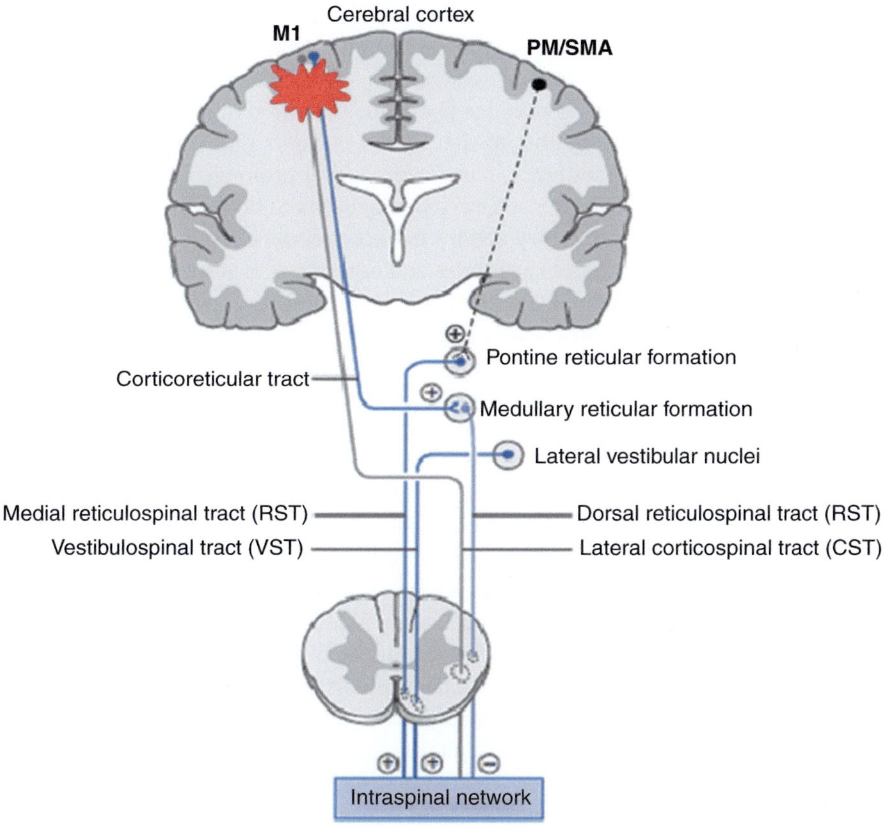

Fig. 1.2 Schematic diagram illustrating the descending pathways contributing to the medial reticulospinal tract in the pathophysiology of spasticity. The pontine reticular formation receives cortical input primarily from the ipsilateral premotor (PM) cortex and supplementary motor area (SMA), and via the medial reticulospinal tract (RST) provides excitatory descending input to the spinal circuitry. The medullary reticular formation receives cortical input primarily from the contralateral primary motor cortex (M1), and via the dorsal RST provides inhibitory descending inputs to the spinal circuitry. Injury to the corticospinal tract (indicated in red) leads to reduced inhibition of the spinal circuitry via the dorsal RST causing an excitatory-inhibitory imbalance. In addition, it is proposed that the contribution of the contralesional hemisphere to the excitatory medial RST becomes gradually upregulated and unopposed further increasing spinal hyperexcitability. (+) excitatory; (–) inhibitory. (From Li et al. [77], with permission (open access))

Consequences of Excitatory-Inhibitory Imbalance in Spinal Circuitry

The descending RST inputs are primarily mediated by the monoamines serotonin (5-HT) and norepinephrine (NE), which have neuromodulatory effects that correlate with the level of behavioral arousal and/or the behavioral state, for example when awake and in fight or flight situations [78]. These neuromodulatory effects, in turn, have been shown to be mediated via persistent inward currents (PIC). A PIC is a depolarizing current generated by voltage-sensitive channels that stay open as long as the membrane potential remains above the threshold of activation. This persistence stands in marked contrast to the inward currents that generate the action potential, which inactivate within 1–2 ms, even during prolonged membrane depolarization [79]. PICs increase the sensitivity of neurons to both excitation and inhibition – they have strong excitatory actions on motoneurons involved in tonic motor activity, for example in antigravity muscles and other muscle groups associated with gross motor activity. These neuromodulatory inputs have been shown to be critical for the production of high forces and have a major influence on input-output behavior of the whole system [80, 81]. Turning off these sustained outputs also requires considerably large inhibitory inputs [82]. In contrast to their strong excitatory actions on motoneurons, monoamines inhibit many of the synaptic inputs to interneurons [78]. This inhibition is largely presynaptic and focused on sensory afferents that mediate both high- and low-threshold cutaneous inputs [83], and high-threshold muscle afferents [84]. The differential role of monoaminergic actions on motoneurons and interneurons occurs via their action on different receptor subtypes – facilitation of PICs in motoneurons appears to occur via 5HT2 and NE alpha 1 receptors, whereas inhibition occurs via 5HT1b/d and NE alpha 2 receptors [85]. In effect, monoamines increase the sensitivity of motoneurons to both excitation and inhibition in a movement-dependent manner [86]. Accumulating evidence indicates that the movement-related motor excitability is related to coactivation of the sympathetic nervous system and to modulation of afferent inputs [79].

When descending pathways are interrupted following CNS injury, the overall excitability of the spinal motoneuronal pool is initially reduced, producing weakness and flaccidity. However, the acute loss of descending brainstem inhibition of presynaptic afferent inputs, especially cutaneous inputs, is thought to increase intrinsic motoneuron excitability via the development of PICs [87, 88]. At first, these low-threshold polysynaptic inputs do not produce long-lasting reflexes because of lack of motoneuron excitability in a monoamine-deficient state. Over time, the PICs become supersensitive to the residual monoamines below the level of the injury [89], which more than compensate for the monoamine deficiency, leading to the development of large PICs and hyperexcitable motoneurons which trigger sustained motoneuron discharges associated with long-lasting reflexes and muscle spasms to innocuous stimulation, such as gently rubbing the skin or passive movement [88]. In fact, indirect measurements of PIC amplitude from paired motor unit recordings in human subjects suggest that PICs in motor neurons contribute to muscle spasms after spinal cord injury [90]. Pharmacologically blocking the PICs on the motoneurons, without inhibiting the synaptic inputs, can eliminate the long-lasting reflexes [91].

However, in individuals with stroke, PIC estimates have not been found to be larger in spastic-paretic motoneurons, compared with contralateral, and age-matched healthy control motoneurons. Instead, following voluntary isometric contractions, the majority of the low-threshold motor units in spastic-paretic muscles exhibit spontaneous discharges, suggesting that firing changes are likely due to low-level depolarizing synaptic drive to the resting motoneuron pool [92, 93], which can account for hyperreflexia. However, voluntary activation of the spastic-paretic motoneuron pool results in saturation in firing profiles of the individual motor units, and an inability to modulate firing rates [94], suggesting lack of synaptic drive for voluntary muscle activation or paresis. The contradiction in the PIC estimates of the spastic-paretic motorneurons can be reconciled by considering that the net excitability of the alpha motor neuron is achieved via a complex and poorly quantified afferent pool that influences the central state of the cells, which is influenced by the function of both lesioned and nonlesioned areas contributing to the tracts. This is in contrast to the more simplistic view of hyperreflexia described historically (Fig. 1.3) [95, 96].

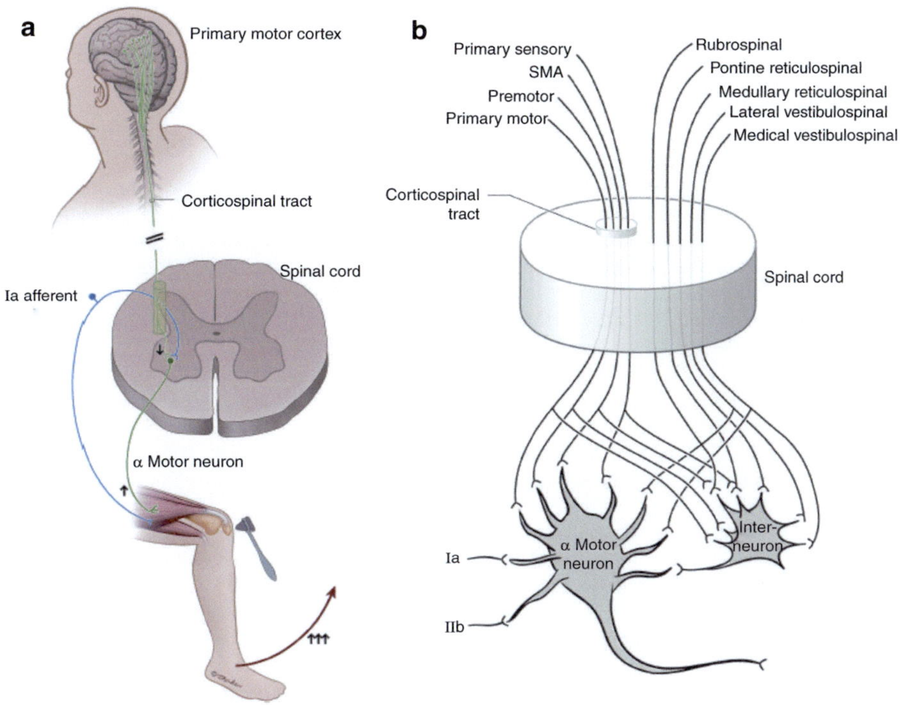

Fig. 1.3 Schematic illustration of the spinal stretch reflex. (**a**) The classically described spinal reflex arc demonstrating hyperreflexia (indicated by the arrows) after corticospinal tract injury. (**b**) Contemporary summary of the afferent pool of the alpha motor neuron showing significant contributions from the spinal interneuron pool whose inputs include projections received from the corticospinal tract. (From Florman et al. [95], with permission (open access))

Conclusion

Injury to the central nervous system results in both negative symptoms such as paresis and positive symptoms such as spasticity. While findings from both animal studies and studies with human subjects support the role of the dorsal reticulospinal tract in producing hyperexcitability of the spinal stretch reflexes, a more contemporary view is that the overall state of excitability of the spinal afferent pool is influenced by cortical input from both lesioned and nonlesioned areas and their descending pathways.

References

1. Walshe FM. Contributions of John Hughlings JACKSON to neurology. A brief introduction to his teachings. Arch Neurol. 1961;5:119–31.
2. Lance JW. Symposium synopsis. In: Feldman RG, Young RR, Koella WP, editors. Spasticity: disordered motor control. Chicago: Year Book Medical Publishers; 1980.
3. Pandyan AD, Gregoric M, Barnes MP, Wood D, Van Wijck F, Burridge J, et al. Spasticity: clinical perceptions, neurological realities and meaningful measurement. Disabil Rehabil. 2005;27(1–2):2–6.
4. Li S, Francisco GE, Rymer WZ. A new definition of poststroke spasticity and the interference of spasticity with motor recovery from acute to chronic stages. Neurorehabil Neural Repair. 2021;35(7):601–10. https://doi.org/10.1177/15459683211011214.
5. Schindler-Ivens SM, Shields RK. Soleus H-reflex recruitment is not altered in persons with chronic spinal cord injury. Arch Phys Med Rehabil. 2004;85(5):840–7.
6. Sinkjaer T, Toft E, Larsen K, Andreassen S, Hansen HJ. Non-reflex and reflex-mediated ankle joint stiffness in multiple sclerosis patients with spasticity. Muscle Nerve. 1993;16(1):69–76.
7. Willerslev-Olsen M, Lorentzen J, Sinkjaer T, Nielsen JB. Passive muscle properties are altered in children with cerebral palsy before the age of 3 years and are difficult to distinguish clinically from spasticity. Dev Med Child Neurol. 2013;55(7):617–23.
8. Nam KE, Lim SH, Kim JS, Hong BY, Jung HY, Lee JK, et al. When does spasticity in the upper limb develop after a first stroke? A nationwide observational study on 861 stroke patients. J Clin Neurosci. 2019;66:144–8.
9. Sommerfeld DK, Eek EU, Svensson AK, Holmqvist LW, von Arbin MH. Spasticity after stroke: its occurrence and association with motor impairments and activity limitations. Stroke. 2004;35(1):134–9.
10. Dornak T, Justanova M, Konvalinkova R, Riha M, Muzik J, Hoskovcova M, et al. Prevalence and evolution of spasticity in patients suffering from first-ever stroke with carotid origin: a prospective, longitudinal study. Eur J Neurol. 2019;26(6):880–6.
11. Plantin J, Pennati GV, Roca P, Baron JC, Laurencikas E, Weber K, et al. Quantitative assessment of hand spasticity after stroke: imaging correlates and impact on motor recovery. Front Neurol. 2019;10:836.
12. Sunnerhagen KS, Opheim A, Alt MM. Onset, time course and prediction of spasticity after stroke or traumatic brain injury. Ann Phys Rehabil Med. 2019;62(6):431–4.
13. Pundik S, McCabe J, Skelly M, Tatsuoka C, Daly JJ. Association of spasticity and motor dysfunction in chronic stroke. Ann Phys Rehabil Med. 2019;62(6):397–402.
14. Milinis K, Young CA. Trajectories of outcome in neurological conditions. Systematic review of the influence of spasticity on quality of life in adults with chronic neurological conditions. Disabil Rehabil. 2016;38(15):1431–41.

15. Lundstrom E, Smits A, Borg J, Terent A. Four-fold increase in direct costs of stroke survivors with spasticity compared with stroke survivors without spasticity: the first year after the event. Stroke. 2010;41(2):319–24.
16. Lundstrom E, Terent A, Borg J. Prevalence of disabling spasticity 1 year after first-ever stroke. Eur J Neurol. 2008;15(6):533–9.
17. Picelli A, Tamburin S, Gajofatto F, Zanette G, Praitano M, Saltuari L, et al. Association between severe upper limb spasticity and brain lesion location in stroke patients. Biomed Res Int. 2014;2014:162754.
18. Cheung DK, Climans SA, Black SE, Gao F, Szilagyi GM, Mochizuki G. Lesion characteristics of individuals with upper limb spasticity after stroke. Neurorehabil Neural Repair. 2016;30(1):63–70.
19. Holstege G, Bandler R, Saper CB. The emotional motor system. Prog Brain Res. 1996;107:3–6.
20. Lemon RN, Griffiths J. Comparing the function of the corticospinal system in different species: organizational differences for motor specialization? Muscle Nerve. 2005;32(3):261–79.
21. Lemon RN. Descending pathways in motor control. Annu Rev Neurosci. 2008;31:195–218.
22. Morecraft RJ, Ge J, Stilwell-Morecraft KS, McNeal DW, Pizzimenti MA, Darling WG. Terminal distribution of the corticospinal projection from the hand/arm region of the primary motor cortex to the cervical enlargement in rhesus monkey. J Comp Neurol. 2013;521(18):4205–35.
23. Kuypers HGJM. Anatomy of the descending pathways. In: Brooks VB, editor. Handbook of physiology. Bethesda: American Physiological Society; 1981.
24. Kuypers HG. A new look at the organization of the motor system. Prog Brain Res. 1982;57:381–403.
25. Wall PD, Lidierth M. Five sources of a dorsal root potential: their interactions and origins in the superficial dorsal horn. J Neurophysiol. 1997;78(2):860–71.
26. Cheema SS, Rustioni A, Whitsel BL. Light and electron microscopic evidence for a direct corticospinal projection to superficial laminae of the dorsal horn in cats and monkeys. J Comp Neurol. 1984;225(2):276–90.
27. Prochazka A. Sensorimotor gain control: a basic strategy of motor systems? Prog Neurobiol. 1989;33(4):281–307.
28. Brooks JX, Cullen KE. Predictive sensing: the role of motor signals in sensory processing. Biol Psychiatry Cogn Neurosci Neuroimaging. 2019;4(9):842–50.
29. Prut Y, Perlmutter SI, Fetz EE. Distributed processing in the motor system: spinal cord perspective. In: Nicolelis MAL, editor. Advances in neural population coding. Amsterdam: Elsevier; 2001. p. 267–78.
30. Morecraft RJ, Ge J, Stilwell-Morecraft KS, Rotella DL, Pizzimenti MA, Darling WG. Terminal organization of the corticospinal projection from the lateral premotor cortex to the cervical enlargement (C5-T1) in rhesus monkey. J Comp Neurol. 2019;527(16):2761–89.
31. Lacroix S, Havton LA, McKay H, Yang H, Brant A, Roberts J, et al. Bilateral corticospinal projections arise from each motor cortex in the macaque monkey: a quantitative study. J Comp Neurol. 2004;473(2):147–61.
32. Qin W, Yang M, Li F, Chen C, Zhen L, Tian S. Influence of positional changes on spasticity of the upper extremity in poststroke hemiplegic patients. Neurosci Lett. 2019;712:134479.
33. Kline TL, Schmit BD, Kamper DG. Exaggerated interlimb neural coupling following stroke. Brain. 2007;130(Pt 1):159–69.
34. Maier MA, Armand J, Kirkwood PA, Yang HW, Davis JN, Lemon RN. Differences in the corticospinal projection from primary motor cortex and supplementary motor area to macaque upper limb motoneurons: an anatomical and electrophysiological study. Cereb Cortex. 2002;12(3):281–96.
35. Lemon RN, Mantel GW, Muir RB. Corticospinal facilitation of hand muscles during voluntary movement in the conscious monkey. J Physiol. 1986;381:497–527.
36. Lemon RN, Baker SN, Davis JA, Kirkwood PA, Maier MA, Yang HS. The importance of the cortico-motoneuronal system for control of grasp. Novartis Found Symp. 1998;218:202–15; discussion 15–8.
37. Lawrence DG, Kuypers HG. The functional organization of the motor system in the monkey. I. The effects of bilateral pyramidal lesions. Brain. 1968;91(1):1–14.

38. Morecraft RJ, Ge J, Stilwell-Morecraft KS, McNeal DW, Hynes SM, Pizzimenti MA, et al. Vulnerability of the medial frontal corticospinal projection accompanies combined lateral frontal and parietal cortex injury in rhesus monkey. J Comp Neurol. 2015;523(4):669–97.
39. Morecraft RJ, Ge J, Stilwell-Morecraft KS, McNeal DW, Hynes SM, Pizzimenti MA, et al. Frontal and frontoparietal injury differentially affect the ipsilateral corticospinal projection from the nonlesioned hemisphere in monkey (Macaca mulatta). J Comp Neurol. 2016;524(2):380–407.
40. Evarts EV, Tanji J. Reflex and intended responses in motor cortex pyramidal tract neurons of monkey. J Neurophysiol. 1976;39(5):1069–80.
41. Alstermark B, Lundberg A. The C3-C4 propriospinal system: target-reaching and food-taking. In: Jami L, Pierrrot-Deseilligny E, Zytnicki D, editors. Muscle afferents and spinal control of movement Oxford. UK: Pergamon Press; 1992. p. 327–54.
42. Porter R, Lemon RN. Corticospinal function and voluntary movement. Oxford: Oxford University Press; 1993.
43. Jankowska E, Padel Y, Tanaka R. Disynaptic inhibition of spinal motoneurones from the motor cortex in the monkey. J Physiol. 1976;258(2):467–87.
44. Maier MA, Illert M, Kirkwood PA, Nielsen J, Lemon RN. Does a C3-C4 propriospinal system transmit corticospinal excitation in the primate? An investigation in the macaque monkey. J Physiol. 1998;511(Pt 1):191–212.
45. Bacon SJ, Smith AD. A monosynaptic pathway from an identified vasomotor centre in the medial prefrontal cortex to an autonomic area in the thoracic spinal cord. Neuroscience. 1993;54(3):719–28.
46. Wolpaw JR. The complex structure of a simple memory. Trends Neurosci. 1997;20(12):588–94.
47. Eyre JA, Miller S, Clowry GJ, Conway EA, Watts C. Functional corticospinal projections are established prenatally in the human foetus permitting involvement in the development of spinal motor centres. Brain. 2000;123(Pt 1):51–64.
48. Martin JH, Kably B, Hacking A. Activity-dependent development of cortical axon terminations in the spinal cord and brain stem. Exp Brain Res. 1999;125(2):184–99.
49. Magoun HW, Rhines R. An inhibitory mechanism in the bulbar reticular formation. J Neurophysiol. 1946;9:165–71.
50. Woolsey CN. Discussion on experimental hypertonia in the monkey: interruption of pyramidal or pyramidal-extra pyramidal cortical projections. Trans Am Neurol Assoc. 1971;96:164–6.
51. Engberg I, Lundberg A, Ryall RW. Reticulospinal inhibition of interneurones. J Physiol. 1968;194(1):225–36.
52. Engberg I, Lundberg A, Ryall RW. Reticulospinal inhibition of transmission in reflex pathways. J Physiol. 1968;194(1):201–23.
53. Putnam TJ. Treatment on unilateral paralysis agitans by section of the lateral pyramidal tract. Arch Neurol Psychiatr. 1940;44:950–76.
54. Sheean G. The pathophysiology of spasticity. Eur J Neurol. 2002;9(Suppl 1):3–9; dicussion 53–61.
55. Burke D, Knowles L, Andrews C, Ashby P. Spasticity, decerebrate rigidity and the clasp-knife phenomenon: an experimental study in the cat. Brain. 1972;95(1):31–48.
56. Bucy PC. Studies on the human neuromuscular mechanism. II Effect of ventromedial cordotomy on muscular spasticity in man. Arch Neurol Psychiatr. 1938;40:639–62.
57. Hyndman OR, Jarvis FJ. Gastric crises of tabes dorsalis: treatment by anterior chordotomy in eight cases. Arch Surg. 1940;40(5):997–1013.
58. Fregosi M, Contestabile A, Hamadjida A, Rouiller EM. Corticobulbar projections from distinct motor cortical areas to the reticular formation in macaque monkeys. Eur J Neurosci. 2017;45(11):1379–95.
59. Darling WG, Ge J, Stilwell-Morecraft KS, Rotella DL, Pizzimenti MA, Morecraft RJ. Hand motor recovery following extensive frontoparietal cortical injury is accompanied by upregulated corticoreticular projections in monkey. J Neurosci. 2018;38(28):6323–39.

60. Fregosi M, Contestabile A, Badoud S, Borgognon S, Cottet J, Brunet JF, et al. Changes of motor corticobulbar projections following different lesion types affecting the central nervous system in adult macaque monkeys. Eur J Neurosci. 2018;48(4):2050–70.
61. Herbert WJ, Powell K, Buford JA. Evidence for a role of the reticulospinal system in recovery of skilled reaching after cortical stroke: initial results from a model of ischemic cortical injury. Exp Brain Res. 2015;233(11):3231–51.
62. Ortiz-Rosario A, Berrios-Torres I, Adeli H, Buford JA. Combined corticospinal and reticulospinal effects on upper limb muscles. Neurosci Lett. 2014;561:30–4.
63. Chollet F, DiPiero V, Wise RJ, Brooks DJ, Dolan RJ, Frackowiak RS. The functional anatomy of motor recovery after stroke in humans: a study with positron emission tomography. Ann Neurol. 1991;29(1):63–71.
64. Weiller C, Chollet F, Friston KJ, Wise RJ, Frackowiak RS. Functional reorganization of the brain in recovery from striatocapsular infarction in man. Ann Neurol. 1992;31(5):463–72.
65. Fries W, Danek A, Scheidtmann K, Hamburger C. Motor recovery following capsular stroke. Role of descending pathways from multiple motor areas. Brain. 1993;116(Pt 2):369–82.
66. Cramer SC, Nelles G, Benson RR, Kaplan JD, Parker RA, Kwong KK, et al. A functional MRI study of subjects recovered from hemiparetic stroke. Stroke. 1997;28(12):2518–27.
67. Seitz RJ, Hoflich P, Binkofski F, Tellmann L, Herzog H, Freund HJ. Role of the premotor cortex in recovery from middle cerebral artery infarction. Arch Neurol. 1998;55(8):1081–8.
68. Schulz R, Braass H, Liuzzi G, Hoerniss V, Lechner P, Gerloff C, et al. White matter integrity of premotor-motor connections is associated with motor output in chronic stroke patients. Neuroimage Clin. 2015;7:82–6.
69. Pantano P, Formisano R, Ricci M, Di Piero V, Sabatini U, Di Pofi B, et al. Motor recovery after stroke. Morphological and functional brain alterations. Brain. 1996;119(Pt 6):1849–57.
70. Rehme AK, Eickhoff SB, Rottschy C, Fink GR, Grefkes C. Activation likelihood estimation meta-analysis of motor-related neural activity after stroke. NeuroImage. 2012;59(3):2771–82.
71. Backhaus W, Braass H, Higgen FL, Gerloff C, Schulz R. Early parietofrontal network upregulation relates to future persistent deficits after severe stroke-a prospective cohort study. Brain Commun. 2021;3(2):fcab097.
72. Brihmat N, Tarri M, Gasq D, Marque P, Castel-Lacanal E, Loubinoux I. Cross-modal functional connectivity of the premotor cortex reflects residual motor output after stroke. Brain Connect. 2020;10(5):236–49.
73. Harrington RM, Chan E, Rounds AK, Wutzke CJ, Dromerick AW, Turkeltaub PE, et al. Roles of lesioned and nonlesioned hemispheres in reaching performance poststroke. Neurorehabil Neural Repair. 2020;34(1):61–71.
74. Tscherpel C, Hensel L, Lemberg K, Vollmer M, Volz LJ, Fink GR, et al. The differential roles of contralesional frontoparietal areas in cortical reorganization after stroke. Brain Stimul. 2020;13(3):614–24.
75. Chen YT, Li S, Magat E, Zhou P, Li S. Motor overflow and spasticity in chronic stroke share a common pathophysiological process: analysis of within-limb and between-limb EMG-EMG coherence. Front Neurol. 2018;9:795.
76. Owen M, Ingo C, Dewald JPA. Upper extremity motor impairments and microstructural changes in bulbospinal pathways in chronic hemiparetic stroke. Front Neurol. 2017;8:257.
77. Li S, Chen YT, Francisco GE, Zhou P, Rymer WZ. A unifying pathophysiological account for post-stroke spasticity and disordered motor control. Front Neurol. 2019;10:468.
78. Jacobs BL, Fornal CA. Serotonin and motor activity. Curr Opin Neurobiol. 1997;7(6):820–5.
79. Heckmann CJ, Gorassini MA, Bennett DJ. Persistent inward currents in motoneuron dendrites: implications for motor output. Muscle Nerve. 2005;31(2):135–56.
80. Lee RH, Kuo JJ, Jiang MC, Heckman CJ. Influence of active dendritic currents on input-output processing in spinal motoneurons in vivo. J Neurophysiol. 2003;89(1):27–39.

81. Binder MD, Powers RK, Heckman CJ. Nonlinear input-output functions of motoneurons. Physiology (Bethesda). 2020;35(1):31–9.
82. Kuo JJ, Lee RH, Johnson MD, Heckman HM, Heckman CJ. Active dendritic integration of inhibitory synaptic inputs in vivo. J Neurophysiol. 2003;90(6):3617–24.
83. Clarke RW, Eves S, Harris J, Peachey JE, Stuart E. Interactions between cutaneous afferent inputs to a withdrawal reflex in the decerebrated rabbit and their control by descending and segmental systems. Neuroscience. 2002;112(3):555–71.
84. Jankowska E. Interneuronal relay in spinal pathways from proprioceptors. Prog Neurobiol. 1992;38(4):335–78.
85. Hochman S, Garraway SM, Machacek DW, Shay BL. 5-HT receptors and the neuromodulatory control of spinal cord function. In: Cope TC, editor. Motor neurobiology of the spinal cord. London: CRC Press; 2001. p. 47–87.
86. Heckman CJ, Kuo JJ, Johnson MD. Synaptic integration in motoneurons with hyper-excitable dendrites. Can J Physiol Pharmacol. 2004;82(8–9):549–55.
87. D'Amico JM, Condliffe EG, Martins KJ, Bennett DJ, Gorassini MA. Recovery of neuronal and network excitability after spinal cord injury and implications for spasticity. Front Integr Neurosci. 2014;8:36.
88. Bennett DJ, Sanelli L, Cooke CL, Harvey PJ, Gorassini MA. Spastic long-lasting reflexes in the awake rat after sacral spinal cord injury. J Neurophysiol. 2004;91(5):2247–58.
89. Harvey PJ, Li X, Li Y, Bennett DJ. 5-HT2 receptor activation facilitates a persistent sodium current and repetitive firing in spinal motoneurons of rats with and without chronic spinal cord injury. J Neurophysiol. 2006;96(3):1158–70.
90. Gorassini MA, Knash ME, Harvey PJ, Bennett DJ, Yang JF. Role of motoneurons in the generation of muscle spasms after spinal cord injury. Brain. 2004;127(Pt 10):2247–58.
91. Li Y, Gorassini MA, Bennett DJ. Role of persistent sodium and calcium currents in motoneuron firing and spasticity in chronic spinal rats. J Neurophysiol. 2004;91(2):767–83.
92. Mottram CJ, Suresh NL, Heckman CJ, Gorassini MA, Rymer WZ. Origins of abnormal excitability in biceps brachii motoneurons of spastic-paretic stroke survivors. J Neurophysiol. 2009;102(4):2026–38.
93. Mottram CJ, Wallace CL, Chikando CN, Rymer WZ. Origins of spontaneous firing of motor units in the spastic-paretic biceps brachii muscle of stroke survivors. J Neurophysiol. 2010;104(6):3168–79.
94. Mottram CJ, Heckman CJ, Powers RK, Rymer WZ, Suresh NL. Disturbances of motor unit rate modulation are prevalent in muscles of spastic-paretic stroke survivors. J Neurophysiol. 2014;111(10):2017–28.
95. Florman JE, Duffau H, Rughani AI. Lower motor neuron findings after upper motor neuron injury: insights from postoperative supplementary motor area syndrome. Front Hum Neurosci. 2013;7:85.
96. Ditunno JF, Little JW, Tessler A, Burns AS. Spinal shock revisited: a four-phase model. Spinal Cord. 2004;42(7):383–95.

Spasticity Versus Spastic Movement Disorder

2

Volker Dietz

> *...it is not merely the nature of the motions of the living substance which we must interpret in terms of force, but also the conformation of the organism itself, whose permanence or equilibrium is explained by the interaction or balance of forces.*
> *– D'Arcy Wentwoth Thompson, On Growth and Form, 1917.*

- Spastic movement disorder is the consequence of vascular, inflammatory, or traumatic damage to the central nervous system (CNS), characterized by impaired performance of natural, functional movements.
- Neural phenomena such as exaggerated tendon tap reflexes explain spastic movement disorder only to a limited degree. Additional neural characteristics include attenuation or loss of polysynaptic reflex activity associated with reduced modulation of limb muscle activation during movement.
- CNS damage also leads to secondary non-neural alterations in mechanical muscle fiber properties, which lead to the development of muscle stiffness. These changes may support the body during the stance phase, and partially compensate for the paresis, but contribute to the spastic movement disorder.
- A better understanding of the pathophysiological basis of spastic movement disorder can assist in selecting the right therapeutic strategy.

V. Dietz (✉)
Spinal Cord Injury Center, University Hospital Balgrist, Zürich, Switzerland
e-mail: volker.dietz@balgrist.ch

P. Raghavan (ed.), *Spasticity and Muscle Stiffness*,
https://doi.org/10.1007/978-3-030-96900-4_2

Introduction

Spastic Movement Disorder develops as a consequence of damage to sensorimotor areas within the central nervous system (CNS). It is almost always associated with some degree of weakness or paresis leading to the syndrome of spastic paresis. The clinical diagnosis of spastic paresis is based on a number of physical signs elicited during the clinical examination, such as exaggerated tendon tap reflexes and resistance to muscle stretch (muscle tone or tension) in the sitting/lying positions, i.e., on a passive patient. Lance [1] defined spastic muscle hypertonia as the resistance of a muscle to stretch that is activated by tonic stretch reflex activity. Early after damage to the CNS, tendon tap reflexes are exaggerated even though the muscle tone of the affected limb is flaccid. However, passive stretching of a paretic muscle during clinical examination (e.g., the Ashworth test), in contrast to that on the unaffected limb, may produce increased resistance. Such passive resistance may not be due to hyperreflexia per se, but due to mechanical changes in the muscles [2]. This is elaborated further in Chaps. 4, 5, and 6.

Furthermore, the clinical signs and symptoms after acute damage to the CNS change over time due to neuronal reorganization [3], and depend on the location of the lesion [4]. After an acute cerebral infarction or traumatic spinal cord injury, flaccidity can persist for weeks during which the tendon tap reflex (or its electrophysiological correlate, the H-reflex) can still be elicited [5]. Afterwards the transition to spastic movement disorder occurs over weeks and months, during which there is an increase in the H-reflex to M-wave ratio (H/M ratio). The M-wave reflects muscle contractility. Interestingly, the increased H/M ratio is more due to decline in the M-wave amplitude rather than due to an increase in the H-reflex, suggesting that non-neural changes, such as loss of muscle fibers due to atrophy and/or reduced motor conduction through the muscle, may contribute more to the spastic movement disorder than has been previously presumed [5]. In fact, the spastic movement disorder *during* gait appears to be due to lack of normal suppression and modulation of the size of the reflexes, and is usually more pronounced after spinal compared to cerebral lesions, particularly in the antigravity muscles, i.e., arm flexor and leg extensor muscles [6]. Lack of reflex modulation suggests that impaired processing of afferent input in combination with secondary changes in muscles contributes to the spastic movement disorder during complex functional movements, such as locomotion [7].

Pathophysiology

Clinical Aspects

In the hospital or clinic, examination of reflexes and resistance to stretch are performed under passive conditions on the relaxed patient [8]. Spasticity, in clinical terms, is characterized by exaggerated tendon tap reflexes in the affected limb(s) compared to the unaffected limb(s), presence of pyramidal signs (e.g., positive

Babinski sign), and increased resistance to stretch. The disinhibition of short-latency reflex activity, corresponding to the tendon tap reflexes, is suggested to be due to reduced presynaptic inhibition of afferent (group I) fibers [9, 10]. After a few months, changes in mechanical muscle properties develop, especially in the antigravity muscles of the limbs (leg extensors, [11]; and arm flexors, [12] which contribute to muscle stiffness) (for review see [2, 13]). These structural changes are fully established around one year after the acute lesion [14].

Functional Aspects

After CNS damage, a patient's functional behavior suffers not due to the abnormality in tendon reflexes but due to the spastic movement disorder. This is of critical relevance for any therapeutic approach aimed at restoring function. During the passive clinical examination, patients with CNS damage may appear to show overactivation of limb muscles compared to healthy subjects. However, during active functional movement, muscle activity in upper and lower limbs is reduced compared to that of the unaffected limbs or that of healthy subjects [11, 12, 15, 16]. The muscle activity shows reduced modulation and is of smaller amplitude. The reduced muscle activation is due to both the loss of supraspinal drive and attenuated polysynaptic reflex activity [7, 17]. The long-latency polysynaptic reflexes are known to modulate EMG activity, especially in the antigravity muscles (arm flexors and leg extensors) during functional movements [7], thereby enabling adaptation of muscle activation patterns to external demands. In contrast, the short-latency reflexes are not involved in muscle activation during functional movements – neither in healthy individuals nor in patients with spastic movement disorder. Consequently, there is no relationship between muscle activation during leg [18] and arm movements [12, 19, 20] and the clinically exaggerated tendon tap reflexes.

During stepping, the reciprocal mode of leg muscle activation remains preserved in spastic limb muscles. The exaggerated short-latency reflex activity is associated with attenuation of the functionally essential polysynaptic (or long-latency) reflex activity which results in overall reduced leg muscle activation. The tension to support the body develops within the stretching period of the leg extensor muscles during the stance phase of gait that shows low amplitude tonic EMG activity [18]. This is achieved by modulating leg muscle activation in healthy subjects. In contrast, patients with spastic movement disorder develop the tension required for body support during stepping using alternative compensatory mechanisms [2, 15].

Structural non-neural changes in muscle mechanical properties (e.g., loss of sarcomeres, changes in muscle extracellular matrix) take place within the first weeks [2], as a secondary consequence of the CNS damage, and can partially compensate for muscle paresis (Fig. 2.1). The consequence of these electrophysiological [11, 14] and histological [21–23] changes results in the development of muscle stiffness, allowing the patient to support the weight of the body during stepping to achieve limited mobility. This new mode of development of muscle stiffness, however, does

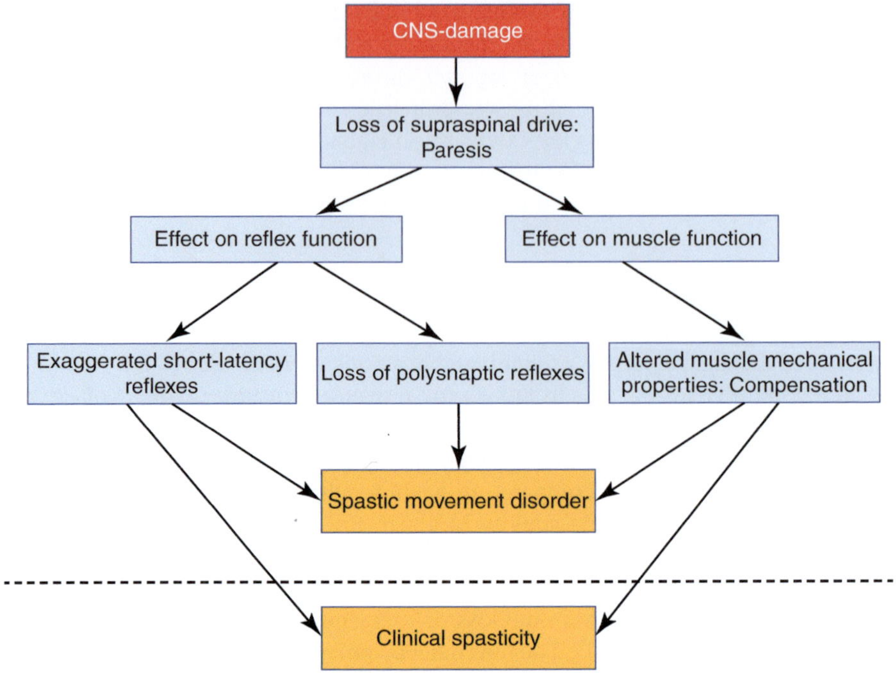

Fig. 2.1 Physiological mechanisms underlying the syndrome of spastic paresis

not allow the performance of fast movements because of the lack of modulation of muscle activation. After severe spinal or supraspinal damage associated with severe paresis and immobilization, these muscle changes can lead to excessive muscle stiffness and painful spasms [5].

In patients with spastic paresis both the efferent and the afferent aspects of movement performance are impaired. This is reflected in defective neural coupling between the arms and legs. Interlimb coupling is an integral part of the organization of locomotion and is responsible for arm swing during gait [7]. In healthy subjects, stimulation of the tibial nerve during mid-stance leads to responses in the proximal arm muscles of both sides. However, stimulation of the unaffected leg in poststroke subjects leads to stronger responses in both arms compared with stimulation of the affected leg [17]. These results can be explained by impaired processing of afferent input from the affected leg [24]. Thus, defective neural coupling also contributes to impaired movement performance.

Taken together, it can be concluded that in patients with spastic movement disorder, even when muscle activity is enhanced in the passive condition, e.g., during the clinical examination, it is reduced during active functional movements compared to healthy subjects. Consequently, the pathophysiological signs assessed during the passive clinical examination cannot explain the spastic movement disorder. Pathophysiological studies show no qualitative differences between spinal and cerebral damage [15, 25].

Implications for Treatment

As established above, exaggerated short-latency reflexes contribute little to the spastic movement disorder that hampers the patient's movement. However, most antispastic drugs reduce reflex muscle overactivity. In fact such blocking is associated with increased paresis (e.g., with Clonidine, [26]) leading to more pronounced impairment of upper and lower limb function in mobile patients [27, 28]. Research in animal models suggests that loss of afferent input, such as due to immobility, can lead to major structural changes in connectivity of the spinal cord interneuronal circuits [29].

Functional training which restores appropriate feedback signals from peripheral receptors (below the CNS damage) can induce directed and meaningful neuroplasticity associated with stronger physiological arm and leg muscle activation [30] (Fig. 2.2). Such functional training, e.g., stepping training, can lead to improvement of movement performance that is accompanied by stronger muscle activation, and consequently a reduction in spastic movement disorder. Furthermore, training of natural interactions between the paretic and unaffected limbs has a positive

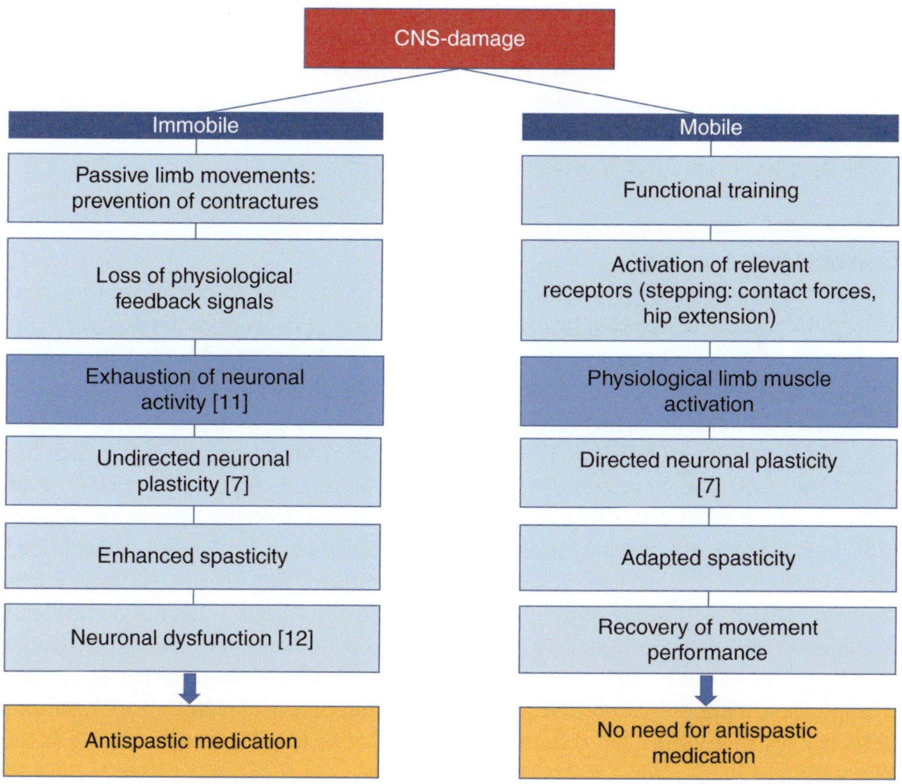

Fig. 2.2 Changes in neuronal function after central nervous system (CNS) damage

influence on recovery of function [17]. During training of stepping movements, the hip joint and body load-related receptors have to become activated to achieve the beneficial effects on function [31]. This is achieved by reloading the body as much as possible by inducing sufficient hip extension movements. Furthermore, longer training times have been shown to have positive effects on function and on spastic movement disorder [32].

The use of rehabilitation technology can support repetitive functional movements and allow for longer training times [33, 34]. In the early 90s, the concept of functional training of arm and leg movements in patients with cerebral and spinal lesions became established. Clinical and electrophysiological studies have shown that functional training can evoke and train a locomotor pattern [26, 31, 35]; for review see [36, 37]. This training approach was based on rodent and cat experimental studies [38], and led to improved functional ability and adaptation of muscle tone/tension to the actual functional requirements of the task. The success of such therapy, however, depends on the intensity and duration of training [32]. The increasing availability of rehabilitation technology makes longer training times possible [33]. The first robot to assist stepping movements, the "Lokomat", was developed for training of paraplegic patients [33, 34, 39]. The device supported and assisted functional movements which could be optimized and adapted to the individual patient. For functional arm training, the robot "ARMin" was developed, and a beneficial effect of training with this device was reported in poststroke subjects [40]. At present, there are a large number of robotic devices on the market to assist in the neurorehabilitation of arm and leg movements.

Conclusion

The application of antispastic drugs in mobile patients can hamper the recovery and performance of functional movements [26]. This is due to the fact that functional training requires muscle activation, which is invariably reduced with antispastic drugs [28]. In severely affected, immobilized (e.g., complete paraplegic) patients, neuronal dysfunction develops below the level of lesion about one year after the injury [41, 42]. This neuronal dysfunction may be due to undirected sprouting of spinal cord fibers as a consequence of the loss of physiological feedback signals [28]. In these patients, antispastic drugs (e.g., the intrathecal application of baclofen) can prevent the occurrence of spasms and facilitate nursing [43]. These drugs dampen exaggerated reflex activity and reduce spastic muscle tone, but do not lead to improvement in motor function [15, 44–46]. The application of antispastic drugs should be accompanied by physiotherapy to avoid muscle contractures [47]. The therapy should not only comprise passive stretching of muscles as this does little to influence spasticity [48], but should also include active training of movements as far as possible [49].

References

1. Lance JW. Pathophysiology of spasticity and clinical experience with baclofen. In: Lance JW, Feldman RG, Young RR, Koella WP, editors. Spasticity: disordered motor control. Chicago: Year Book; 1980. p. 185–204.
2. O'Dwyer NJ, Ada L. Reflex hyperexcitability and muscle contracture in relation to spastic hypertonia. Curr Opin Neurol. 1996;9(6):451–5.
3. Carr LJ, Harrison LM, Evans AL, Stephens JA. Patterns of central motor reorganization in hemiplegic cerebral palsy. Brain. 1993;116(Pt 5):1223–47.
4. Nathan PW. Effects on movement of surgical incisions into the human spinal cord. Brain. 1994;117(Pt 2):337–46.
5. Hiersemenzel LP, Curt A, Dietz V. From spinal shock to spasticity: neuronal adaptations to a spinal cord injury. Neurology. 2000;54(8):1574–82.
6. Faist M, Ertel M, Berger W, Dietz V. Impaired modulation of quadriceps tendon jerk reflex during spastic gait: differences between spinal and cerebral lesions. Brain. 1999;122(Pt 3):567–79.
7. Dietz V. Proprioception and locomotor disorders. Nat Rev Neurosci. 2002;3(10):781–90.
8. Thilmann AF, Fellows SJ, Garms E. The mechanism of spastic muscle hypertonus. Variation in reflex gain over the time course of spasticity. Brain. 1991;114(Pt 1A):233–44.
9. Burke D, Ashby P. Are spinal "presynaptic" inhibitory mechanisms suppressed in spasticity? J Neurol Sci. 1972;15(3):321–6.
10. Faist M, Mazevet D, Dietz V, Pierrot-Deseilligny E. A quantitative assessment of presynaptic inhibition of Ia afferents in spastics. Differences in hemiplegics and paraplegics. Brain. 1994;117(Pt 6):1449–55.
11. Dietz V, Quintern J, Berger W. Electrophysiological studies of gait in spasticity and rigidity. Evidence that altered mechanical properties of muscle contribute to hypertonia. Brain. 1981;104(3):431–49.
12. Ibrahim IK, Berger W, Trippel M, Dietz V. Stretch-induced electromyographic activity and torque in spastic elbow muscles. Differential modulation of reflex activity in passive and active motor tasks. Brain. 1993;116(Pt 4):971–89.
13. Lieber RL, Steinman S, Barash IA, Chambers H. Structural and functional changes in spastic skeletal muscle. Muscle Nerve. 2004;29(5):615–27.
14. Sinkjaer T, Toft E, Larsen K, Andreassen S, Hansen HJ. Non-reflex and reflex- mediated ankle joint stiffness in multiple sclerosis patients with spasticity. Muscle Nerve. 1993;16(1):69–76.
15. Dietz V, Sinkjaer T. Spastic movement disorder: impaired reflex function and altered muscle mechanics. Lancet Neurol. 2007;6(8):725–33.
16. Dietz V. Behavior of spinal neurons deprived of supraspinal input. Nat Rev Neurol. 2010;6(3):167–74.
17. Kloter E, Wirz M, Dietz V. Locomotion in stroke subjects: interactions between unaffected and affected sides. Brain. 2011;134(Pt 3):721–31.
18. Berger W, Horstmann G, Dietz V. Tension development and muscle activation in the leg during gait in spastic hemiparesis: independence of muscle hypertonia and exaggerated stretch reflexes. J Neurol Neurosurg Psychiatry. 1984;47(9):1029–33.
19. Dietz V, Trippel M, Berger W. Reflex activity and muscle tone during elbow movements in patients with spastic paresis. Ann Neurol. 1991;30(6):767–79.
20. Powers RK, Campbell DL, Rymer WZ. Stretch reflex dynamics in spastic elbow flexor muscles. Ann Neurol. 1989;25(1):32–42.
21. Dietz V, Ketelsen UP, Berger W, Quintern J. Motor unit involvement in spastic paresis. Relationship between leg muscle activation and histochemistry. J Neurol Sci. 1986;75(1):89–103.
22. Foran JR, Steinman S, Barash I, Chambers HG, Lieber RL. Structural and mechanical alterations in spastic skeletal muscle. Dev Med Child Neurol. 2005;47(10):713–7.

23. Gracies JM. Pathophysiology of spastic paresis. I: paresis and soft tissue changes. Muscle Nerve. 2005;31(5):535–51.
24. Lemon RN. Descending pathways in motor control. Annu Rev Neurosci. 2008;31:195–218.
25. Dietz V, Sinkjaer T. Spasticity. Handb Clin Neurol. 2012;109:197–211.
26. Dietz V, Colombo G, Jensen L, Baumgartner L. Locomotor capacity of spinal cord in paraplegic patients. Ann Neurol. 1995;37(5):574–82.
27. Dietz V. State of the art: Spastik. Pharma Focus ZNS. 2014;11:48–50.
28. Dietz V, Fouad K. Restoration of sensorimotor functions after spinal cord injury. Brain. 2014;137(Pt 3):654–67.
29. Kapitza S, Zorner B, Weinmann O, Bolliger M, Filli L, Dietz V, et al. Tail spasms in rat spinal cord injury: changes in interneuronal connectivity. Exp Neurol. 2012;236(1):179–89.
30. Beauparlant J, van den Brand R, Barraud Q, Friedli L, Musienko P, Dietz V, et al. Undirected compensatory plasticity contributes to neuronal dysfunction after severe spinal cord injury. Brain. 2013;136(Pt 11):3347–61.
31. Dietz V, Muller R, Colombo G. Locomotor activity in spinal man: significance of afferent input from joint and load receptors. Brain. 2002;125(Pt 12):2626–34.
32. Kwakkel G, Wagenaar RC, Twisk JW, Lankhorst GJ, Koetsier JC. Intensity of leg and arm training after primary middle-cerebral-artery stroke: a randomised trial. Lancet. 1999;354(9174):191–6.
33. Riener R, Lünenburger L, Maier IC, Colombo G, Dietz V. Locomotor training in subjects with sensori-motor deficits: an overview of the robotic gait orthosis lokomat. J Healthc Eng. 2010;1(2):197–216.
34. Colombo G, Wirz M, Dietz V. Driven gait orthosis for improvement of locomotor training in paraplegic patients. Spinal Cord. 2001;39(5):252–5.
35. Hesse S, Bertelt C, Jahnke MT, Schaffrin A, Baake P, Malezic M, et al. Treadmill training with partial body weight support compared with physiotherapy in nonambulatory hemiparetic patients. Stroke. 1995;26(6):976–81.
36. Dietz V, Harkema SJ. Locomotor activity in spinal cord-injured persons. J Appl Physiol. 2004;96(5):1954–60.
37. Dietz V. Body weight supported gait training: from laboratory to clinical setting. Brain Res Bull. 2008;76(5):459–63.
38. Barbeau H, Rossignol S. Enhancement of locomotor recovery following spinal cord injury. Curr Opin Neurol. 1994;7(6):517–24.
39. Wirz M, Colombo G, Dietz V. Long-term effects of locomotor training in spinal humans. J Neurol Neurosurg Psychiatry. 2001;71(1):93–6.
40. Klamroth-Marganska V, Blanco J, Campen K, Curt A, Dietz V, Ettlin T, et al. Three-dimensional, task-specific robot therapy of the arm after stroke: a multicentre, parallel-group randomised trial. Lancet Neurol. 2014;13(2):159–66.
41. Dietz V, Muller R. Degradation of neuronal function following a spinal cord injury: mechanisms and countermeasures. Brain. 2004;127(Pt 10):2221–31.
42. Dietz V, Grillner S, Trepp A, Hubli M, Bolliger M. Changes in spinal reflex and locomotor activity after a complete spinal cord injury: a common mechanism? Brain. 2009;132(Pt 8):2196–205.
43. Dietz V. Klinik der Spastik – spastische Bewegungsstörung. Nervenarzt. 2013;84:1508–11.
44. Thach W, Montgomery E. Motor systems. In: Pearlman A, Collins R, editors. Neurobiology disease. Oxford: Oxford University Press; 1990. p. 168–96.
45. Landau WM. Spasticity: what is it? What is it not? In: Feldman RG, Young RR, Koells WP, editors. Spasticity: disordered motor control. Chicago: Year Book Publ; 1980. p. 17–24.
46. Dietz V, Sinkjaer T. Secondary changes after CNS damage: the significance of spastic muscle tone in rehabilitation. In: Dietz V, Ward N, editors. Oxford textbook of neurorehabilitation. Oxford: Oxford University Press; 2015. p. 76–88.

47. Ansari NN, Naghdi S. The effect of Bobath approach on the excitability of the spinal alpha motor neurones in stroke patients with muscle spasticity. Electromyogr Clin Neurophysiol. 2007;47(1):29–36.
48. Katalinic OM, Harvey LA, Herbert RD, Moseley AM, Lannin NA, Schurr K. Stretch for the treatment and prevention of contractures. Cochrane Database Syst Rev (Online). 2010;(9):CD007455.
49. Hoffman HB, Blakey GL. New design of dynamic orthoses for neurological conditions. NeuroRehabilitation. 2011;28(1):55–61.

Clinical Assessment of the Syndrome of Spastic Paresis

3

Marjolaine Baude, Mouna Ghedira, Maud Pradines, and Jean-Michel Gracies

For our organs of sense, after all, are a kind of instrument.
– Erwin Schrodinger, What is life?, 1943.

- The syndrome of spastic paresis consists of two superimposed disorders: a neural disorder and a non-neural or muscle disorder, which can be assessed by a clinical five-step assessment, based on the pathophysiology of events that follow lesions to central motor pathways.
- Step 1 assesses the functional spastic movement disorder in the upper and lower limbs (using the Modified Frenchay Scale for the upper limb, and ambulation speed for the lower limb).
- Steps 2–4 evaluate the various forms of resistance encountered during passive and active movements. The Tardieu Scale is used to evaluate passive movements from a position of minimal stretch of the muscle group to completion of full range of motion of the joint.
- Step 5 assesses rapid alternating movements to determine fatiguability.
- Several coefficients of impairment can be calculated based on the five-step assessment to assist in developing comprehensive treatment strategies.

M. Baude (✉)
BIOTN Research Unit, UPEC University, Créteil, France
e-mail: marjolaine.baude@aphp.fr

M. Ghedira · M. Pradines · J.-M. Gracies
Service de Rééducation Neurolocomotrice, CHU Henri Mondor, Créteil, France

P. Raghavan (ed.), *Spasticity and Muscle Stiffness*,
https://doi.org/10.1007/978-3-030-96900-4_3

Introduction

In 1954, Tardieu defined *spasticity* as an increase in stretch reflexes that could be assessed by the speed of joint movement required to elicit the reflexes [1]. This concept was not immediately adopted by the medical community. However, in 1979, Lance and colleagues defined spasticity as a *velocity-dependent increase in stretch reflexes* [2]. See also Chap. 1 for additional definitions. An error in this definition is that the stretch reflex threshold in spastic paresis may not be *velocity-dependent* [3]. However, the *amplitude* of muscle activation in response to stretch is velocity-dependent, both in healthy subjects [4] and in patients with spastic paresis [5, 6]. However, studies show that the *enhancement* of the stretch reflex amplitude in spastic paresis is inversely related to speed [6, 7]. An adjusted definition of spasticity was therefore proposed in 2005, as an *increase in the velocity-dependent stretch reflexes, measured at rest* [8, 9]. See Chap. 2 for the difference between spasticity measured at rest and spastic movement disorder which occurs during movement.

Assessment of Spasticity

Ashworth-Derived Scales

In 1964, Ashworth created an ordinal 5-point scale (Table 3.1) to rate the resistance to passive movement, i.e., *tone*, in patients presenting with upper motor neuron syndrome, which was first used to evaluate the efficacy of carisoprodol as an *anti-spastic* drug in multiple sclerosis [10]. Later, the Ashworth scale was considered as a tool to evaluate *spasticity* – instead of tone – and its use markedly increased from the 1990s onward [11], as botulinum toxin treatment became popular.

The Ashworth scale, which neither specified the speed of stretch nor the angle at which resistance had to be felt at each grade, was later refined to a 6-point Modified Ashworth Scale (Table 3.2) to increase the sensitivity at the lower end of the scale [12]. The Modified Ashworth Scale better described grades 1, 1+, and 2 by adding *range of motion (ROM)* criteria over which the increased resistance had to be felt with respect to the *maximally expected* joint ROM (However *ROM* remained vaguely defined; hence see added italics in Table 3.2).

Table 3.1 The Ashworth Scale [10]

Grade	Description
0	No increase in tone
1	Slight increase in tone giving a catch when the limb is moved in flexion or extension
2	More marked increase in tone but limb easily flexed
3	Considerable increase in tone – passive movement is difficult
4	Limb rigid in flexion or extension

Table 3.2 The Modified Ashworth Scale [12]

Grade	Description
0	No increase in muscle tone
1	Slight increase in muscle tone, manifested by a catch and release or by minimal resistance *at the end* of the ROM when the affected part(s) is moved in flexion or in extension
1+	Slight increase in muscle tone, manifested by a catch, followed by minimal resistance throughout the reminder (*less than half*) of the ROM
2	More marked increase in muscle tone throughout *most of* the ROM, but affected part(s) is easily moved
3	Considerable increase in muscle tone, passive movement is difficult
4	Affected part(s) rigid in flexion or extension

ROM Range of Motion

There is strong evidence since, that the amount of resistance to passive movement is not an appropriate measure of spasticity [13, 14]. In the Ashworth scale, only grades 1 and 1+ refer to true spasticity, as these grades describe specific clinical features of stretch reflexes, in particular the "catch and release". However, see Chap. 4 for the large amount of variability even at these grades on quantitative measurement of the catch during the clinically graded Ashworth scale. Grades 2, 3, and 4 are more problematic as they describe forms of global resistance to passive movement, which may result from nonreflex-related components, such as increase in muscle viscous-elastic components, inadvertent voluntary contractions, dystonic activity, and contractures as described in Chaps. 5 and 6.

Perhaps more importantly, the Ashworth and Modified Ashworth scales do not specify the exact range of movement over which the resistance is rated, even though passive and active resistance to muscle stretch is highly dependent on the amount of imposed muscle stretch during joint rotation [15, 16]. This can lead to major inter-rater variability as some raters may assess a low grade because they evaluate resistance during the initial part of the available range, whereas others may arrive at a higher grade because they rate the resistance mostly at the end of the range ([17]; also see Chap. 4). Finally, although instructions for the Ashworth scale recommend that the passive joint range of motion be completed over one second, the speed at which the joint should be moved is not specified, which may also have a major impact on the resistance experienced by the examiner, i.e., whether the resistance is due to the active reflex (spasticity) or due to passive nonreflex velocity-dependent resistance or stiffness [5, 7, 18–22].

Furthermore, a number of studies have pointed to a lack of validity and reliability of the Ashworth scales, as Ashworth ratings were found not to be comparable to laboratory measures of spasticity or clinical tendon taps in paretic populations [15, 23–26]. The Ashworth scales grade the resistance to movement – spasticity included – and do not differentiate between the neural or the non-neural nature of the resistance [25–28]. Thus, these scores do not distinguish spasticity from muscle stiffness, soft tissue contracture or spastic dystonia [11, 13]. However, Ashworth-derived scores are still recommended by regulatory agencies for the rating of "spasticity" and used for that purpose [29–32], despite an increasing number of articles that clearly dispute its validity as a spasticity evaluation tool [33, 34].

The Tardieu Scale

From the 1950s to the late 1970s, Tardieu developed and gradually refined a clinical examination method based on angular measurements [35]. Continuing on Tardieu's steps, the scale today known as the "Tardieu Scale" was first published in 2000 [36]. The scale involves two clinical maneuvers, both of which consist of measuring an angle from the theoretical position of minimal stretch of the tested muscle group (not the standard anatomical zero of the joint; see Fig. 3.1).

The first maneuver aims to estimate the maximal passive extensibility of soft tissue and is performed at the slowest velocity, V1 (Table 3.3). The test is thus only administered after ensuring that the patient – and in particular the tested muscle

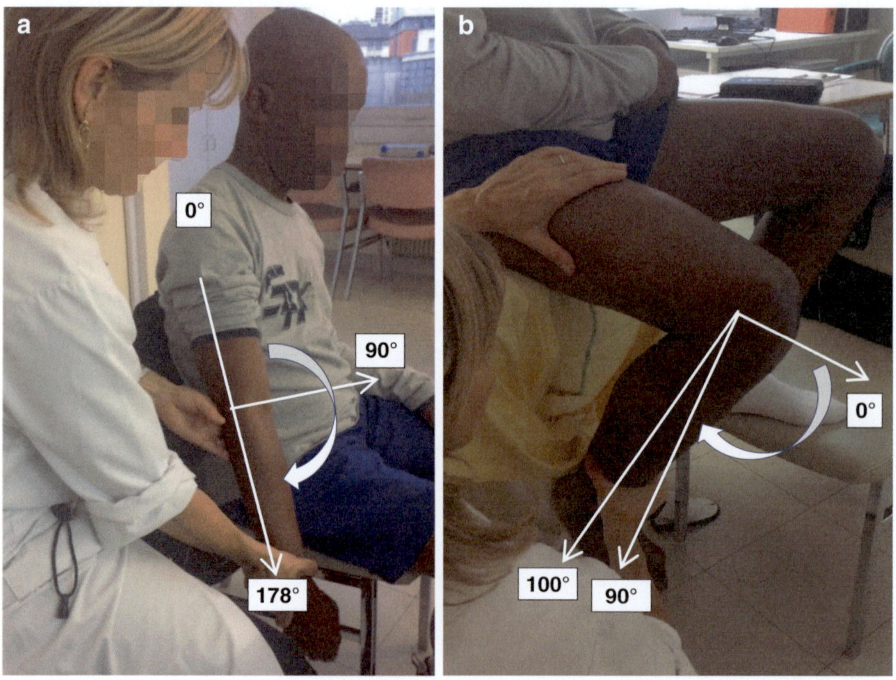

Fig. 3.1 Start and end positions to assess passive resistance to movement using the Tardieu Scale. (**a**) Examiner performing passive elbow extension to assess the resistance in the elbow flexors, and (**b**) passive knee flexion to assess resistance in the knee extensors. The zero position in the Tardieu scale is the theoretical position of minimal stretch of the tested muscle groups

Table 3.3 The Tardieu Scale

X **= Spasticity angle (threshold)**
Angle of arrest at slow speed X_{V1} *minus* angle of catch at fast speed X_{V3}
Y **= Spasticity grade (gain)**
0. No resistance throughout passive movement
1. Slight resistance throughout passive movement, no catch elicited
2. Clear catch at precise angle, interrupting passive movement, followed by release
3. Fatigable clonus (<10 s when maintaining pressure) occurring at a precise angle, followed by release
4. Unfatigable clonus (>10 s when maintaining pressure) occurring at a precise angle
Catch without release: graded 0 if $X_{V1} = X_{V3}$; "unrateable" spasticity otherwise
Catch with "minimal" release: graded 2 if X_{V3} is consistent and consistently less than X_{V1}
Angle 0° = position of minimal stretch of the tested muscle
For grades 0 and 1, spasticity angle $X = 0°$ by definition

From Gracies et al. [37]

group – is in the optimal resting position. The measurements must always be made in the same position, e.g., seated or supine, for comparison [15, 36, 37]. One can visually assess – without a goniometer – the angle of arrest of a slow and strong pull on the muscle (yielding the maximal passive range of motion or "functional muscle length" or "maximal clinical muscle extensibility") for each tested muscle group. It is important to *exert the slowest and strongest possible stretch* on the muscle group and its associated soft tissue to move the limb segment as far as possible without causing pain or jeopardizing soft tissue integrity. The rationale behind using extreme slowness is to minimize recruitment of stretch reflex afferents, which might create a spastic reaction that would impact the measured amplitude [5, 7]. The rationale behind using strong stretching force (maximal force for the examiner, compatible with preserving soft tissue integrity) is to optimally overcome the spastic dystonia present in the assessed muscle group, such that this type of overactivity should have minimal involvement in explaining the angle of arrest [16, 38, 39]. The measured angle of maximal passive range of motion has been termed X_{V1} [36, 37]. In effect, X_{V1}, which we like to call *maximal clinical muscle extensibility*, represents the angle that passive movement against the tested antagonist should theoretically reach, if the disorder was limited to non-neural muscle tissue shortening and not to neural events. Obviously, various underlying nonmuscular joint alterations may also impact X_{V1}, such as arthritis, capsulitis, or immobilization-induced joint retractions [40]. However, pure joint limitations should not be responsible for large reductions in X_{V1} [40]. X_{V1} may also reflect extensibility losses in fascia, aponeuroses, skin, vessels, etc. [41, 42]. Depending on the degree of contracture and spastic dystonia, X_{V1} may be more or less remote from the expected maximal anatomical angle at the tested joint, a "normal" angle that may be called X_N (using standard anatomical values, rather than an estimation based on the ipsilesional side of hemiparetic patients, which is often altered as well [21]).

The second clinical maneuver aims to assess the response of the tested muscles to fast stretch at high velocity, V3 (spasticity), which may reflect both motoneuronal excitability [8, 9, 43, 44] and increased transmission of the stretching forces to the spindles [45, 46]. This maneuver is therefore also performed after ensuring that the muscles are in the optimal resting position prior to testing [36, 37]. One may use a few brisk movements in the opposite direction to that used for testing immediately prior to the test, to ensure that the muscle is at rest [37]. The test maneuver then involves stretching the muscle group of interest as fast as possible until a catch is felt. If the catch repeatedly and reliably occurs before maximal clinical muscle extensibility (X_{V1}) is reached *and is followed by a clear release*, that can be visually measured without a goniometer, then the angle of catch represents the threshold of transient resistance that is due to an elicited stretch reflex [5]. Occasionally the catch is not followed by a clear release but still reliably occurs at an angle that is different from, and smaller than, the maximal clinical muscle extensibility X_{V1}. The absence of clear release may then be explained by the velocity-dependent viscoelastic passive resistance from the tested muscle group [22, 47], or by strong residual spastic dystonia in the tested muscle group. If the catch is followed by a release and then a recatch, this is called a clonus. The angle of catch that is obtained using this maneuver is called X_{V3} (V3, fastest possible velocity for the examiner; [36]). Depending on the presence or absence of a catch or a clonus, the Tardieu Scale also provides a spasticity grade, Y, an ordinal variable [37]. The two parameters, X_{V3} and Y, may have physiological relevance as one may represent the threshold and the other the gain of the stretch reflex [48]. The *Tardieu Scale* consists in determining X_{V1}, X_{V3}, and Y.

The reliability of the Tardieu Scale was first demonstrated in children with cerebral palsy [49] and then in adults with spastic paresis as far as the determination of angles (not the spasticity grade) was concerned [50]. Baude et al. in 2015 also showed excellent intra- and inter-rater reliability of X_{V1}, X_{V3}, and Y in eight key muscle groups in adult patients with chronic hemiparesis using the five-step assessment – see below [51].

The Syndrome of Spastic Paresis

The term *spastic paresis* describes the clinical syndrome caused by lesions involving the corticospinal pathways [52]. This syndrome involves two disorders: a non-neural muscle disorder called *spastic myopathy* that combines muscle shortening and loss of extensibility (See Chaps. 4, 5 and 6) [52]; and a neural disorder comprising four main components: (i) *Spastic dystonia* defined as unwanted, involuntary muscle activity at rest, in the absence of any phasic stretch or voluntary effort, but which is sensitive to tonic stretch [39]; (ii) *Spastic cocontraction*, defined as unwanted, involuntary muscle activity in the antagonist, elicited by voluntary effort directed to the agonist, aggravated by antagonist stretch [38]; (iii) *Spasticity*, which is an enhancement of the velocity-dependent responses to phasic stretch, detected and measured at rest [8, 9]; and (iv) *Stretch-sensitive paresis*, which refers to decreased central command to the agonist that is aggravated by antagonist stretch [8, 9, 52, 53]. The pathophysiology of spastic paresis has recently been revisited and clarified [38]; this will be briefly described here and is summarized in Table 3.4.

Table 3.4 Main features of spastic paresis with their deforming and disabling properties and their clinical measurability

	Symptom name	Condition of detection	Trigger	Deforming capacity	Disabling level	Measurability at bedside
Muscle disorder	Spastic myopathy	Rest	N/A	High	High	Estimation possible
Neural disorder						
Paresis	Stretch-sensitive paresis	Effort	N/A	None	Moderate	No
Muscle overactivity types	Spasticity	Rest	Phasic stretch	None	Low	Yes
	Spastic dystonia	Rest	None	High	High	No
	Spastic cocontraction	Effort	Effort directed to agonist	None	High	No
	Extrasegmental cocontraction (synkinesis)	Effort	Effort	Moderate	Moderate	No
	Nociceptive (FRA) spasms	Rest or effort	FRA stimulation	High	Moderate	No

FRA flexor reflex afferents

The Non-Neural Muscle Disorder: Spastic Myopathy

After a lesion to the central motor pathways, immobilization of muscles in a shortened position leads to mechanical changes in muscle tissue [8], which result in muscle shortening and stiffness as described in Chap. 6. In most current health systems, immobility typically begins with the onset of paresis (at which time the muscle tissue is initially normal), and persists as paresis lingers [42, 54–56]. A muscle disorder then develops due to modifications in gene transcription in the muscle fibers immobilized in a shortened position, with deleterious quantitative and qualitative changes [54–56]. The existence of a causative factor (immobilization in a shortend position in the context of paresis) and of molecular, histological and then biomechanical, physiological, and lastly clinical (loss of muscle extensibility and muscle stiffness, see below) events constitutes a pathogenic entity termed *spastic myopathy* [52]. This is an evolving form of a mostly avoidable disorder that is superimposed on the neural disorder [41, 52, 57]. Clinically, spastic myopathy manifests as a loss of extensibility of the muscle or muscle stiffness as a result of increased muscle viscoelasticity, especially under conditions of high tension or high speed. Spastic myopathy is thus the first factor that leads to deformity in patients with spastic paresis and that limits passive and active movement [8].

The Neural Disorder

The neural disorder comprises of two components that are superimposed around each joint and act synergistically to challenge active movement: muscle overactivity in antagonists and stretch-sensitive paresis in agonists [8, 9, 53].

Muscle Overactivity in Antagonists

Spastic muscle overactivity comprises different forms of increased involuntary recruitment of motor units, which often co-exist.

Spastic Dystonia In 1966, based on animal experiments that involved ablating various motor cortical areas, Denny-Brown defined the term spastic dystonia as involuntary tonic activity in the context of otherwise exaggerated stretch reflexes [58]. This phenomenon was later confirmed in humans [59]. Sustained involuntary muscle activity in the absence of stretch or voluntary command contributes to burdensome and disabling body deformities in patients with spastic paresis. Following Denny-Brown's work, a refined definition of spastic dystonia was proposed as *excessive, chronic, tonic muscle activation of supraspinal origin, detected and measured at rest, that is potentially reduced after maintained stretch of the dystonic muscle* [9, 38, 39]. In the most shortened muscles, spastic dystonia thus superimposes on spastic myopathy to represent the second major factor leading to deformity in patients with spastic paresis.

Spastic Cocontraction Spastic cocontraction is defined as *excessive degree of antagonistic activation elicited by voluntary agonist command, aggravated by antagonist stretch* [9, 60]. This type of overactivity is revealed and exclusively measured during a *voluntary command directed to the agonist*; it is mainly of supraspinal origin and is aggravated by stretch of the cocontracting muscle [8, 9, 60]. Spastic cocontraction is a critical factor limiting active movement and sometimes produces the opposite movement to that intended in subjects with spastic paresis [8, 9, 60].

Spasticity Already described in this chapter.

Stretch-Sensitive Paresis in Agonists

Stretch-sensitive paresis is defined as *a reduction in the voluntary recruitment of agonist motor units that is worsened by stretching of the antagonist* [8, 9, 53]. In the most severe cases, i.e., when the antagonist is prominently shortened and spastic myopathy has set in, full antagonist stretch may completely abolish the ability to bring agonist motor neurons to firing threshold, leading to full agonist plegia in a particular joint position [53]. The worsening of the agonist command by antagonist stretch represents yet another incentive for clinicians to prevent severe spastic myopathy in patients with paresis of central origin.

The Five-Step Assessment

Expanding on the Tardieu Scale, a step-wise clinical assessment aiming to reflect as many aspects of spastic paresis as clinically possible was developed in 2010, called the Five-Step Assessment (FSA; [37]). The FSA was further expanded in 2015 with the calculation of specific *Coefficients of Impairment,* the first of them aims to estimate the muscle disorder, and the others aim to estimate the neural contribution separately from the muscle disorder [37, 52]. Each step of the FSA is quantitative. Step 1 corresponds to functional evaluation of the limb and the other four correspond to technical measurements. In practice, complete evaluation may take around 60 min: 40 min for the upper limb and 20 min for the lower limb.

Functional Step: Step 1

Upper Limb In the upper limb, functional evaluation of spastic paresis may utilize the Modified Frenchay Scale (MFS) [37, 51, 61], derived from the Frenchay Arm Test [62]. The MFS measures active upper limb function in individuals with hemiparesis based on a video review of 10 everyday tasks, each rated on a 10-point visual analog scale. Six tasks are bimanual and four are unimanual, performed with the paretic hand. Figure 3.2 displays the instructions for each task and the rating system. Figure 3.3 shows patient and rater positioning as well as the equipment required. The tasks are always attempted in the same order, as objects are always placed from left to right on the table, regardless of whether the subject presents with left or right hemiparesis. Unimanual tasks are performed strictly with the paretic hand, with no help whatsoever from the nonparetic hand.

Figure 3.4 provides suggestions to facilitate rating on the MFS. Each task is rated between zero (no movement) and 10 (task is accomplished perfectly), in increments of 0.5 points. The score for a task that is barely accomplished is 5. Use the following guidance for rating tasks between 0 and 5 and 5 and 10:

- Between 0 and 5 (task not achieved), use 2 for a task that appears closer to not being achieved than to being achieved and 3 in the opposite case.
- Between 3 and 5, the concept of primary components of the overall movement task can be used. When only one primary component (e.g., hand opening, elbow extension or elbow supination) is just short of making the task achievable, i.e., reaching a 5, half a point can be deducted from 5, to give a score of 4.5, or one full point can be deducted depending on how close the performance is to being achievable.
- Between 5 and 10 (task achieved), use 6 for a task that is slowly but *securely* accomplished even though the movements may not be smooth, 7 for a task that is performed *smoothly* but is still slow, and 8 for a task that is performed *fast* but is still clearly far from normal (close to normal would be a 9).

Modified Frenchay Scale

1. Open and close jam jar using both hands (Paretic hand holds jar)

No movement Normal

2. Reach, pick up and release big bottle using paretic hand <u>only</u>

No movement Normal

3. Reach, pick up and release small bottle using paretic hand <u>only</u>

No movement Normal

4. Reach, pick up glass and bring to mouth using paretic hand <u>only</u>

No movement Normal

5. Rule line with ruler using both hands (paretic hand holds ruler)

No movement Normal

6. Clip 3 clothe-pins on paper-pad edge using both hands (paretic hand holds and clips pins)

No movement Normal

7. Reach, pick up comb and mimic combing using paretic hand <u>only</u>

No movement Normal

8. Put toothpaste on toothbrush using both hands (paretic hand holds and presses on tube)

No movement Normal

9. Pick up knife and fork using both hands and mimic cutting (paretic hand holds fork)

No movement Normal

10. Sweep floor with broom using both hands

No movement Normal

Scoring: 0, no movement; 5, task barely accomplished; 10, normal performance

Fig. 3.2 Instructions for performing and scoring each task on the Modified Frenchay Scale

- In case the person did not comply with the instructions, the task is not ratable and may be scored as NA ("Not Applicable"). The overall MFS score is the mean of the 10 task scores. The reliability of the MFS in chronic hemiparesis in adults is excellent, both in terms of intra- and inter-rater reliability [63].

Lower Limb The syndrome of spastic paresis in the lower limb has been evaluated using walking speed over 10 meters or maximal walking speed over 2 min, both of which have excellent ecological validity [64–71]. Among the various possible test-

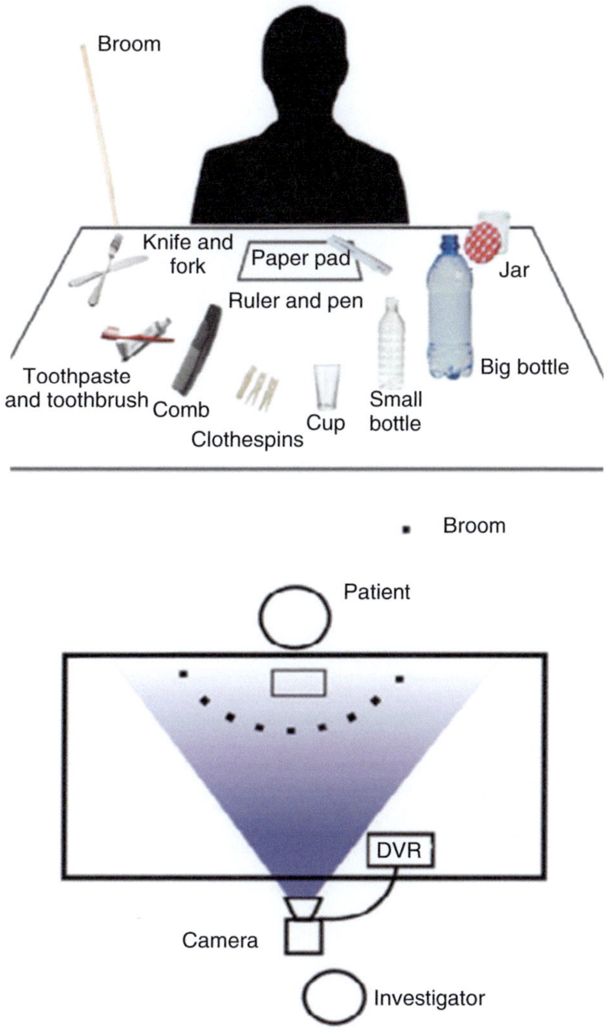

Fig. 3.3 Patient and rater positioning and equipment required for the Modified Frenchay Scale

ing modes (barefoot or with shoes, with or without assistive device(s), at comfortable or fast speed, including or not including sit-to-stand, u-turn, and stand-to-sit), use the mode that is more sensitive to change because it imposes a greater strain on the neuromotor system [72] and provides minimal assistance to the patient. For example, the recommendation is to test gait *barefoot without assistive devices* every time if it is possible, at maximal rather than at comfortable speed, and including sit-to-stand, u-turns, and stand-to-sit (modified Timed Up and Go test). A 10 meter walk test at maximal speed, barefoot, starting and ending seated, has both the highest level of reliability [73] and the highest sensitivity to change (more sensitive than

Suggestions to facilitate rating of the Modified Frenchay Scale

Examples given for unimanual tasks

0: **No movement**

1: Movement initiated with ≥ 1 movement component
e.g., tasks 2, 3, 4: onset of shoulder flexion/abduction

2. ≥ 2 movement component initated
e.g., tasks 2, 3, 4: onset of shoulder flexion and elbow extension;
Overall, task still closer to not being achieved than to being achieved

2.5: ≥ 3 movement component initated
e.g., tasks 2. 3. 4: onset of shoulder flexion, elbow extension and supination;
Overall, task midway between being achieved and not

3: ≥ 4 components initated but incomplete
e.g., tasks 2, 3, 4: onset of shoulder flexion, elbow extension, elbow supination and hand opening;
Overall, task closer to being achieved than not to

3.5: ≥ 3 movement components incomplete
e.g., tasks 2, 3, 4: elbow extension, supination and hand opening

4: ≥ 2 movement components incomplete
e.g., tasks 2, 3, 4: supination and hand opening

4.5: 1 movement component incomplete
e.g., tasks 2, 3, 4: hand opening

5: Task barely accomplished

6: Sense of difficulty: task secured but with difficulty, slowly

7: Sense of smoothness: task accomplished with some smoothness but still slow

8: Sense of speed: task fast completed, whike still clearly different from normal

9: Almost normal

10: Normal performance

NA: non applicable

Fig. 3.4 Suggestions to facilitate rating of the Modified Frenchay Scale

comfortable speed barefoot tests or tests with shoes) after therapeutic interventions involving neurorehabilitation (Guided Self-rehabilitation Contracts) or repeat injections of neuromuscular blocking agents [34, 74].

In addition to quantifying gait speed, step length, and cadence, such gait tests lend themselves to visual observation that can lead to improved understanding of specific gait patterns. When observing proximal lower limb activity in spastic paresis, it is possible to define various gait patterns [75].

- In the "anterior pattern", overactivity or stiffness in the quadriceps predominates over that in the hip extensors [52]. Anterior patterns are characterized by relatively preserved step length but slow speed of the swing phase on the paretic side (leading to a particularly slowed gait cadence), a lack of hip extension at late stance (due to rectus femoris shortening/overactivity), preserved knee re-extension at late swing, and knee flexion that remains below the degree of hip flexion in a test of rapid alternating hip flexion. Anterior patterns are commonly seen following ischemic middle cerebral artery lesions in adult patients and typically point to the need to reduce quadriceps resistance to knee flexion.

- At the other end of the spectrum, "posterior patterns" are produced when overactivity or stiffness in the hip extensors (hamstrings and gluteus maximus) predominate over that in the quadriceps [52]. Posterior patterns are characterized by markedly reduced step length on the paretic side (while cadence is relatively preserved), preserved hip extension at late stance, insufficient knee re-extension at late swing (due to hamstrings shortening/overactivity), and knee flexion greater than hip flexion in a test of rapid alternating hip flexion (backward "leg recall"). Posterior patterns are commonly seen after spinal cord lesions (traumatic or inflammatory) and in cerebral palsy, although in cerebral palsy the patterns are often mixed and typically point to the need to reduce mainly hip extensor resistance to hip flexion.

Technical Steps: Steps 2–5

Step 2

Step 2 consists of assessing the maximum passive range of motion at the slowest velocity (X_{V1}) on the Tardieu scale. The difference between the total possible range of motion at the joint (X_N) and the maximum passive range of motion at the slowest velocity (X_{V1}), normalized to the total possible range of motion at the joint ($X_N - X_{V1})/X_N$ is defined as the *coefficient of shortening*, which estimates the loss of functional muscle length or muscle shortening [52].

Step 3

Step 3 consists of assessing the catch angle at fast velocity (X_{V3}) on the Tardieu scale. The difference between the maximum passive range of motion at the slowest velocity (X_{V1}) and the catch angle (X_{V3}), normalized to the maximum passive range of motion at the slowest velocity ($X_{V1} - X_{V3})/X_{V1}$ is defined as the *coefficient of spasticity*, which estimates the extent of spasticity separately from the functional length of the muscle [52].

Step 4

The objective of Step 4 is to assess the capacity of agonist activation to overcome passive and active resistance in the antagonist muscle group. Ask the patient to accomplish one active movement of maximal range of motion. While goniometry does not improve the reliability in assessing X_{V1} and X_{V3} [49], a goniometer is recommended to measure the active angle X_A. The angle of active range of motion represents the balance between the forces generated by agonist activation and the resistance from passive (stiffness/increased visco-elasticity) and active (spastic cocontraction) phenomena opposing the agonist muscle group. The measured angle is the maximal active range of motion (X_A) over one single movement. The difference between the maximum passive range of motion at the slowest possible velocity (X_{V1}) and the maximum active range of motion (X_A), normalized to the maximum passive range of motion at the slowest velocity ($X_{V1} - X_A)/X_{V1}$ is the *coefficient of weakness*, which estimates the impairment of active command, regardless of the maximal passive extensibility of the opposing muscle [52].

Step 5

The objective of Step 5 is to assess the ability to overcome the passive (non-neural) and active (neural) resistance repeatedly [37]. The patient is asked to accomplish as many alternating movements of a joint as possible in 15 s, keeping the range of motion as large as possible on each repetition. The amplitude of the last active movement of the series and the mean movement frequency are recorded. The amplitude of the last movement within the 15-s period of maximal active repetitions (X_{A15}) represents the change or decrement from a single maximal active range of motion (X_A) and reflects performance fatigability. The difference between the maximum active range of motion (X_A) and the amplitude of the movement at the end of 15 s (X_{A15}), normalized to the maximum active range of motion ($X_A - X_{A15})/X_A$ is the *coefficient of fatigability*, which quantifies the movement decrement over 15 s, regardless of the maximum active range of motion achieved over a single movement [52]. Figures 3.5 and 3.6 show the evaluation forms for the upper and lower limb.

Five-Step Assessment in Spastic Paresis - Upper limb												
Modified Frenchay		Movement	Tested muscles	Clinical measures					Coefficients (coeff.) of impairment			
Modified Frenchay Scale		Shoulder		X_{V1}	X_{V3}	Y	X_A	X_{A15}	Coeff.of shortening	Coeff. of spasticity	Coeff. of weakness	Coeff. of fatigability
Jar		Flexion - elbow straight	LD, TM, Rh-MT>60°, PM>90°									
Big bottle		Flexion - elbow bent	LD, TM, Rh-MT>60°, PM>90°, LHT									
Small bottle		Extension	AD, SS, CB									
Cup		Vertical abduction/lateral elevation	LD, PM, Rh, MT									
Paper pad		Horizontal abduction	PM, Tm, IS									
Comb		External rotation - shoulder neutral	SS, PM									
Clothe pins		External rotation - shoulder flexed	SS, PM + LD, TM									
Toothpaste		Internal rotation	IS, Tm, PD									
Fork and knife		Elbow										
Broom		Extension shoulder neutral	BB, B, BR									
MEAN		Extension shoulder flexed	BB, B, BR									
Notes:		Flexion - shoulder neutral	TB without LHT									
		Flexion - flexed shoulder	TB with LHT									
		Supination - elbow flexed	PQ									
		Supination - elbow straight	PQ + PT									
		Pronation - elbow flexed	Supinator + BB									
		Pronation - elbow straight	Supinator									
		Wrist										
		Extension - elbow flexed	FCR, FCU, FDS, FDP									
		Extension - elbow straight	FCR, FCU, FDS, FDP									
		Flexion - elbow flexed	ECU, EDC									
		Flexion - elbow straight	ECU, EDC, ECRB, ECRL									
		Fingers										
		Extension PIII/PII - wrist and MCP neutral	FDP II, III, IV, V									
		Extension PII/MC - wrist and MCP neutral	FDS, FDP II-V, PIO, DIO									
		Extension PI/MC - wrist flexed	PIO, DIO, lumbricals									
		Extension I - wrist neutral	FPL, FPB									
		Extension I - wrist flexed	FPB									
		Thumb de-opposition (long abduction)	Opponens pollicis									
		Thumb short abduction	Adductor pollicis									

Fig. 3.5 Five-Step Assessment in Spastic Paresis in the Upper Limb. X_{V1} maximal passive range of motion at slow speed; X_{V3} angle of catch or clonus at fast speed; *Y* grade of spasticity; X_A maximal active range of motion; X_{A15} residual amplitude of active motion after 15 seconds of maximal amplitude active movements; *PI* first phalanx; *PII* second phalanx; *PIII* third phalanx; *MCP* metacarpophalangeal; *MC* metacarpal; *AD* anterior deltoid; *BB* biceps brachii; *B* brachialis; *BR* brachio-radialis; *CB* coracobrachialis; *DIO* dorsal interossei; *ECRB* extensor carpi radialis brevis; *ECRL* extensor carpi radialis longus; *ECU* extensor carpi ulnaris; *EDC* extensor digitorum communis; *FCR* flexor carpi radialis; *FCU* flexor carpi ulnaris; *FDP* flexor digitorum profundus; *FDS* flexor digitorum superficialis; *FBP* flexor pollicis brevis; *FPL* flexor pollicis longus; *IS* infraspinatus; *LD* latissimus dorsi; *LHT* long head of triceps; *MT* middle trapezius; *PD* posterior detoid; *PIO* palmar interossei; *PL* palmaris longus; *PM* pectoralis major; *PQ* pronator quadratus; *PT* pronator teres; *Rh* rhomboids; *SS* subscapularis; *TB* triceps brachii; *TM* teres major; *Tm* teres minor

Five-Step Assessment in Spastic Paresis - Lower limb

10 meter Walk Test		Number of steps	Seconds	Speed (m/s)	Step length (m)	Cadence (steps/min)	Notes:
Shoes + splint + cane	Comfortable						
	Rapid						
Shoes + splint - no cane	Comfortable						
	Rapid						
Shoes - no splint + cane	Comfortable						
	Rapid						
Shoes - no splint - no cane	Comfortable						
	Rapid						
Barefoot + cane	Comfortable						
	Rapid						
Barefoot no cane	Comfortable						
	Rapid						

Step-wise technical assessment		Soleus		Soleus + gastrocnemius		Gluteus maximus		Gluteus maximus + hamstrings		Vastus muscles		Vastus + rectus femoris		Flexor hip adductors		Extensor hip adductors		Internal hip rotators		External hip rotators	
		Left	Right	Left	Right	Left	Right	Left	Right	Left	Right	Left	Right	Left	Right	Left	Right	Left	Right	Left	Right
Passive range of motion	X_{V1}																				
Angle of catch	X_{V3}																				
Spasticity grade	Y																				
Active range of motion	X_A																				
Active range of motion at 15 sec	X_{A15}																				
Nb of max ampl mvts in 15 sec	N_{15}																				
Coefficient of shortening	C_{SH}																				
Coefficient of spasticity	C_{SP}																				
Coefficient of weakness	C_W																				
Coefficient of fatigability	C_F																				

Fig. 3.6 Five-Step Assessment in Spastic Paresis in the Lower Limb. X_{V1} maximal passive range of motion at slow speed; X_{V3} angle of catch or clonus at fast speed; Y grade of spasticity; X_A maximal active range of motion; X_{A15} residual amplitude of active motion at the end of 15 seconds of maximal amplitude active movements; *Nb* number; *ampl* amplitude; *mvts* movements

Conclusion

A useful assessment of the syndrome of spastic paresis should follow, as closely as possible, the current understanding of the pathophysiology of the neural and non-neural (muscle) components of the disorder. Clear and accurate definitions of common words that are often used should also be kept in mind. *Tone* is not *spasticity*; nor is it spastic *cocontraction*, *spastic dystonia*, *stretch-sensitive paresis* or *spastic myopathy*. The era of *one-name-fits-all* should come to a close, as longstanding oversimplifications do not inform therapeutic strategies to treat the problem accurately. This chapter summarizes a comprehensive understanding of the pathophysiology of the syndrome of spastic paresis, which can be used to validate and measure its various components.

References

1. Tardieu G, Shentoub S, Delarue R. Research on a technic for measurement of spasticity. Rev Neurol (Paris). 1954;91(2):143–4.
2. Lance JW. Symposium synopsis. In: Feldman RG, Young RR, Koella WP, editors. Spasticity: disordered motor control. Chicago: Yearbook Medical; 1980. p. 485–94.
3. Powers RK, Campbell DL, Rymer WZ. Stretch reflex dynamics in spastic elbow flexor muscles. Ann Neurol. 1989;25(1):32–42.
4. Berardelli A, Hallett M, Kaufman C, Fine E, Berenberg W, Simon SR. Stretch reflexes of triceps surae in normal man. J Neurol Neurosurg Psychiatry. 1982;45(6):513–25.
5. Ashby P, Burke D. Stretch reflexes in the upper limb of spastic man. J Neurol Neurosurg Psychiatry. 1971;34(6):765–71.
6. Fellows SJ, Ross HF, Thilmann AF. The limitations of the tendon jerk as a marker of pathological stretch reflex activity in human spasticity. J Neurol Neurosurg Psychiatry. 1993;56(5):531–7.
7. Thilmann AF, Fellows SJ, Garms E. Pathological stretch reflexes on the "good" side of hemiparetic patients. J Neurol Neurosurg Psychiatry. 1990;53(3):208–14.
8. Gracies JM. Pathophysiology of spastic paresis. I: paresis and soft tissue changes. Muscle Nerve. 2005;31(5):535–51.
9. Gracies JM. Pathophysiology of spastic paresis. II: emergence of muscle overactivity. Muscle Nerve. 2005;31(5):552–71.
10. Ashworth B. Preliminary trial of carisoprodol in multiple sclerosis. Practitioner. 1964;192:540–2.
11. Patrick E, Ada L. The Tardieu Scale differentiates contracture from spasticity whereas the Ashworth Scale is confounded by it. Clin Rehabil. 2006;20(2):173–82.
12. Bohannon RW, Smith MB. Interrater reliability of a modified Ashworth scale of muscle spasticity. Phys Ther. 1987;67(2):206–7.
13. Fleuren JF, Voerman GE, Erren-Wolters CV, Snoek GJ, Rietman JS, Hermens HJ, Nene AV. Stop using the Ashworth Scale for the assessment of spasticity. J Neurol Neurosurg Psychiatry. 2010;81(1):46–52.
14. Pandyan AD, Johnson GR, Price CI, Curless RH, Barnes MP, Rodgers H. A review of the properties and limitations of the Ashworth and modified Ashworth Scales as measures of spasticity. Clin Rehabil. 1999;13(5):373–83.
15. Fleuren JF, Nederhand MJ, Hermens HJ. Influence of posture and muscle length on stretch reflex activity in poststroke patients with spasticity. Arch Phys Med Rehabil. 2006;87(7):981–8.
16. Tardieu C, Tardieu G, Gagnard L, Leconte S. Differences between tension-length diagrams of the sural triceps and the anterior tibial muscles in cats. J Physiol (Paris). 1967;59(1 Suppl):302–3.

17. Brashear A, Zafonte R, Corcoran M, Galvez-Jimenez N, Gracies JM, Gordon MF, McAfee A, Ruffing K, Thompson B, Williams M, Lee CH, Turkel C. Inter- and intrarater reliability of the Ashworth Scale and the Disability Assessment Scale in patients with upper-limb poststroke spasticity. Arch Phys Med Rehabil. 2002;83(10):1349–54.
18. Burke D, Gillies JD, Lance JW. Hamstrings stretch reflex in human spasticity. J Neurol Neurosurg Psychiatry. 1971;34(3):231–5.
19. Dietz V, Quintern J, Berger W. Electrophysiological studies of gait in spasticity and rigidity. Evidence that altered mechanical properties of muscle contribute to hypertonia. Brain. 1981;104(3):431–49.
20. Singer B, Dunne J, Allison G. Reflex and non-reflex elements of hypertonia in triceps surae muscles following acquired brain injury: implications for rehabilitation. Disabil Rehabil. 2001;23(17):749–57.
21. Singer B, Dunne J, Singer KP, Allison G. Evaluation of triceps surae muscle length and resistance to passive lengthening in patients with acquired brain injury. Clin Biomech (Bristol, Avon). 2002;17(2):152–61.
22. Singer BJ, Dunne JW, Singer KP, Allison GT. Velocity-dependent passive plantar flexor resistive torque in patients with acquired brain injury. Clin Biomech (Bristol, Avon). 2003;18(2):157–65.
23. Nielsen JF, Sinkjaer T. A comparison of clinical and laboratory measures of spasticity. Mult Scler. 1996;1(5):296–301.
24. Priebe MM, Sherwood AM, Thornby JI, Kharas NF, Markowski J. Clinical assessment of spasticity in spinal cord injury: a multidimensional problem. Arch Phys Med Rehabil. 1996;77(7):713–6.
25. Vattanasilp W, Ada L. The relationship between clinical and laboratory measures of spasticity. Aust J Physiother. 1999;45(2):135–9.
26. Vattanasilp W, Ada L, Crosbie J. Contribution of thixotropy, spasticity, and contracture to ankle stiffness after stroke. J Neurol Neurosurg Psychiatry. 2000;69(1):34–9.
27. Bakheit AM, Maynard VA, Curnow J, Hudson N, Kodapala S. The relation between Ashworth scale scores and the excitability of the alpha motor neurones in patients with post-stroke muscle spasticity. J Neurol Neurosurg Psychiatry. 2003;74(5):646–8.
28. Pandyan AD, Price CI, Barnes MP, Johnson GR. A biomechanical investigation into the validity of the modified Ashworth Scale as a measure of elbow spasticity. Clin Rehabil. 2003;17(3):290–3.
29. Calabrò RS, Naro A, Russo M, Milardi D, Leo A, Filoni S, Trinchera A, Bramanti P. Is two better than one? Muscle vibration plus robotic rehabilitation to improve upper limb spasticity and function: a pilot randomized controlled trial. PLoS One. 2017;12(10):e0185936.
30. Marinelli L, Balestrino M, Mori L, Puce L, Rosa GM, Giorello L, Currà A, Fattapposta F, Serrati C, Gandolfo C, Abbruzzese G, Trompetto C. A randomised controlled cross-over double-blind pilot study protocol on THC:CBD oromucosal spray efficacy as an add-on therapy for post-stroke spasticity. BMJ Open. 2017;7(9):e016843.
31. Villafañe JH, Taveggia G, Galeri S, Bissolotti L, Mullè C, Imperio G, Valdes K, Borboni A, Negrini S. Efficacy of short-term robot-assisted rehabilitation in patients with hand paralysis after stroke: a randomized clinical trial. Hand (NY). 2018;13(1):95–102.
32. Wein T, Esquenazi A, Jost WH, Ward AB, Pan G, Dimitrova R. OnabotulinumtoxinA for the treatment of poststroke distal lower limb spasticity: a randomized trial. PM R. 2018;10(7):693–703.
33. Delgado MR, Bonikowski M, Carranza J, Dabrowski E, Matthews D, Russman B, Tilton A, Velez JC, Grandoulier AS, Picaut P. Safety and efficacy of repeat open-label abobotulinumtoxinA treatment in pediatric cerebral palsy. J Child Neurol. 2017;32(13):1058–64.
34. Gracies JM, Esquenazi A, Brashear A, Banach M, Kocer S, Jech R, Khatkova S, Benetin J, Vecchio M, McAllister P, Ilkowski J, Ochudlo S, Catus F, Grandoulier AS, Vilain C, Picaut P, International AbobotulinumtoxinA Adult Lower Limb Spasticity Study Group. Efficacy and safety of abobotulinumtoxinA in spastic lower limb: randomized trial and extension. Neurology. 2017;89(22):2245–53.

35. Tardieu G. Evaluation et caractères distinctifs des diverses raideurs d'origine cérébrale. Chapitre VB1b Les feuillets de l'infirmité motrice cérébrale. Paris: Association nationale des IMC; 1966. p. 1–28.
36. Gracies JM, Marosszeky JE, Renton R, Sandanam J, Gandevia SC, Burke D. Short-term effects of dynamic lycra splints on upper limb in hemiplegic patients. Arch Phys Med Rehabil. 2000;81(12):1547–55.
37. Gracies JM, Bayle N, Vinti M, Alkandari S, Vu P, Loche CM, Colas C. Five-step clinical assessment in spastic paresis. Eur J Phys Rehabil Med. 2010;46(3):411–21.
38. Baude M, Nielsen JB, Gracies JM. The neurophysiology of deforming spastic paresis: a revised taxonomy. Ann Phys Rehabil Med. 2018 Nov 28. pii:S1877-0657(18)31479-9.
39. Lorentzen J, Pradines M, Gracies JM, Bo NJ. On Denny-Brown's 'spastic dystonia' – what is it and what causes it? Clin Neurophysiol. 2018;129(1):89–94.
40. Trudel G, Laneuville O, Coletta E, Goudreau L, Uhthoff HK. Quantitative and temporal differential recovery of articular and muscular limitations of knee joint contractures; results in a rat model. J Appl Physiol (1985). 2014;117(7):730–7.
41. de Bruin M, Smeulders MJ, Kreulen M, Huijing PA, Jaspers RT. Intramuscular connective tissue differences in spastic and control muscle: a mechanical and histological study. PLoS One. 2014;9(6):e101038.
42. Tabary JC, Tabary C, Tardieu C, Tardieu G, Goldspink G. Physiological and structural changes in the cat's soleus muscle due to immobilization at different lengths by plaster casts. J Physiol. 1972;224(1):231–44.
43. Gorassini M, Bennett DJ, Kiehn O, Eken T, Hultborn H. Activation patterns of hindlimb motor units in the awake rat and their relation to motoneuron intrinsic properties. J Neurophysiol. 1999;82(2):709–17.
44. Gorassini MA, Knash ME, Harvey PJ, Bennett DJ, Yang JF. Role of motoneurons in the generation of muscle spasms after spinal cord injury. Brain. 2004;127(Pt 10):2247–58.
45. Gioux M, Petit J. Effects of immobilizing the cat peroneus longus muscle on the activity of its own spindles. J Appl Physiol (1985). 1993;75(6):2629–35.
46. Rosant C, Nagel MD, Pérot C. Adaptation of rat soleus muscle spindles after 21 days of hindlimb unloading. Exp Neurol. 2006;200(1):191–9.
47. Jalal N, Zidi M. Influence of experimental conditions on visco-hyperelastic properties of skeletal muscle tissue using a Box-Behnken design. J Biomech. 2019;85:204–9.
48. Katz RT, Rymer WZ. Spastic hypertonia: mechanisms and measurement. Arch Phys Med Rehabil. 1989;70(2):144–55.
49. Gracies JM, Burke K, Clegg NJ, Browne R, Rushing C, Fehlings D, Matthews D, Tilton A, Delgado MR. Reliability of the Tardieu Scale for assessing spasticity in children with cerebral palsy. Arch Phys Med Rehabil. 2010;91(3):421–8.
50. Ben-Shabat E, Palit M, Fini NA, Brooks CT, Winter A, Holland AE. Intra- and inter-rater reliability of the Modified Tardieu Scale for the assessment of lower limb spasticity in adults with neurologic injuries. Arch Phys Med Rehabil. 2013;94(12):2494–501.
51. Baude M, Loche CM, Gault-Colas C, Pradines M, Gracies JM. Intra- and inter-rater reliability of a stepped clinical assessment of chronic spastic paresis in adults. Ann Phys Rehabil Med. 2015;58(S1):e4–5.
52. Gracies JM. Coefficients of impairment in deforming spastic paresis. Ann Phys Rehabil Med. 2015;58(3):173–8.
53. Vinti M, Bayle N, Hutin E, Burke D, Gracies JM. Stretch-sensitive paresis and effort perception in hemiparesis. J Neural Transm (Vienna). 2015;122(8):1089–97.
54. Baptista IL, Leal ML, Artioli GG, Aoki MS, Fiamoncini J, Turri AO, Curi R, Miyabara EH, Moriscot AS. Leucine attenuates skeletal muscle wasting via inhibition of ubiquitin ligases. Muscle Nerve. 2010;41(6):800–8.
55. Giger JM, Bodell PW, Zeng M, Baldwin KM, Haddad F. Rapid muscle atrophy response to unloading: pretranslational processes involving MHC and actin. J Appl Physiol (1985). 2009;107(4):1204–12.

56. Kelleher AR, Gordon BS, Kimball SR, Jefferson LS. Changes in REDD1, REDD2, and atrogene mRNA expression are prevented in skeletal muscle fixed in a stretched position during hindlimb immobilization. Physiol Rep. 2014;2(2):e00246.
57. Diong J, Harvey LA, Kwah LK, Clarke JL, Bilston LE, Gandevia SC, Herbert RD. Gastrocnemius muscle contracture after spinal cord injury: a longitudinal study. Am J Phys Med Rehabil. 2013;92(7):565–74.
58. Denny-Brown D. The cerebral control of movement. Liverpool: Liverpool University Press; 1966. p. 124–3, 171–84.
59. Laplane D, Talairach J, Meininger V, Bancaud J, Bouchareine A. Motor consequences of motor area ablations in man. J Neurol Sci. 1977;31:29–49.
60. Vinti M, Couillandre A, Hausselle J, Bayle N, Primerano A, Merlo A, Hutin E, Gracies JM. Influence of effort intensity and gastrocnemius stretch on co-contraction and torque production in the healthy and paretic ankle. Clin Neurophysiol. 2013;124(3):528–35.
61. Gracies JM, Hefter H, Simpson D, Moore P. Botulinum toxin in spasticity. In: Moore P, Naumann M, editors. Handbook of botulinum toxin. Oxford: Blackwell Science; 2002. p. 221–74.
62. Wade DT, Langton-Hewer R, Wood VA, Skilbeck CE, Ismail HM. The hemiplegic arm after stroke: measurement and recovery. J Neurol Neurosurg Psychiatry. 1983;46(6):521–4.
63. Baude M, Mardale V, Loche CM, Hutin E, Gracies JM, Bayle N. Intra- and inter-rater reliability of the Modified Frenchay Scale to measure active upper limb function in hemiparetic patients. Ann Phys Rehabil Med. 2016;59S:e59–60.
64. Dalgas U, Kjølhede T, Gijbels D, Romberg A, Santoyo C, de Noordhout BM, Knuts K, Feys P. Aerobic intensity and pacing pattern during the six-minute walk test in patients with multiple sclerosis. J Rehabil Med. 2014;46(1):59–66.
65. Dean CM, Richards CL, Malouin F. Walking speed over 10 metres overestimates locomotor capacity after stroke. Clin Rehabil. 2001;15(4):415–21.
66. Flansbjer UB, Holmbäck AM, Downham D, Patten C, Lexell J. Reliability of gait performance tests in men and women with hemiparesis after stroke. J Rehabil Med. 2005;37(2):75–82.
67. Gijbels D, Eijnde BO, Feys P. Comparison of the 2- and 6-minute walk test in multiple sclerosis. Mult Scler. 2011;17(10):1269–72.
68. Moseley AM, Lanzarone S, Bosman JM, van Loo MA, de Bie RA, Hassett L, Caplan B. Ecological validity of walking speed assessment after traumatic brain injury: a pilot study. J Head Trauma Rehabil. 2004;19(4):341–8.
69. Roth EJ, Merbitz C, Mroczek K, Dugan SA, Suh WW. Hemiplegic gait. Relationships between walking speed and other temporal parameters. Am J Phys Med Rehabil. 1997;76(2):128–33.
70. van Loo MA, Moseley AM, Bosman JM, de Bie RA, Hassett L. Inter-rater reliability and concurrent validity of walking speed measurement after traumatic brain injury. Clin Rehabil. 2003;17(7):775–9.
71. van Loo MA, Moseley AM, Bosman JM, de Bie RA, Hassett L. Test-re-test reliability of walking speed, step length and step width measurement after traumatic brain injury: a pilot study. Brain Inj. 2004;18(10):1041–8.
72. Beuter A, Edwards R, de Geoffroy A, Mergler D, Hundnell K. Quantification of neuromotor function for detection of the effects of manganese. Neurotoxicology. 1999;20(2–3):355–66.
73. Hutin E, Ghédira M, Loche CM, Mardale V, Hennegrave C, Gracies JM, Bayle N. Intra- and inter-rater reliability of the 10-meter ambulation test in hemiparesis is better barefoot at maximal speed. Top Stroke Rehabil. 2018;25(5):345–50.
74. Pradines M, Ghedira M, Portero R, Masson I, Marciniak C, Hicklin D, Hutin E, Portero P, Gracies JM, Bayle N. Ultrasound structural changes in triceps surae after a 1-year daily self-stretch program: a prospective randomized controlled trial in chronic hemiparesis. Neurorehabil Neural Repair. 2019;33(4):245–59. https://doi.org/10.1177/1545968319829455.
75. Chambéron M, Radot C, Baude M, Colas C, Gracies JM. Anterior vs posterior patterns of hip flexion impairment in spastic paresis. Toxicon. 2017;123:S14–5.

Quantitative Measurement of Resistance to Passive Joint Motion in Chronic Stroke Survivors

4

Jourdan K. Ewoldt, Preeti Raghavan, and Nina L. Suresh

The physical interactions between our system and others must, as a rule, themselves possess a certain degree of physical orderliness… they too must obey strict physical laws to a certain degree of accuracy.
– Erwin Schrodinger, What is life?, 1943.

- This chapter describes how the "catch", which reflects the resistance to joint rotation during the Modified Ashworth Scale (MAS) and the Tardieu Scale, varies as a function of joint rotation speed, and assesses the contribution of the reflex response to the catch.
- Clinical assessments of spasticity, including the MAS, were performed by a trained clinician on chronic stroke survivors. Separately, the elbow joint was moved passively at three different speeds during which the elbow angle and activity of the medial and lateral biceps muscles were measured using an electrogoniometer and electromyography (EMG), respectively.
- Large variability in the catch angle and the EMG responses as a function of joint rotation speed were noted among stroke survivors with the same clinical MAS

J. K. Ewoldt
Department of Mechanical Engineering, Boston University, Boston, MA, USA
e-mail: jewoldt@bu.edu

P. Raghavan
Departments of Physical Medicine and Rehabilitation and Neurology, The Johns Hopkins University School of Medicine, Baltimore, MD, USA
e-mail: praghavan@jhmi.edu

N. L. Suresh (✉)
Department of Physical Medicine and Rehabilitation, Shirley Ryan Ability Lab, Chicago, IL, USA
e-mail: nsuresh@sralab.org

P. Raghavan (ed.), *Spasticity and Muscle Stiffness*,
https://doi.org/10.1007/978-3-030-96900-4_4

score. Participants with a higher clinical MAS score showed an increased occurrence of catches earlier during elbow joint rotation (i.e., larger catch angle).
- Not all participants who demonstrated a catch showed an EMG response in the biceps, suggesting the contribution of other muscles and/or the presence of a non-neural or mechanical component to the resistance. In participants who showed an EMG response, the catch angle decreased as a function of joint rotation speed (i.e., the catch angle became smaller with increased speed) due to a constant latency between EMG onset and the catch.
- Quantification of the resistance to passive elbow joint rotation before and after botulinum toxin (BoNT) injections in the elbow flexors of chronic stroke survivors, provided as part of clinical care, showed that reduction in the EMG response with BoNT did not necessarily reduce the passive resistance or catch angle, suggesting that overactivity in muscles other than those injected or non-neural changes in the muscles injected likely contributed to the passive resistance.

Introduction

Spasticity, as originally defined by Lance [1], is characterized by a velocity-dependent increase in tonic stretch reflexes with exaggerated tendon jerks, resulting from hyperexcitability of the stretch reflex (see Chap. 1). Spasticity develops in 30–40% of stroke survivors [2, 3], and left uncontrolled may limit functional recovery, impede everyday tasks, cause pain [4, 5], and increase financial [6] and caregiver [7] burden after stroke. Physical rehabilitation and pharmacologic treatments are the currently accepted treatments for spasticity. Pharmacologic treatments using botulinum toxin [8, 9], a neuromuscular blocking agent (see Chap. 12), and baclofen [10], a GABA agonist (see Chaps. 10 and 11), work by targeting neural hyperexcitability and the ensuing muscle overactivity. Physical interventions including stretching [11] to preserve muscle length and structure, and neuromuscular electrical stimulation [12] to inhibit interneurons, have also been found to decrease poststroke spasticity. Starting these interventions early has been shown to improve clinical outcomes [8, 13, 14] (see Chap. 8).

To deliver the appropriate pharmacologic and/or rehabilitation therapy, the baseline degree of spasticity and its change over the course of treatment should be assessed. The clinical assessment of spasticity generally involves grading the perceived resistance elicited in a muscle group in response to passive joint rotation [15, 16]. The Modified Ashworth Scale (MAS) is commonly used for this purpose [16] (see Chap. 3). During the MAS assessment at the elbow joint the clinician rotates the joint from the position of maximal flexion to the position of maximal extension in the direction of gravitational force over one second. The qualitative assessment grades spasticity based on the perceived "catch", which is a brief resistance encountered during joint rotation, and any perceived resistance after the initial catch [15]. On the other hand, the Tardieu Scale more closely follows Lance's original definition of spasticity by determining the resistance to joint rotation at different speeds [17] (see Chap. 3 for details).

While these clinical assessments have been used extensively to characterize spasticity and are widely accepted, studies have shown that they have poor to moderate inter-rater reliability [18–21], which could be attributed to differences in clinicians' perception of the resistance during these assessments. The lack of reliability could also be because of variability in clinician-applied limb acceleration and speed, and because the mechanisms underlying the perceived resistance are different across patients. Quantifying the neural and biomechanical responses to joint rotation can allow for a more standardized and uniform assessment of spasticity across raters and can provide greater insight as to the source of the resistance in individual patients.

The biomechanical response to stretch in patients with spasticity, including the resistance and dynamics of spastic catches, has been quantified in experiments where a motor is used to apply a stretch while recording force, torque, and/or deceleration [22–32]. The quantification of resistance and spastic catch was then correlated with a clinician's assessments of spasticity, using the MAS and/or the Tardieu Scale, performed separately. One system, the NeuroFlexor, uses various rotation speeds to determine the velocity-dependent responses, allowing the neural, viscous, and elastic components of the passive resistance to be estimated separately [33–35]. Sophisticated systems have also been developed that quantify both the neural and biomechanical responses by simultaneously acquiring EMG and torque signals, where the signals are acquired during a passive joint rotation initiated by a device instead of a clinician [35–38]. Some studies have used these systems to demonstrate a decrease in viscosity and an increase in the reflex response threshold after treatment with botulinum toxin injections [39, 40].

Few studies have quantified the neural and biomechanical responses to clinician-applied joint rotation. One study quantified the biomechanical response to passive stretch applied to lower limb muscles in children with cerebral palsy, using an electrogoniometer, force sensors, and surface EMG, and found weak correlations between the clinical assessments and the objective data [36]. This study showed that a comprehensive understanding of the source of the catch requires both biomechanical and EMG data. However, other studies that quantified the spastic catch during clinical assessment used torque and angle sensors but did not quantify the reflex response simultaneously using EMG [41, 42]. Hence the origin of the catch could not be determined. Thus, while these above-mentioned studies quantified important aspects of spasticity, they did not quantify both the neural and biomechanical responses during clinician-applied joint rotation in the upper limbs of chronic stroke survivors.

Quantification of Neural and Biomechanical Responses During Elbow Joint Rotation

In general, the resistance perceived by clinicians during the assessment of spasticity can be attributed to either alterations in the neurally-mediated reflex response and/or in the passive mechanical properties of the affected muscles acting across the targeted joint. It is essential to obtain information regarding reflex muscle activation to determine the extent to which the resistance may be potentially reduced by pharmacologic therapies for spasticity targeting increased neural excitability (e.g., tizanidine, baclofen, see Chap. 10) or reflex-mediated muscle overactivity (e.g., botulinum toxin, see Chap. 12). More recently, pharmacologic therapy targeting passive mechanical resistance (e.g., using hyaluronidase injections, see Chaps. 6 and 13) has been used. In addition, quantification of the catch angle and the joint rotation speed provides precise information regarding the relationship of the resistance to joint rotation speed. Hence the acquisition of EMG signals and joint motion information during spasticity assessments can provide a better understanding of the origins of the perceived resistance and the inter- and intra-rater variability of these assessments, and can also provide more precise guidance as to the efficacy of clinical interventions.

We build on previously published data describing quantitative measurements of the elicited reflex response, as well as the catch angle and angular joint rotation speed during elbow joint rotations by a trained clinician, emulating the MAS and Tardieu clinical assessments of spasticity [43]. Previous work demonstrated the variability in the catch angle and EMG responses in a cohort of chronic stroke survivors who scored a 1+ on the MAS. Here, we present the results from a larger cohort of patients with a wider range of clinical MAS scores. Our cohort consisted of 14 chronic stroke survivors who were recruited at the Shirley Ryan Ability Lab (Chicago, IL, USA). Individuals currently receiving botulinum toxin injections and/or oral baclofen were excluded from the study. Study participants gave informed consent through protocols approved by the Institutional Review Board under the Office for the Protection of Human Subjects at Northwestern University. Table 4.1 shows the demographic and stroke characteristics of the subjects, as well as the clinical assessments performed. The upper extremity Fugl-Meyer score (UEFM) ranged from 12 to 55/66 on the affected side and was 66/66 on the contralateral (unaffected) side for all participants. The clinical MAS score was recorded prior to the instrumented joint rotations described below. Deep tendon reflexes (DTRs) ranged from 2 to 3+ on the affected side and 1 to 3+ on the contralateral side.

Study participants were seated upright in a chair with their arms supported, enabling the clinician to perform passive elbow joint rotations on each arm. Surface EMG electrodes (Delsys, Boston, MA) were placed on the medial and lateral biceps of the affected and contralateral upper limbs to measure muscle activity during elbow joint rotations as shown in Fig. 4.1a. An electrogoniometer (Biometrics Ltd., Ladysmith, VA) was centered on the lateral side of each elbow joint to measure the angular position of the elbow during extension and flexion relative to the starting position at maximum elbow flexion.

The clinician rotated the elbow joint five times each at three designated speed categories: as slow as possible (V1, a 5–10 s rotation), in the direction of gravity over one second as for the MAS (V2), and as fast as possible (V3, in less than 1 second). The order of the speed of joint rotations was randomized. The rotations were first performed on the affected side and then on the contralateral side, and the joint angle and EMG signals from both sides were recorded. The elbow joint was rotated from a position of full flexion to the position of maximal extension, ~0°. The position of maximal extension depended on the passive extension possible for each subject. The clinician held the elbow in the position of maximal extension for ~20 s after each rotation to allow the biceps muscle activity to return to baseline levels.

Table 4.1 Demographic characteristics and clinical assessments at the elbow joint from the affected arm of participants

Subject	Age	Stroke type	Years poststroke	UEFM	Clinical MAS score	DTRs	Passive ROM (°)	Active ROM (°)	Catch angle[a] (°)	EMG Sum[a] (V)
1	54	Hemorrhagic	5	17	1+	2	151	118	65.4 ± 10.0	90.9 ±53.8
2	63	Hemorrhagic	16	19	1+	3	147	86	42.7 ± 21.5	130.9 ± 92.8
3	67	Hemorrhagic	11	17	2	3	155	133	36.4 ± 23.9	114.1 ± 67.9
4	70	Unknown	12	18	2	3+	130	85	67.2 ± 19.2	130.9 ± 72.7
5	51	Ischemic	5	54	1+	2+	151	142	83.9 ± 7.5	1.0 ±1.5
6	56	Ischemic	6.7	51	1	2+	148	144	4.1 ± 11.5	2.7 ± 2.2
7	59	Ischemic	4	55	1+	3+	148	148	52.5 ± 29.4	0.4 ± 0.5
8	63	Ischemic	3	27	1+	3+	139	111	54.0 ± 19.1	9.0 ± 3.7
9	40	Ischemic	2	12	2	3+	137	121	53.0 ± 32.8	14.7 ± 9.7
10	69	Unknown	19	13	3	2+	135	104	60.4 ± 12.4	119.6 ± 20.5
11	50	Ischemic	4	36	2	3+	150	145	33.6 ± 70.4	2.2 ± 4.0
12	66	Ischemic and hemorrhagic	23	10	1+	3+	152	87	62.1 ± 13.8	57.6 ± 54.3
13	62	Unknown	29.4	13	1	2+	128	89	18.1 ± 21.6	126.0 ± 53.5
14	46	Unknown	11	27	2	4+	152	149	40.0 ± 26.8	16.3 ± 3.9

UEFM upper extremity Fugl-Meyer score/66, *MAS* Modified Ashworth Scale, *DTRs* deep tendon reflexes, *ROM* total range of motion for elbow flexion-extension

[a]Mean catch angle and EMG sum across all trials for all joint rotation speeds for each participant. The average catch angle and EMG sum on the contralateral side for all subjects were 0.9° ± 6.3° and 0.9 ± 2.0 V, respectively

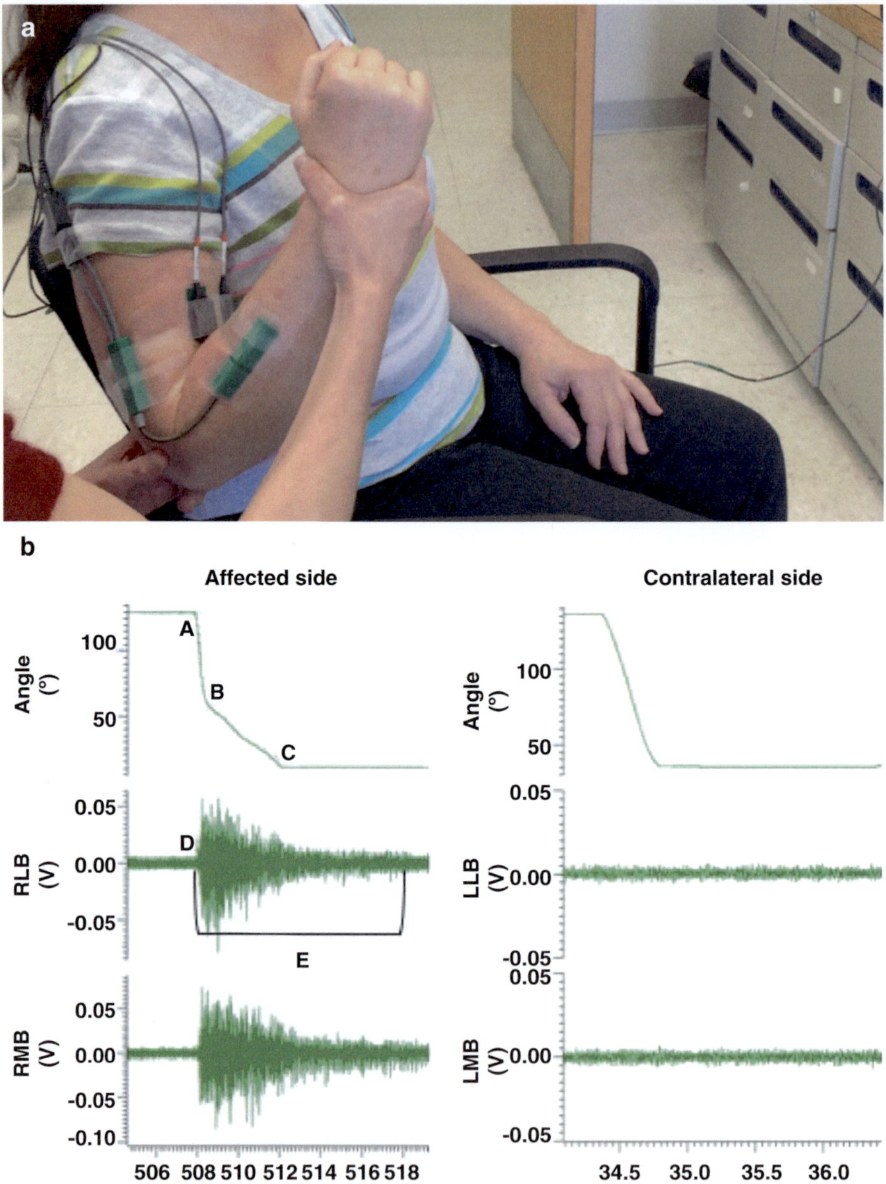

Fig. 4.1 Set up for quantitative measurement of resistance to passive elbow joint rotation. (**a**) Elbow in maximum flexion with surface electrogoniometer and electromyography (EMG) electrodes on the medial and lateral biceps and the electrogoniometer centered at the elbow joint as the clinician prepares to perform the MAS. (**b**) Sample signals from the electrogoniometer, right lateral biceps (RLB), and right medial biceps (RMB) from top to bottom on the affected and contralateral sides. A: beginning of joint rotation, B: catch angle detection, C: end of joint rotation, D: EMG onset, E: duration of EMG response used to calculate the EMG response sum

Determination of Catch Angle and EMG Response

The signals from the electrogoniometer and EMG were digitized and stored on a computer for later off-line analysis. The derivative of the electrogoniometer signal was taken to obtain the angular speed of joint rotation as a function of time. The beginning of elbow joint rotation was identified from the goniometer signals as the time at which the angular speed increased above a preset threshold of 50°/s, based on prior experimental data, and the catch was identified as the point at which the angular speed decreased below this threshold during joint rotation. Thus, a larger catch angle occurred sooner during elbow joint rotation from flexion to extension. If no catch was detected, the catch was marked at the end of rotation as 0°. The catch latency was defined as the time between the beginning of the joint rotation and the detection of the catch using signals derived from the electro-goniometer.

The mean baseline EMG signal recorded from the medial and lateral biceps muscles was averaged for the initial segment immediately prior to the onset of joint rotation and subtracted from the EMG signal during joint rotation. The beginning of the EMG response for each muscle was found as the time at which the amplitude of the EMG signal increased by more than three standard deviations above the mean baseline EMG signal (EMG threshold). The end of the neural response occurred when the EMG activity stayed below the EMG threshold for at least one second. The EMG response sum was calculated by taking the area under the curve of the rectified EMG signal for the entire EMG response duration. Figure 4.1b shows exemplary data recorded from both arms on one subject during a single elbow joint rotation trial. The data were pooled for subjects based on their MAS scores, and descriptive statistical analyses were performed using Graph Pad Prism 8.0 between the MAS score groups using unpaired Student t-tests assuming unequal variance. We report EMG data on the medial biceps only as the EMG response was larger for the medial biceps, but the results were similar for both the medial and the lateral biceps muscles.

Occurrence of a Catch

The affected limb exhibited a catch in most of the trials, while the contralateral upper limb of all subjects consistently showed little or no catch at all applied joint rotation speeds, with less than 3% of all trials exhibiting a catch. The frequency of occurrence of a catch in the affected upper limb showed an increasing trend with the clinical MAS score. Across all joint rotation speeds, a catch was detected in 11% of trials in subjects with an MAS score of 1, in 67% of trials in subjects with an MAS score of 1+, in 96% of trials in subjects with an MAS score of 2, and in 100% of trials in subjects with an MAS score of 3 (Fig. 4.2a).

The mean angle of the elbow at which the catch occurred (across all limb speeds) on the affected upper limb is shown in Fig. 4.2b. There were no significant

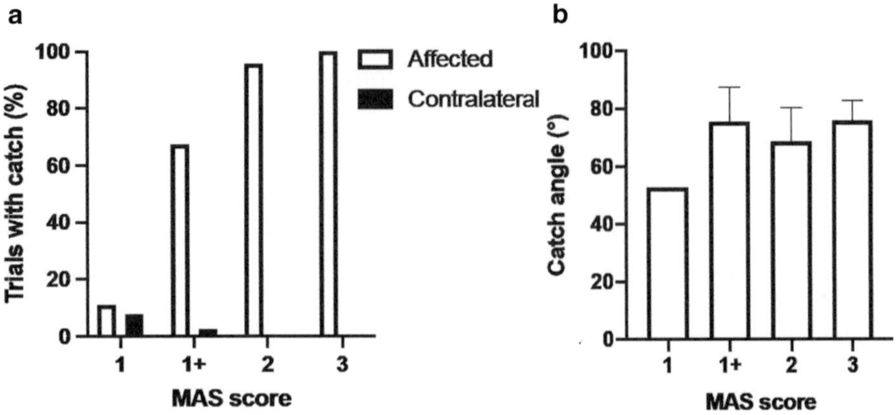

Fig. 4.2 Frequency of occurrence of a catch and catch angle across Modified Ashworth Score (MAS) categories. (**a**) Percentage of trials across all rotation speeds in which a catch or sudden resistance was identified grouped by clinical MAS score for the affected and contralateral upper limbs. (**b**) Catch angle of the affected upper limb grouped by clinical MAS score. Error bars represent the standard deviation

differences between the MAS score groups. Note that participants with an MAS score of 1 demonstrated the lowest mean catch angle at 52.8° ± 0.0° (on trials that demonstrated a catch), i.e., the resistance was perceived later during arm extension. The mean catch angle was 75.6° ± 11.8° for participants with an MAS score of 1+, 68.5° ± 11.9° for those with an MAS score of 2, and 76.0° ± 6.8° with an MAS score of 3. In general, the catch occurred slightly earlier during elbow extension in subjects with a higher MAS score. The lack of significant gradation in the mean catch angle across the various MAS score categories may be due to averaging across a wide range of joint rotation speeds. Hence, we also characterized the catch angle and the magnitude of the EMG response as a function of joint rotation speed, as reported and discussed below.

EMG Onset Angle

The EMG onset angle is the angle of joint rotation at which the EMG onset occurs. For subjects that recorded a reflex EMG response, the EMG onset angle was lowest in the group with an MAS score of 1 and highest in one subject with an MAS score of 3, as for the catch angle. The average EMG onset angle was 35.3° ± 20.0° for those with an MAS score of 1, 78.6° ± 21.6° for those with an MAS score of 1+, 88.4° ± 12.8° for an MAS score of 2, and 89.7° ± 1.2° for the subject with an MAS score of 3. Above a joint rotation speed of 100°/s, the angle of EMG onset remained in a relatively constant range of 80–100° as a function of limb speed. Thus, we observed no consistent relationship between joint rotation speed and the EMG onset angle.

Catch Angle and Reflex EMG Response as a Function of Joint Rotation Speed

Clinicians used a wide range of rotation speeds that did not fit neatly into the three discrete speed categories, V1, V2 and V3. Hence data across the joint rotation speeds are pooled together. Figure 4.3 shows the covariation in catch angle (top row) and the reflex EMG response (bottom row) as a function of joint rotation speed from the affected and contralateral arms grouped according to the MAS score as originally assessed by the study clinician. In general, the contralateral arm exhibited neither a consistent catch nor a reflex EMG response. Within each MAS group, some subjects exhibited a catch but not an EMG response. For example, in Fig. 4.3a (MAS score = 1) subject S6A did not exhibit a catch consistently at any joint rotation speed, and showed a minimal EMG response. In Fig. 4.3b (MAS score = 1+) subjects S5A, S7A, and S8A, and in Fig. 4.3c (MAS score = 2 or 3) subjects S9A, S11A, and S14A exhibited a catch with a minimal EMG response across all joint rotation speeds. It is possible that muscles other than the biceps, from which data were not recorded, may have contributed to the catch. It is also possible that the catch originated from non-neural passive mechanical properties of the muscle (see Chap. 6).

Furthermore, few subjects demonstrated the expected velocity-dependent increase in the catch angle and/or the reflex EMG response. The amplitude of the EMG response trended with the clinical MAS scores, but there were no significant differences across the MAS score categories. Interestingly, in all tested subjects, and even in the subjects who showed a velocity-dependent increasing trend in the EMG response amplitude, the catch angle decreased, or occurred later during joint rotation when the joint was rotated faster. To understand this finding, it is necessary to examine the relationship between the onset of the EMG response and the catch angle.

Timing of the Onset of the EMG Response and the Catch Angle

We recorded a higher angle of EMG onset compared to the catch angle, and a shorter EMG latency compared to the catch latency, in most of the recorded responses on the affected side. This suggests that for trials with an EMG response, the muscle was activated before the catch during the joint rotation at all joint rotation speeds. Both the EMG latency and the catch latency decreased with increasing joint rotation speed. Despite the decrease in EMG latency with increased speed, the angle of EMG onset was rather constant, indicating that the muscle becomes activated at a certain angular threshold (the point in joint rotation when the muscle is stretched) during the joint rotation. This angular threshold will be reached sooner during faster joint rotations, and hence shows a shorter EMG onset latency.

Figure 4.4 shows the time difference between the EMG response and the recorded catch angle for subjects with an MAS score of 2 or 3. Note that the catch angle occurred at a fixed time latency after the EMG response for trials in which an EMG

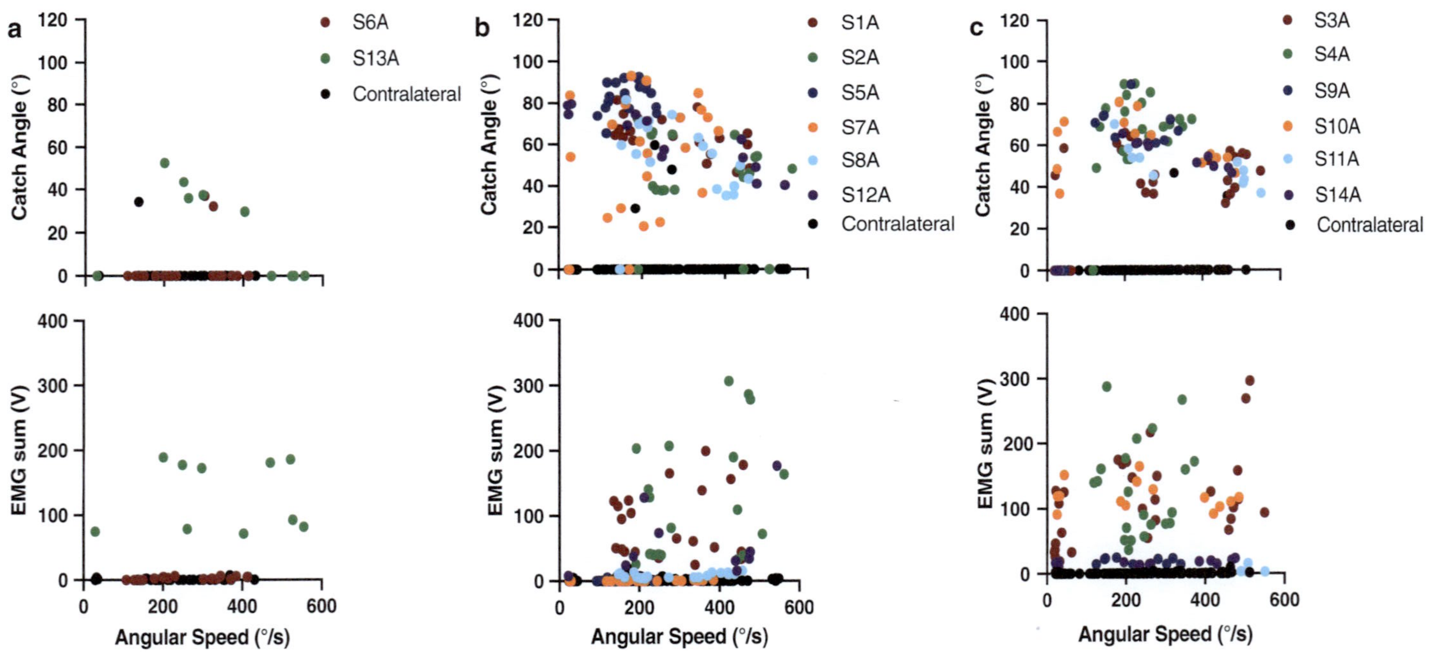

Fig. 4.3 Catch angle and reflex EMG response as a function of joint rotation speed grouped by Modified Ashworth Score (MAS). (**a**) MAS score = 1, (**b**) MAS score = 1+, and (**c**) MAS score = 2 or 3. Top row: Catch angle as a function of elbow joint rotation speed for each subject. Bottom row: EMG sum as a function of elbow joint rotation speed for each subject. "A" refers to the affected side. Contralateral data across the subjects in each category are combined

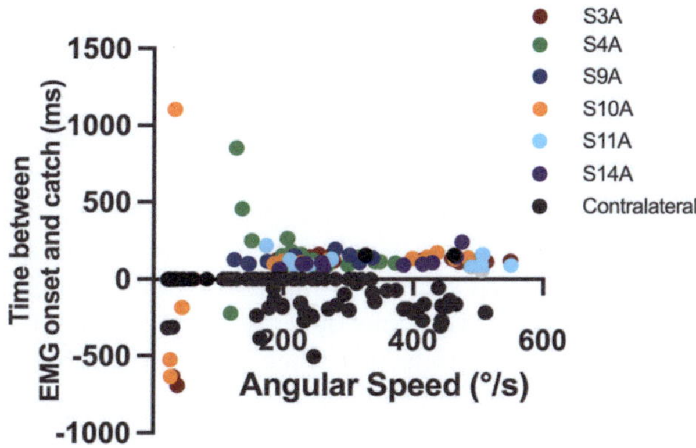

Fig. 4.4 Time difference between the EMG latency and the catch latency as a function of speed of elbow joint rotation for subjects with MAS scores of 2 or 3

response was recorded. In general, at faster joint rotations, the angular displacement will be greater over a fixed time. Since the latency between the onset of muscle activation and the catch angle remains constant, this results in a catch angle that is smaller, or occurs when the arm is in a more extended position with increased joint rotation speed. Thus, the smaller catch angle at higher joint rotation speeds (shown in Fig. 4.3) can be explained by a relatively constant time difference between the EMG response and the catch angle. This consistent time difference or electromechanical delay of the catch after the onset of the EMG reflex response was between 150 and 200 ms.

In some subjects (e.g., Fig. 4.4, S10A), the latency between the EMG onset and the catch is negative, indicating that the catch occurs before the EMG response, particularly when the joint is moved slowly. This suggests that the catch may be due to passive mechanical resistance from the muscle upon initiation of the movement (see Chap. 6). The negative latency which is seen at various speeds on the contralateral side, upon examination of the raw data records, was found to be due to voluntary muscle activation rather than a reflex response.

Origins of the Resistance to Passive Joint Motion

Taken together, the quantification of the neural and biomechanical responses to passive joint movement reveals a large variability in the catch angle, which is largely dependent on the speed of joint rotation and the variability in the elicitation and magnitude of the reflex response. These factors could contribute to the low intra- and inter-rater reliability of the MAS score. Furthermore, the existence of a minimal reflex response, both in magnitude and duration in some patients with clinically defined spasticity, would suggest that pharmacologic therapies to reduce neural excitability or muscle overactivity in such cases may not alleviate the catch or resistance to passive joint rotation.

Quantification of the Resistance to Passive Joint Rotation After BoNT Injections in Chronic Stroke Survivors

Two chronic stroke survivors (unrelated to the cohort reported above), underwent quantitative testing of neural and biomechanical responses using the same protocol described above, before and after BoNT injections to upper arm muscles. The BoNT injections were administered by their respective physicians, and the dose and muscles to be injected were determined as part of their clinical care plan. Quantitative testing was performed immediately prior to the BoNT injections and every 2 weeks thereafter until postinjection week 6. Subject BoNT1 was injected with abobotulinumtoxinA (Dysport®) in the left biceps brachii (200 units) as well as in the brachialis (100 units). Subject BoNT2 was injected with onabotulinumtoxinA (Botox®) in the left biceps (50 units). The clinical assessments performed at the various time points are summarized in Table 4.2.

Figure 4.5 shows the covariation in the EMG response (EMG sum) and the catch angle elicited as a function of time post injection. Note that both participants exhibited a measurable catch along with a considerable EMG response to elbow joint rotation prior to the BoNT injections (Pre-BoNT). The EMG response greatly diminished in the post-BoNT sessions for both participants suggesting adequate dosing. However, for subject BoNT1, the catch angle range in the post-BoNT testing sessions remained in the same range as that observed in the pre-BoNT session, suggesting that reduction in the EMG activity with BoNT did not reduce or eliminate the catch, although the injections did lead to a reduction in the MAS score (Table 4.2). The EMG response reduced but did not go down to zero.

Table 4.2 Clinical assessments performed before and after botulinum toxin (BoNT) injections

Subject	Assessments	Pre injection	Post Week 2	Post Week 4	Post Week 6
BoNT1	Active elbow flexion/extension (°)	132.9/78.3	133.4/81.3	136.2/73.4	134.0/61.2
	Passive elbow flexion/extension (°)	149.5/70.1	149.2/64.7	145.7/63.8	148.9/55.0
	MAS affected/contralateral	3/0	2/0	1+/0	2/0
	DTRs affected/contralateral	3+/2+	3+/2+	3+/2+	3+/2+
	UEFM affected/contralateral	14/66	16/66	16/66	14/66
BoNT2	Active elbow flexion/extension (°)	126.4/79.5	120.3/82.4	131.6/76.6	123.6/78.3
	Passive elbow flexion/extension (°)	134.3/33.5	135.4/43.5	144.0/36.3	138.7/38.3
	MAS affected/contralateral	3/0	2/0	2/0	3/0
	DTRs affected/contralateral	3/2	3/2	3/2	3/2
	UEFM affected/contralateral	14/66	14/66	13/66	14/66

MAS Modified Ashworth Scale, *DTRs* deep tendon reflexes, *UEFM* upper extremity Fugl-Meyer score/66

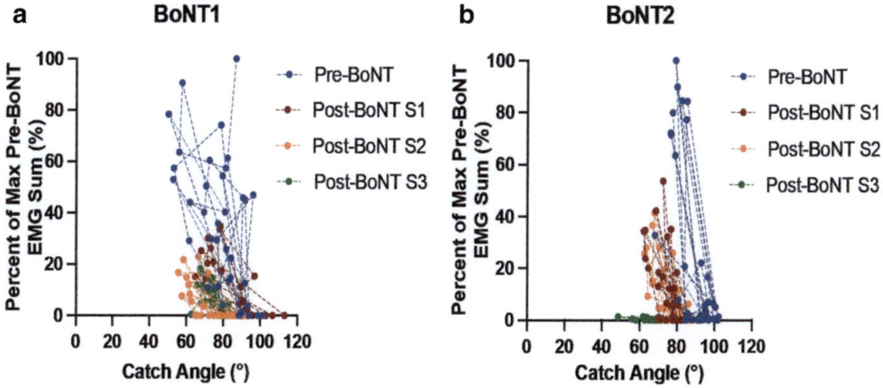

Fig. 4.5 Covariation in the EMG response and the catch angle as a function of time post injection in a session prior to the botulinum toxin injections (Pre-BoNT) and at postinjection testing sessions at week 2 (S1), week 4 (S2), and week 6 (S3) for (**a**) Subject BoNT1 and (**b**) Subject BoNT2

For subject BoNT2, the catch angle did become smaller but was not eliminated despite complete reduction in the EMG response and there was minimal change in the MAS score, suggesting that the reduction in muscle overactivity was not sufficient to change the clinical presentation. These data suggest that while both subjects showed an EMG response to passive elbow joint rotation, the catch or resistance elicited may have originated from elbow flexor muscles that were not injected, or from non-neural passive mechanical resistance.

The passive range of motion increased to a larger extent in subject BoNT2 (~10°), consistent with the improvement in the catch angle, but reverted closer to the baseline by week 6. Further analyses to quantify the severity of the catch, the duration of the EMG response, and the relationship between the EMG response and duration as a function of joint rotation speed are warranted to provide greater insight into the origin of the resistance to joint rotation.

Conclusions

Quantitative measurement of muscle activity and passive resistance during clinician-applied joint rotation demonstrates large variability in the catch angles and in the EMG responses elicited as a function of joint rotation speed among stroke survivors with the same clinical MAS score. As expected, participants with higher clinical MAS scores showed an increased occurrence of catches earlier during elbow joint rotation. However, not all participants who demonstrated a catch showed an EMG response in the biceps, suggesting that some of the resistance may originate from other muscles contributing to the movement, or from non-neural passive mechanical properties of the muscle. Furthermore, in participants who showed an EMG response, the catch angle decreased as a function of joint rotation speed due to a constant latency between the onset of EMG and the catch. Elicitation of an

EMG response and its reduction with BoNT injections did not necessarily reduce the elicited catch or passive resistance, suggesting contribution from muscles other than those injected, or from non-neural muscle changes.

Acknowledgments This work was supported in part by American Heart Association: Scientist Development Grant #16SDG30980033. We would like to acknowledge the assistance of Emily Lazarro, Andres Cardona, Giselle Jamarillo, and Dr. Elliot Roth.

References

1. Lance JW. The control of muscle tone, reflexes, and movement: Robert Wartenbeg lecture. Neurology. 1980;30(12):1303–13.
2. Sommerfeld DK, Eek EUB, Svensson AK, Holmqvist LW, Von Arbin MH. Spasticity after stroke: its occurrence and association with motor impairments and activity limitations. Stroke. 2004;35(1):134–9. https://doi.org/10.1161/01.STR.0000105386.05173.5E.
3. Watkins CL, Leathley MJ, Gregson JM, Moore AP, Smith TL, Sharma AK. Prevalence of spasticity post stroke. Clin Rehabil. 2002;16(5):515–22. https://doi.org/10.1191/0269215502cr512oa.
4. Wissel J, Schelosky LD, Scott J, Christe W, Faiss JH, Mueller J. Early development of spasticity following stroke: a prospective, observational trial. J Neurol. 2010;257(7):1067–72. https://doi.org/10.1007/s00415-010-5463-1.
5. Collin C, Wade DT, Davies S, Horne V. The Barthel ADL Index: a reliability study. Int Disabil Stud. 1988;10(2):61–3.
6. Lundström E, Smits A, Borg J, Terént A. Four-fold increase in direct costs of stroke survivors with spasticity compared with stroke survivors without spasticity: the first year after the event. Stroke. 2010;41(2):319–24. https://doi.org/10.1161/STROKEAHA.109.558619.
7. Denno MS, Gillard PJ, Graham GD, Dibonaventura MD, Goren A, Varon SF, Zorowitz R. Anxiety and depression associated with caregiver burden in caregivers of stroke survivors with spasticity. Arch Phys Med Rehabil. 2013;94(9):1731–6. https://doi.org/10.1016/j.apmr.2013.03.014.
8. Rosales RL, Efendy F, Teleg ES, Delos Santos MM, Rosales MC, Ostrea M, Tanglao MJ, Ng AR. Botulinum toxin as early intervention for spasticity after stroke or non-progressive brain lesion: a meta-analysis. J Neurol Sci. 2016;371:6–14. https://doi.org/10.1016/j.jns.2016.10.005.
9. Santamato A, Cinone N, Panza F, Letizia S, Santoro L, Lozupone M, Daniele A, Picelli A, Baricich A, Intiso D, Ranieri M. Botulinum toxin type A for the treatment of lower limb spasticity after stroke. Drugs. 2019;79(2):143–60. https://doi.org/10.1007/s40265-018-1042-z.
10. Creamer M, Cloud G, Kossmehl P, Yochelson M, Francisco GE, Ward AB, Wissel J, Zampolini M, Abouihia A, Berthuy N, Calabrese A, Loven M, Saltuari L. Intrathecal baclofen therapy versus conventional medical management for severe poststroke spasticity: results from a multicentre, randomised, controlled, open-label trial (SISTERS). J Neurol Neurosurg Psychiatry. 2018;89(6):642–50. https://doi.org/10.1136/jnnp-2017-317021.
11. Coroian F, Jourdan C, Bakhti K, Palayer C, Jaussent A, Picot MC, Mottet D, Julia M, Bonnin H-Y, Laffont I. Upper limb isokinetic strengthening versus passive mobilization in patients with chronic stroke: a randomized controlled trial. Arch Phys Med Rehabil. 2018;99(2):321–8. https://doi.org/10.1016/j.apmr.2017.08.490.
12. Stein C, Fritsch CG, Robinson C, Sbruzzi G, Plentz RDM. Effects of electrical stimulation in spastic muscles after stroke: systematic review and meta-analysis of randomized controlled trials. Stroke. 2015;46(8):2197–205. https://doi.org/10.1161/STROKEAHA.115.009633.
13. Rosales RL, Balcaitiene J, Berard H, Maisonobe P, Goh KJ, Kumthornthip W, Mazlan M, Latif LA, Delos Santos MMD, Chotiyarnwong C, Tanvijit P, Nuez O, Kong KH. Early abob-

otulinumtoxina (Dysport®) in post-stroke adult upper limb spasticity: ONTIME pilot study. Toxins. 2018;10(7):1–12. https://doi.org/10.3390/toxins10070253.

14. Sunnerhagen KS, Opheim A, Alt Murphy M. Onset, time course and prediction of spasticity after stroke or traumatic brain injury. Ann Phys Rehabil Med. 2019;62(6):431–4. https://doi.org/10.1016/j.rehab.2018.04.004.
15. Nielsen M, Willersley-Olsen M, Lorentzen J. Chapter 2: Pathophysiology of spasticity. Elsass Fonden; Denmark. 2015.
16. Bohannon RW, Smith MB. Interrater reliability of a modified Ashworth Scale of muscle spasticity. Phys Ther. 1987;67(2):206–7. https://doi.org/10.1093/ptj/67.2.206.
17. Haugh AB, Pandyan AD, Johnson GR. A systematic review of the Tardieu Scale for the measurement of spasticity. Disabil Rehabil. 2006;28(15):899–907. https://doi.org/10.1080/09638280500404305.
18. Ansari NN, Naghdi S, Moammeri H, Jalaie S. Ashworth Scales are unreliable for the assessment of muscle spasticity. Physiother Theory Pract. 2006;22(3):119–25. https://doi.org/10.1080/09593980600724188.
19. Craven BC, Morris AR. Modified Ashworth Scale reliability for measurement of lower extremity spasticity among patients with SCI. Spinal Cord. 2010;48(3):207–13. https://doi.org/10.1038/sc.2009.107.
20. Yan X, He L, Zheng Y. Inter-rater reliability of Modified Ashworth Scale and Modified Tardieu Scale in children with spastic cerebral palsy. Chin J Rehabil Med. 2015;30(1):18–21. https://doi.org/10.3969/j.issn.1001-1242.2015.01.005.
21. Ansari NN, Naghdi S, Hasson S, Rastgoo M, Amini M, Forogh B. Clinical assessment of ankle plantarflexor spasticity in adult patients after stroke: inter-and intra-rater reliability of the Modified Tardieu Scale. Brain Inj. 2013;27(5):605–12. https://doi.org/10.3109/02699052.2012.750744.
22. Katz RT, Rovai GP, Brait C, Rymer WZ. Objective quantification of spastic hypertonia: correlation with clinical findings. Arch Phys Med Rehabil. 1992;73(4):339–47. https://doi.org/10.1016/0003-9993(92)90007-J.
23. O'Dwyer NJ, Ada L, Neilson PD. Spasticity and muscle contracture following stroke. Brain. 1996;119(5):1737–49. https://doi.org/10.1093/brain/119.5.1737.
24. Pandyan AD, Price CIM, Barnes MP, Johnson GR. A biomechanical investigation into the validity of the modified Ashworth Scale as a measure of elbow spasticity. Clin Rehabil. 2003;17(3):290–4. https://doi.org/10.1191/0269215503cr610oa.
25. Patrick E, Ada L. The Tardieu Scale differentiates contracture from spasticity whereas the Ashworts Scale is confounded by it. Clin Rehabil. 2006;20(2):173–81. https://doi.org/10.1191/0269215506cr922oa.
26. Vattanasilp W, Ada L. The relationship between clinical and laboratory measures of spasticity. Aust J Physiother. 1999;45(2):135–9. https://doi.org/10.1016/S0004-9514(14)60345-7.
27. Heung HL, Tang ZQ, Shi XQ, Tong KY, Li Z. Soft rehabilitation actuator with integrated post-stroke finger spasticity evaluation. Front Bioeng Biotechnol. 2020;8(February):1–10. https://doi.org/10.3389/fbioe.2020.00111.
28. Bui HT, Gagnon C, Audet O, Mathieu J, Leone M. Measurement properties of a new wireless electrogoniometer for quantifying spasticity during the pendulum test in ARSACS patients. J Neurol Sci. 2017;375:181–5. https://doi.org/10.1016/j.jns.2017.01.065.
29. Germanotta M, Taborri J, Rossi S, Frascarelli F, Palermo E, Cappa P, Castelli E, Petrarca M. Spasticity measurement based on tonic stretch reflex threshold in children with cerebral palsy using the pediAnklebot. Front Hum Neurosci. 2017;11(May):1–11. https://doi.org/10.3389/fnhum.2017.00277.
30. Li X, Shin H, Li S, Zhou P. Assessing muscle spasticity with myotonometric and passive stretch measurements: validity of the myotonometer. Sci Rep. 2017;7(February):1–7. https://doi.org/10.1038/srep44022.
31. Xu D, Wu YN, Gaebler-Spira D, Gao F, Clegg NJ, Delgado MR, Zhang LQ. Neural and non-neural contributions to ankle spasticity in children with cerebral palsy. Dev Med Child Neurol. 2020;62(9):1040–6. https://doi.org/10.1111/dmcn.14506.

32. Shin W-S, Chang H, Kim SJ, Kim J. Characterization of spastic ankle flexors based on visco-elastic modeling for accurate diagnosis. Int J Control Autom Syst. 2019;18(1):102–13. https://doi.org/10.1007/s12555-019-0245-8.
33. Plantin J, Pennati GV, Roca P, Baron J-C, Laurencikas E, Weber K, Godbolt AK, Borg J, Lindberg PG. Quantitative assessment of hand spasticity after stroke: imaging correlates and impact on motor recovery. Front Neurol. 2019;10. https://doi.org/10.3389/fneur.2019.00836.
34. Pennati GV, Plantin J, Borg J, Lindberg PG. Normative NeuroFlexor data for detection of spasticity after stroke: a cross-sectional study. J Neuroeng Rehabil. 2016;13(1). https://doi.org/10.1186/s12984-016-0133-x.
35. Wang R, Herman P, Ekeberg Ö, Gäverth J, Fagergren A, Forssberg H. Neural and non-neural related properties in the spastic wrist flexors: an optimization study. Med Eng Phys. 2017;47:198–209. https://doi.org/10.1016/j.medengphy.2017.06.023.
36. Lynn BO, Erwin A, Guy M, Herman B, Davide M, Ellen J, Anne C, Kaat D. Comprehensive quantification of the spastic catch in children with cerebral palsy. Res Dev Disabil. 2013;34(1):386–96. https://doi.org/10.1016/j.ridd.2012.08.019.
37. Wu YN, Park HS, Chen JJ, Ren Y, Roth EJ, Zhang LQ. Position as well as velocity dependence of spasticity-four-dimensional characterizations of catch angle. Front Neurol. 2018;9(OCT):1–10. https://doi.org/10.3389/fneur.2018.00863.
38. Song SY, Pei Y, Tippett SR, Lamichhane D, Zallek CM, Hsiao-Wecksler ET. Validation of a wearable position, velocity, and resistance meter for assessing spasticity and rigidity. In: Frontiers in Biomedical Devices, BIOMED – 2018 Design of medical devices conference, DMD 2018. 2018. p. 6–9. https://doi.org/10.1115/DMD2018-6906.
39. Lee H-M, Chen J-JJ, Wu Y-N, Wang Y-L, Huang S-C, Piotrkiewicz M. Time course analysis of the effects of botulinum toxin type A on elbow spasticity based on biomechanic and electromyographic parameters. Arch Phys Med Rehabil. 2008;89(4):692–9. https://doi.org/10.1016/j.apmr.2007.08.166.
40. Chen J-JJ, Wu Y-N, Huang S-C, Lee H-M, Wang Y-L. The use of a portable muscle tone measurement device to measure the effects of botulinum toxin type a on elbow flexor spasticity. Arch Phys Med Rehabil. 2005;86(8):1655–60. https://doi.org/10.1016/j.apmr.2005.03.019.
41. Ahmad Puzi A, Sidek SN, Mat Rosly H, Daud N, Md Yusof H. Modified Ashworth Scale (MAS) model based on clinical data measurement towards quantitative evaluation of upper limb spasticity. IOP Conf Ser: Mater Sci Eng. 2017;260(1). https://doi.org/10.1088/1757-899X/260/1/012024.
42. Park JH, Kim Y, Lee KJ, Yoon YS, Kang SH, Kim H, Park HS. Artificial neural network learns clinical assessment of spasticity in Modified Ashworth Scale. Arch Phys Med Rehabil. 2019;100(10):1907–15. https://doi.org/10.1016/j.apmr.2019.03.016.
43. Ewoldt JK, Lazzaro EC, Roth EJ, Suresh NL. Quantification of a single score (1+) in the Modified Ashworth Scale (MAS), a clinical assessment of spasticity. In: 2016 38th Annual International Conference of the IEEE Engineering in Medicine and Biology Society (EMBC). Orlando, FL; 2016. p. 1737–40. https://doi.org/10.1109/EMBC.2016.7591052.

5 Structural Alterations in Muscle in Children with Spastic Cerebral Palsy

Sudarshan Dayanidhi

Living forms are hammered into shape…from the combined action of physical forces – tension, compression and shear.
– D'Arcy Wentworth Thompson, On Growth and Form, 1917.

- Skeletal muscles are highly organized structures composed of muscle cells, i.e., myofibers, arranged longitudinally and cross-sectionally with noncontractile scaffold and structural proteins along the length of the muscle. Myofibers in turn are made up of basic contractile units called sarcomeres, i.e., actin and myosin filaments whose interaction generates force.
- Sarcomere length and force production are intricately associated such that at very long and short sarcomere lengths, there is a reduction in force generating capacity. Muscle growth occurs during development by the addition of sarcomeres both longitudinally and cross-sectionally.
- In children with cerebral palsy, sarcomeres are over-stretched and serial sarcomere number is lower, associated with a limitation in joint range of motion, which suggest reduced ability for muscle growth and weakness. Increase in muscle extracellular matrix content and in passive mechanical stiffness of muscle fibers and fiber bundles are also observed in contractured muscles.
- Satellite cells are resident muscle stem cells that are indispensable for postnatal development, and repair and regeneration of skeletal muscles. Satellite cell population is significantly reduced in contractured muscles, suggesting a role in impaired growth.

S. Dayanidhi (✉)
Biologics Lab, Shirley Ryan AbilityLab, Chicago, IL, USA
e-mail: sdayanidhi@sralab.org

P. Raghavan (ed.), *Spasticity and Muscle Stiffness*,
https://doi.org/10.1007/978-3-030-96900-4_5

- Alterations in metabolic properties of muscle, motor unit recruitment, and neuromuscular junctions are also observed. The treatment of spastic muscle contractures in children requires newer therapies based on the biological changes in muscle to facilitate appropriate muscle growth.

Skeletal Muscle Structure

Skeletal muscles are highly organized structures. They are primarily made up of contractile proteins interacting with noncontractile scaffold and structural proteins. The primary cells of muscles are the multinucleated myofibers, which are organized longitudinally and cross-sectionally to form fascicles, which in turn are organized to create the muscle belly attached to the tendinous structures. Myofibers are made up of myofibrils, which are composed of the primary contractile proteins within sarcomeres, which in turn are organized in series and in parallel and are responsible for the force generating property of muscles [1]. Sarcomeres are repeating, functional units of muscle defined by overlapping actin (thin) and myosin (thick) filaments and the degree of overlap between them, i.e., sarcomere length, is associated with the amount of force generated. The force-length property of sarcomeres predicts that the force generated reduces dramatically at high and low sarcomere lengths [2]. The force produced is maximal at sarcomere lengths at which the overlap between the actin and myosin filaments is optimal. There are also a large number of highly organized noncontractile scaffold proteins that coordinate force transmission from the sarcomeres to the cell membranes, the extracellular matrix, and tendons to create whole scale movement at the joints [3].

Change in Muscle Structure During Postnatal Development

During postnatal development, muscles grow in length along with the bone and grow in girth to increase the force generated, so as to maintain movement across the range of motion permissible at a joint. Most of our understanding of muscle growth is from studies in animals. Mammalian development shows muscle hypertrophy rather than hyperplasia, i.e., muscle development occurs by an increase in the dimensions of the existing myofibers, rather than by an increase in the number of myofibers [4–6]. Williams and Goldspink studied the actual process of muscle growth in a series of seminal studies in mice [7–10]. They showed that sarcomeres have a crucial role to play in both longitudinal and cross-sectional myofiber development. They reported an increase in myofiber cross-sectional area by continued addition of myofibrils [7]. More recent work has confirmed that during the first four weeks of development, there is a fourfold increase in muscle mass, an almost twofold increase in myofibrillar packing, and a sevenfold increase in myofiber cross-sectional area [11]. By eight weeks, the linear increase in myofiber cross-sectional area leads to a 14-fold increase in myofiber volume [6].

Similarly, myofiber length increases by the addition of sarcomeres-in-series such that the force-length relationship is maintained. An increase in length of the myofibers without the addition of new sarcomeres would lead to stretching of the existing sarcomeres, i.e., increase in sarcomere length and consequently a reduction in force production. During the postnatal period, there is a fivefold increase in sarcomere number and myofiber length [8, 9, 11] but sarcomere length is maintained [6]. Less is known about human muscle growth since sarcomere addition is difficult to measure noninvasively. However, since muscle biology is fairly conserved across mammalian species, similar processes are likely in play. A clinical case in a child undergoing distraction osteogenesis showed that bone growth is associated with a corresponding increase in sarcomere number [12]. In this case, a twofold increase in fiber length occurred due to a similar increase in sarcomere number, but there was no change in sarcomere length, demonstrating that the increase in fiber length was not purely due to stretching of existing sarcomeres. During the period of development, there is also an increase in the number of myonuclei in the myofibers, which increase fivefold primarily in the first three weeks of development [6]. Since myonuclei are postmitotic and unable to divide to produce new nuclei, the source of these nuclei is from other mononuclear cells, i.e., the satellite cells or muscle stem cells (more on this later in this chapter), located in the periphery of the myofibers [13]. Correspondingly, the satellite cell number reduces threefold during the period of postnatal development [6], and is maintained in a relatively steady state for the rest of adulthood.

Muscle Adaptation

Muscles are very dynamic and can change their homeostatic state under conditions of stretch and disuse. Serial sarcomere number adaptation is seen not only during postnatal development, but also in mature adults. This adaptive response can be seen by maintaining a muscle in a lengthened or shortened position of immobilization. Maintaining an adult muscle in a position of stretch for 2–4 weeks will stretch the myofibers and increase muscle length. For example, maintaining an ankle in dorsiflexion will stretch the soleus muscle. Initially the serial sarcomere number, i.e., the number of sarcomeres along the length of a myofiber will remain unchanged, and the existing sarcomeres will be at a disadvantage in generating force due to their overlengthened state. However, over the course of several weeks, the muscle will add new sarcomeres to increase its serial sarcomere number, and the sarcomere length will return to optimal [10]. Similarly, if a muscle is maintained in a shortened position, the myofiber length will reduce over several weeks due to the loss of sarcomeres. The serial sarcomere number will reduce but optimal sarcomere length will be maintained [10]. On removal of the stretch or shortened position, the muscle will return to its original state by increasing its serial sarcomere number appropriately. During the postnatal period, as described in the previous section, muscle growth occurs via sarcomere addition. If a growing muscle is prevented from increasing in length by maintaining it in a shortened position for three months immediately after birth, it does not increase its serial sarcomere number during that period. However, if it is then allowed to recover by facilitating movement, subsequent stretch and growth result in a rapid increase in serial sarcomere number comparable to the contralateral side [9, 10]. These experiments demonstrate that the postnatal period is particularly plastic not just for bone-stretch-induced sarcomere addition, but also for adaptation to changes in muscle length. This finding is the basis for using serial casting in children with cerebral palsy to increase the joint range of motion and muscle length, which presumably occurs by the addition of sarcomeres [14].

Clinical Presentation in Children with Cerebral Palsy

Cerebral palsy (CP) is the most common developmental movement disorder, and 70–80% of children with CP develop a spastic movement disorder either unilaterally or bilaterally [15]. Muscle weakness and contractures are commonly seen in the plantar flexors, knee flexors, hip flexors, elbow flexors, and wrist flexors [16–18], which limit the available range of motion at these joints [34]. Contractures are dynamic initially, i.e., they are accompanied by spastic movement disorder but with minimal range of motion limitations. However, this changes as the children age and the range of motion becomes limited at the joints. Population-based studies have shown that spasticity, measured using the Modified Ashworth Scale, increases with age in children till the age of four, after which it decreases [19]. Older children show limitations in range of motion that are presumably associated with changes in the properties of the skeletal muscle [20]. However, even younger children, under the age of three years, show changes in the passive mechanical properties of muscle [21]. Importantly, while spasticity is a contributing factor, elimination of spasticity by selective surgical dorsal rhizotomy does not prevent contracture development [22, 23]. Ten-year and 17-year follow-up studies after surgical dorsal rhizotomy showed that there was a reduction in spasticity and an improvement in passive range of motion in the short term, but the procedure did not prevent the development of contractures in the long term. Similarly, there were short-term gains in range of motion and spasticity reduction in children undergoing botulinum toxin injections, but long-term follow-up 1–3 years later showed a decline in range of motion [24]. These studies suggest that the development of contractures is not simply caused by the presence of spasticity.

Functionally, the natural progression of walking in children with CP over 2–4 years, without surgical intervention, leads to a gradual reduction in permissible joint excursion and a crouch gait pattern [25, 26]. Correspondingly, lower limb passive range of motion decreases from early childhood to adolescence [20], suggesting an inability to align muscle growth with bone growth. Muscle growth and muscle volume in children with CP are significantly reduced compared to typically developing (TD) children [27–30], even at 15 months of age [31]. Longitudinal bone growth is also reduced in children with CP [32]. Specifically, tibial length is reduced in ambulatory children with CP compared to TD children and is lower in children who are more severely affected. In addition, abnormal torsion along the femur and tibia is noted, which occurs either due to failure of typical postnatal developmental changes, such as in femoral anteversion, or is acquired due to muscle force abnormalities [33–35]. Consequently, most of the treatments for children with CP are focused on promoting appropriate muscle and bone growth and preventing muscle contractures [34, 36, 37]. Basic science studies in animals on normal muscle growth and clinical data suggest that there are significant alterations in muscle growth during the postnatal period of development in children with CP.

Sarcomere Alterations in Contractured Muscles

Contractured muscles in children with CP have significant alterations in sarcomere length and number. Sarcomere length measured in vivo in wrist flexors in children with static wrist flexion contractures shows a seemingly contradictory pattern consisting of over-lengthened sarcomeres with reduced permissible range of motion at the joint. The sarcomere length of the flexor carpi ulnaris was increased ~45% compared to noncontractured muscles of control subjects [38]. Intraoperative sarcomere length is also highly correlated with the degree of contracture, i.e., children who have the worst contractures also have the longest sarcomere lengths [39]. Sarcomere lengths measured in contractures in lower limb muscles (gracilis, semitendinosus, and soleus) were also increased by 20–50% [40, 41]. Hamstring contractures in children with spastic CP also result from a stiffer extracellular matrix and increased in vivo sarcomere length [41]. These results suggest an inability to add sarcomeres in series to increase the length of the muscle fiber during growth, resulting in over-lengthening of the existing sarcomeres. Consistent with this, the serial sarcomere number is approximately 40% lower in contractured muscles of children with CP compared to TD children [40]. In TD children, the bone grows and stretches the myofibers, which respond by adding new sarcomeres to increase the length of the myofiber, enhance the capacity for force generation, and maintain joint excursion and range of motion. In contrast, in the case of children with CP, muscle stretch caused by bone growth leads to an increase in myofiber length to some extent by stretching of the existing sarcomeres without a concomitant increase in sarcomere number, and eventually leads to the development of muscle contractures. Transcriptional studies from both upper and lower limb muscle contractures show significant up-regulation of genes related to embryonic and perinatal myosin heavy chain isoforms [42, 43], which are not routinely seen during later postnatal development [11, 44]. This implies that the basic physiologic process of muscle growth by sarcomere addition is altered in spastic muscles, or that the processes are unable to move beyond a primitive state to keep up with maturation.

Extracellular Matrix

Alterations in Extracellular Matrix Content

Extracellular matrix (ECM) is the connective tissue around the muscle fibers, fiber bundles, whole muscle, and the tendon. Traditionally, the ECM of muscle is described as the endomysium (surrounding individual myofibers), perimysium (surrounding fiber bundles), and epimysium (surrounding the whole muscle and tendon). While these descriptions are convenient, they are not very helpful to understand the true organization of the ECM, and how it facilitates force interaction and transmission from the contractile proteins to the tendon and bone [45]. The microstructure and function of the normal ECM is fairly complex, and this section only discusses some aspects relevant to what is known in children with CP. Readers seeking detailed information about the potential role of the ECM in the development of contractures are referred to reviews [3, 45, 46], and to Chap. 6 in this book. Briefly, collagen is the major protein of the ECM with type I and III being predominant, although other types such as type IV (in basal lamina), glycoproteins, proteoglycans, and glycosaminoglycans also play a significant role.

Children with CP have a significant increase in ECM material around myofibers as seen by immunohistochemical evaluation of sections of contractured muscle. Labeling for collagen I and laminin (component of the basal lamina) shows a marked qualitative increase in muscles of children with CP compared to muscles from TD children [41] (Fig. 5.1). Quantitative analyses for collagen using hydroxyproline assays also show a significant increase in ECM content in contractured muscles [41].

Histological evaluation of intramuscular connective tissue in contractured muscles of the upper extremity shows significant thickening of the tertiary perimysium (threefold), i.e., the connective tissue reinforcement of neurovascular tissues penetrating the muscle in CP compared to control muscles [47]. Children with moderate-to-severe spasticity show greater intramuscular collagen content [48]. At the level of gene transcription, contractured muscles in both the upper and lower limbs demonstrate increased gene expression of collagens and laminin that constitute the ECM [42, 43, 49]. In addition, there is increased expression of genes related to the breakdown and maintenance of the ECM, such as metalloproteinases, their inhibitors, and

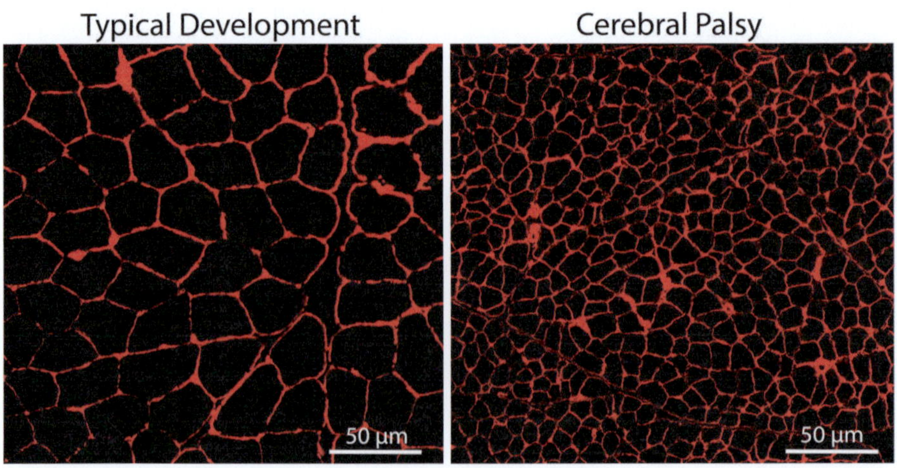

Fig. 5.1 Extracellular matrix of the myofibers. The basal lamina surrounds the myofibers and qualitatively appears to be increased in this child with cerebral palsy. Also note that the size of the myofibers are smaller and more heterogeneous

other associated glycoproteins, suggesting dysregulation of the ECM microenvironment. The interaction of the myofibers and ECM, ECM organization, and their role in whole joint passive resistance and in the development of muscle contractures is addressed in Chap. 6.

Alterations in Passive Muscle Stiffness

One way to test the stiffness of skeletal muscles is to dissect fiber bundles (~20 myofibers) or single fibers from biopsies, secure them with a force transducer on one end and a stable base on the other end, stretch them to various sarcomere lengths, and measure the development of passive stiffness [50]. The use of single fibers and fiber bundles enables the assessment of differences in stiffness due to a change in properties inherent to single fibers (for example, in the large intracellular protein titin which secures the myosin filament to the Z-disc of the sarcomere), or due to the ECM material in fiber bundles. Increased passive stiffness could contribute to the stiffness observed during clinical evaluations of passive range of motion, such as popliteal angle measurement, and contractures.

The stiffness of single fibers of various contractured muscles from the upper extremity has been shown to be slightly higher than that of control muscles. However, the control muscle bundles had dramatically greater stiffness than the bundles from contractured muscles, even though the amount of ECM in contractured muscle bundles was much greater than in controls. These results suggest that although the spastic contractured muscles in the upper extremity have greater ECM content, they generate much less stiffness under conditions of stretch, i.e., their material is not organized in the same way as control muscles [51]. These results could have been influenced by combining different types of muscles from different parts of the body together. However, a subsequent study measured passive stiffness in fibers and bundles from the hamstring muscle group only and revealed that in both gracilis and semitendinosus muscles, a significant increase in bundle stiffness, but not in single fiber stiffness, was noted in contractured muscles of children with CP compared to controls. Importantly, no difference in the mass of the intracellular protein titin in single fibers was observed in the two groups [41]. These studies support the idea that increased ECM content is associated with increased stiffness of muscle fiber bundles. Interestingly, passive stiffness in the gracilis muscle was far greater than that in the semitendinosus muscle, although they were both different from control muscles, illustrating the variability in stiffness between muscles.

In the case of the gastrocnemius and soleus muscles, single fiber stiffness was greater in contractured than in control muscles, but no differences were observed in the fiber bundles. The mass of the protein titin was greater in children with CP; however, the molecular mass of titin was not correlated with the observed fiber stiffness [41]. The studies that measured passive mechanical stiffness and the properties of the ECM show that while there are clear differences in children with CP compared to TD children, the relationship between passive mechanical stiffness and contractures is not clear.

Muscle Stem Cells

Satellite Cells

Satellite cells are the primary resident muscle stem cells responsible for muscle development, repair, and regeneration throughout the lifespan [52]. Satellite cells were named based on their peripheral location in the myofiber, where they are sandwiched between the sarcolemma and the basal lamina [53] (Fig. 5.2a). In contrast, the multiple myonuclei of myofibers are present within the sarcolemma. As mentioned earlier, during postnatal development there is an increase in myonuclear number along with an increase in myofiber dimensions [4]. However, adult (mature) myonuclei are terminally differentiated, i.e., they are unable to divide, proliferate, or regenerate. Consequently, other myogenic tissue-specific stem cells must be present to enable skeletal muscle growth. The source for the postnatal increase in myonuclei are the proliferation, differentiation, and fusion of mononucleated satellite cells in existing myofibers [13, 54]. By definition, an adult tissue stem cell has two properties: the ability to differentiate to create new tissue and the ability to self-renew [55]. Self-renewal is a critical feature that allows all stem cells to maintain their presence and functionality throughout life, without which their population would be depleted as they are used up over time. Satellite cells were visually identified back in the 1960s but it was not until the 2000s, after new molecular markers such as the Pax7 transcription factor were identified [56], that it was convincingly shown that the satellite cells are indeed the primary muscle stem cell capable of differentiation and self-renewal [57–59].

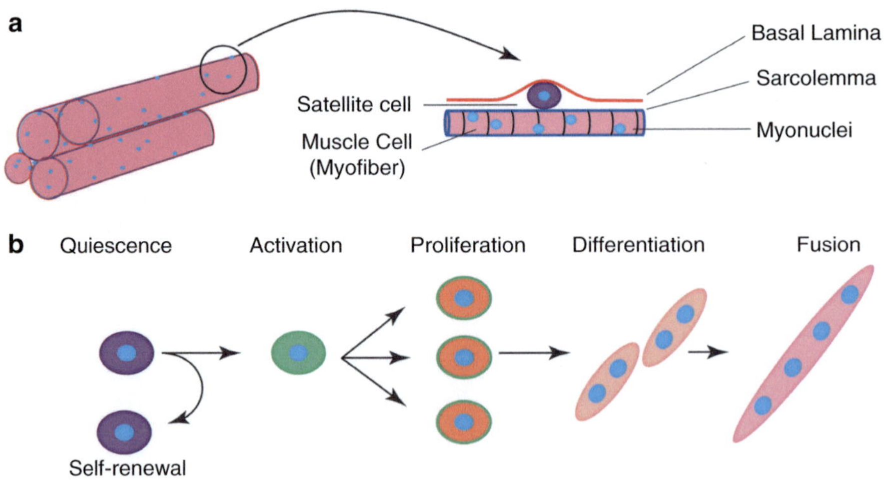

Fig. 5.2 Schematic diagram showing the location and activation of muscle stem cells. (**a**) Satellite cells are the muscle stem cells located in their niche around the fibers between the basal lamina and sarcolemma. (**b**) On activation from quiescence, satellite cells proliferate, differentiate and fuse with the existing myofibers, while maintaining their stem cell state by self-renewal

Satellite cells are normally quiescent. They become activated during growth or in case of repair, and proceed along the myogenic pathway to proliferate, differentiate, and create new myoblasts that fuse with the existing myofibers (Fig. 5.2b). Satellite cells have a large number of activation factors including mechanical stretch, which is important in the postnatal period during bone-mediated muscle growth [60]. Postnatal muscle development is critically dependent on satellite cells [61, 62]. Pax7 null mice demonstrate a dramatic reduction both in myofiber size and satellite cell number during the postnatal period. Using a transgenic mouse that conditionally inactivates Pax7, Lepper et al. showed that myoblasts from the Pax7 lineage fuse into myofibers and are indispensable during the postnatal period [61]. Conditional satellite cell inactivation during the postnatal period results in severely compromised muscle regeneration after injury. A number of studies have conclusively shown that Pax7-expressing satellite cells are critical for the capacity for long-term muscle repair even in adult muscle [63–66]. Satellite cells have similarly been shown to contribute to routine maintenance in uninjured fibers during adulthood and aging [67, 68].

Change in Satellite Cells in Contractured Muscles

It is clear that muscles in children with CP have a reduced capacity for longitudinal and cross-sectional growth during the postnatal period. As mentioned above, there is plenty of evidence showing that satellite cells play a significant role in muscle growth. Consequently, it is possible that impaired muscle growth and contracture formation occur, at least in part, due to satellite cell dysfunction. Flow cytometry of biopsies from hamstring muscle contractures in children with CP shows that they have a significantly reduced (~60%) satellite cell population compared to TD children [69]. However, children with CP also have ECM abnormalities that may systematically bias flow cytometry results making it more difficult to extract satellite cells from muscle. Hence recently, in situ immunohistochemistry has been used to quantify satellite cells using antibodies for satellite cells (anti-Pax7), the basal lamina (anti-Laminin), and a nuclear stain (DAPI) [70]. This method allows quantification of large volumes of tissue in situ without significant tissue manipulation. The satellite cell number quantified from these sections shows a 70% decrease in muscles of children with CP compared to age-appropriate controls. Recently, a significant reduction (~40%) in satellite cell number was also shown in upper extremity biceps muscle contractures [49]. While still preliminary, these studies using different methods, different muscles, and different subjects, demonstrate that it is highly likely that there are significant changes in the satellite cell population in children with CP and suggest possible future avenues for therapeutic intervention using regenerative medicine strategies.

Satellite cells are primary muscle stem cells but they do not act independently of other mononuclear cell types such as fibroblasts and macrophages [71], which are all required and act in a temporally coordinated fashion for muscle repair and regeneration. Recent evidence from animal studies suggests that satellite cells show reciprocal interactions with fibroblasts in the ECM to regulate muscle regeneration after injury, i.e., changes in the ECM can negatively regulate satellite cell function [72]. More recently, Fry et al. showed that activated satellite cells can also regulate ECM composition in response to muscle overload [73]. Depletion of satellite cells leads to increased ECM content and fibrosis with aging [74]. One proposed mechanism is that satellite cell activation is associated with the up-regulation of interstitial collagenases, which allow ECM remodeling and satellite cell migration [75, 76]. Consequently, while it is clear that the satellite cells interact with the ECM, it is not clear what is altered first in the development of muscle contractures (also see Chap. 6). Muscle growth requires numerous interacting factors beyond satellite cells, the alterations of many of which could lead to the development of contractures [77].

As previously discussed, compared with TD children, the muscles of children with CP have increased collagen and ECM content and increased myofiber bundle passive stiffness, consistent with muscle fibrosis [42]. These contractured muscles also have significantly reduced satellite cell numbers [70, 69], suggesting that the increased ECM content may be related to the decreased satellite cell numbers. Reduced satellite cell numbers could lead to the failure of ECM regulation resulting in the development of muscle contractures. Recently, we showed that in satellite cell-depleted transgenic mouse models, sarcomere addition occurs during conditions of stretch but the muscle fiber cross-sectional area remains small and is associated with considerable proliferation of the ECM, consistent with fibrotic changes [78].

Epigenetic factors also appear to play a role in muscle contractures and impaired muscle growth in children with CP. Satellite cells from contractured muscles of children with spastic CP show defects in their ability to differentiate, mature, and fuse to produce myotubes in vitro. These defects appear to be related to epigenetic factors such as DNA hypermethylation, which could be partially rescued by the use of a demethylating agent [79]. This suggests that there could be epigenetic changes in muscle contractures, which could prevent appropriate satellite cell function and muscle growth during development. Interestingly, there is some evidence to suggest that children with CP show epigenetic changes in methylation patterns even in peripheral blood cells, which can distinguish them from children without CP [80]. Knowledge of the exact role of altered epigenetics on muscle development may lead to the development of novel therapies for muscle contractures.

Metabolic Properties

The metabolic properties of muscle have primarily been studied in the context of skeletal muscle fiber types. Human skeletal muscle fibers have three primary fiber types: type 1, type 2A, and type 2X (slowest to fastest/oxidative to more glycolytic), associated with different isoforms of myosin heavy chain, which demonstrates differing metabolic properties [81]. Prior to the discovery of individual myosin heavy chain isoforms, fiber types were classified on the basis of myofibrillar Adenosine Triphosphatase (ATPase) activity which distinguishes between slow (type 1) and fast (type 2) contracting muscle fibers. Lower extremity muscles from children with

CP show a strong preference for one or the other fiber type, with a shift toward type 1 muscle fibers, whereas TD children show a greater balance between fiber types [82]. A similar predominance of one fiber type with a shift toward type 2X has been observed in upper extremity muscles of young adults with contractures using the newer classification technique based on myosin heavy chain isoforms [83]. There are significant alterations in myofiber size, heterogeneity, and fiber type distribution in the muscles of children with CP, and even the newer techniques do not fully capture their metabolic capacity. Our recent work using simple succinate dehydrogenase staining shows that while the hamstring muscles in children with CP are significantly weaker than in TD children, the metabolic activity per unit of both type 1 and type 2A muscle fibers is similar in the two groups (Fig. 5.3) [84]. However, considered as a whole, the muscles of children with CP appear to be in poorer metabolic health. At a transcriptional level, gene expression for oxidative metabolism is

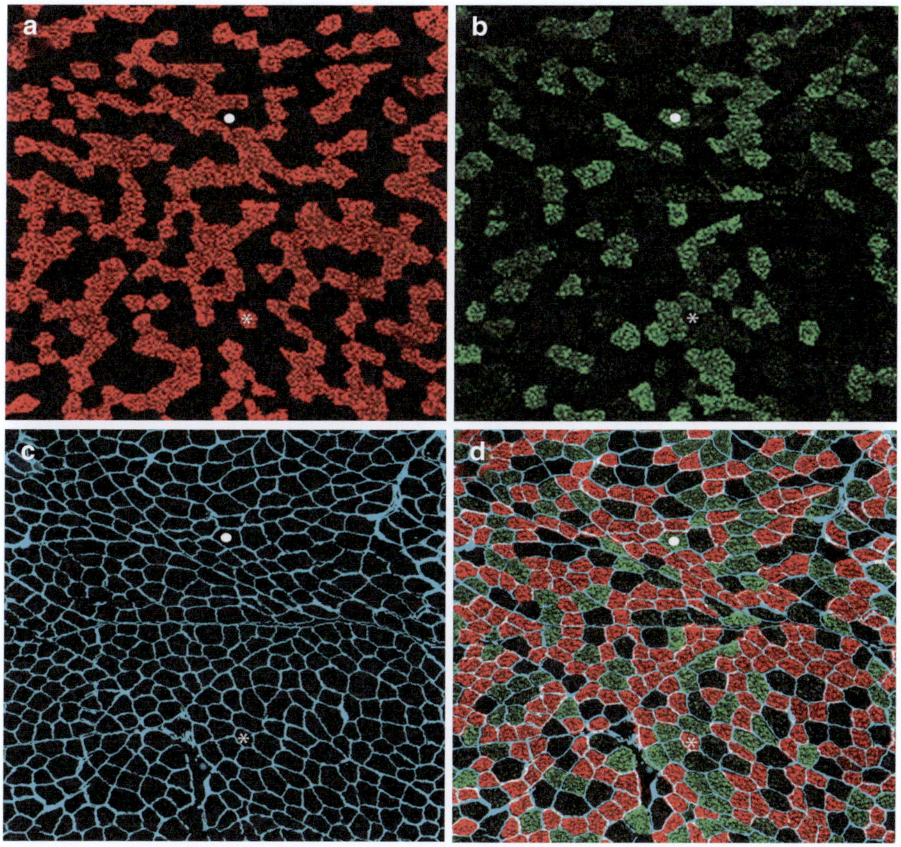

Fig. 5.3 Immunohistochemistry to identify muscle fiber types. (**a**) Type 1 (red), (**b**) Type 2A (bright green), (**c**) Basal lamina, (**d**) Composite image showing all the 3 fiber types including type 2X (dark green). Note that the asterisk shows the same Type 1 fiber, and the white circle shows the same Type 2A fiber across the panels. (Data from Zogby et al. [84])

significantly reduced in both wrist flexor and hamstring muscles of children with CP [43]. The metabolic machinery within the muscle also depends on the delivery of oxygen to the mitochondria through appropriate development of the capillary network. Reduced capillary density has been reported in young adults with wrist flexor contractures compared to control subjects, suggesting that capillary density may have a role in reduced metabolic capacity [83]. Exercise studies have shown that young adults with CP get exhausted at lower exercise intensities, but they are able to dynamically increase muscle vascularization in response to exercise [85].

Alterations in Motor Units and in the Neuromuscular Junction

Motor units are the basic functional units of the CNS; they consist of the alpha motor neuron in the spinal cord and the muscle fibers that its axon innervates. Motor units within a muscle have varying number of muscle fibers, fiber types, and force generating capacity. During force generation, motor units are typically recruited in an orderly fashion starting with those that produce the lowest forces to those that produce the highest, and combined with the modulation of firing rates are able to control the muscle forces generated in a finely tuned manner [86, 87]. Few studies have evaluated the alterations in motor units in spastic muscles of children with CP. Rose and McGill reported that the maximal force generation capacity and maximal motor unit recruitment are significantly reduced in both spastic (gastrocnemius) and nonspastic (tibialis anterior) muscles of children with CP compared to TD children [88]. This suggests that the muscle weakness is, at least in part, associated with the CNS deficit. However, motor unit recruitment and firing rates at low and moderate forces were maintained but required greater percent activation effort, suggesting sufficient capacity for recruitment for submaximal activities.

Alterations in the neuromuscular junction are also reported in children with CP [89, 90]. Specifically, lower limb muscles showed changes in neuromuscular junction structure predominantly in nonambulatory children compared with ambulatory children, and both of these were different from that in control muscles. Although some alterations were noted in the synapse, they did not appear to be due to an immature neuromuscular junction. However, since botulinum toxin creates a temporary blockade at the neuromuscular junction, and is routinely used for treating spasticity, it is difficult to infer if some of the changes in the neuromuscular junction were due to CP or secondary to treatment with botulinum toxin. Recent work also suggests long-term changes in muscle properties following botulinum toxin treatment in spastic muscles [91]. The authors report an association between the number of botulinum toxin injections and a shift in the percentage of type 2 fibers, but it is not clear if the changes were specific to treatment or were a function of impaired growth. At a transcriptional level, no changes were seen in genes related to the neuromuscular junction [43].

Conclusion

Skeletal muscles are composed of contractile proteins organized as sarcomeres, which are arranged in series and in parallel within myofibers, which in turn are integrated with connective tissue and organized in bundles. Children with CP have poor longitudinal and cross-sectional muscle growth and develop contractures. The contractures are associated with increased sarcomere length, decreased serial sarcomere number, and changes in muscle ECM. Muscle stem cells are responsible for postnatal development, repair, and regeneration, and are also significantly reduced in number and altered in function in contractured muscles. Newer therapeutics will utilize avenues to improve muscle stem cell function to promote muscle growth and prevent the development of muscle contractures in children with CP.

References

1. Sweeney HL, Hammers DW. Muscle Contraction. Cold Spring Harb Perspect Biol. 2018;10(2):a023200.
2. Gordon AM, Huxley AF, Julian FJ. The variation in isometric tension with sarcomere length in vertebrate muscle fibres. J Physiol. 1966;184(1):170–92.
3. Patel TJ, Lieber RL. Force transmission in skeletal muscle: from actomyosin to external tendons. Exerc Sport Sci Rev. 1997;25:321–63.
4. Enesco M, Puddy D. Increase in the number of nuclei and weight in skeletal muscle of rats of various ages. Am J Anat. 1964;114:235–44. https://doi.org/10.1002/aja.1001140204.
5. Montgomery RD. Growth of human striated muscle. Nature. 1962;195:194–5.
6. White R, Bierinx A-S, Gnocchi V, Zammit P. Dynamics of muscle fibre growth during postnatal mouse development. BMC Dev Biol. 2010;10(1):21.
7. Goldspink G. The proliferation of myofibrils during muscle fibre growth. J Cell Sci. 1970;6(2):593–603.
8. Griffin GE, Williams PE, Goldspink G. Region of longitudinal growth in striated muscle fibres. Nat New Biol. 1971;232(27):28–9.
9. Williams PE, Goldspink G. Longitudinal growth of striated muscle fibres. J Cell Sci. 1971;9(3):751–67.
10. Williams PE, Goldspink G. The effect of immobilization on the longitudinal growth of striated muscle fibres. J Anat. 1973;116(Pt 1):45–55.
11. Gokhin DS, Ward SR, Bremner SN, Lieber RL. Quantitative analysis of neonatal skeletal muscle functional improvement in the mouse. J Exp Biol. 2008;211(Pt 6):837–43. https://doi.org/10.1242/jeb.014340.
12. Boakes JL, Foran J, Ward SR, Lieber RL. Muscle adaptation by serial sarcomere addition 1 year after femoral lengthening. Clin Orthop Relat Res. 2007;456:250–3. https://doi.org/10.1097/01.blo.0000246563.58091.af.
13. Macconnachie HF, Enesco M, Leblond CP. The mode of increase in the number of skeletal muscle nuclei in the postnatal rat. Am J Anat. 1964;114:245–53. https://doi.org/10.1002/aja.1001140205.
14. McNee AE, Will E, Lin JP, Eve LC, Gough M, Morrissey MC, Shortland AP. The effect of serial casting on gait in children with cerebral palsy: preliminary results from a crossover trial. Gait Posture. 2007;25(3):463–8. https://doi.org/10.1016/j.gaitpost.2006.08.002.

15. Van Naarden BK, Doernberg N, Schieve L, Christensen D, Goodman A, Yeargin-Allsopp M. Birth prevalence of cerebral palsy: a population-based study. Pediatrics. 2016;137(1):1–9. https://doi.org/10.1542/peds.2015-2872.
16. Bunata R, Icenogle K. Cerebral palsy of the elbow and forearm. J Hand Surg Am. 2014;39(7):1425–32. https://doi.org/10.1016/j.jhsa.2013.12.017.
17. Leafblad ND, Van Heest AE. Management of the spastic wrist and hand in cerebral palsy. J Hand Surg Am. 2015;40(5):1035–40. https://doi.org/10.1016/j.jhsa.2014.11.025.
18. Rodda JM, Graham HK, Carson L, Galea MP, Wolfe R. Sagittal gait patterns in spastic diplegia. J Bone Joint Surg Br. 2004;86-B(2):251–8. https://doi.org/10.1302/0301-620x.86b2.13878.
19. Hagglund G, Wagner P. Development of spasticity with age in a total population of children with cerebral palsy. BMC Musculoskelet Disord. 2008;9(1):150.
20. Nordmark E, Hagglund G, Lauge-Pedersen H, Wagner P, Westbom L. Development of lower limb range of motion from early childhood to adolescence in cerebral palsy: a population-based study. BMC Med. 2009;7(1):65. https://doi.org/10.1186/1741-7015-7-65.
21. Willerslev-Olsen M, Lorentzen J, Sinkjær T, Nielsen JBO. Passive muscle properties are altered in children with cerebral palsy before the age of 3 years and are difficult to distinguish clinically from spasticity. Dev Med Child Neurol. 2013;55(7):617–23. https://doi.org/10.1111/dmcn.12124.
22. Tedroff K, Lowing K, Astrom E. A prospective cohort study investigating gross motor function, pain, and health-related quality of life 17 years after selective dorsal rhizotomy in cerebral palsy. Dev Med Child Neurol. 2015;57(5):484–90. https://doi.org/10.1111/dmcn.12665.
23. Tedroff K, Löwing K, Jacobson D, Åström E. Does loss of spasticity matter? A 10-year follow-up after selective dorsal rhizotomy in cerebral palsy. Dev Med Child Neurol. 2011;53(8):724–9. https://doi.org/10.1111/j.1469-8749.2011.03969.x.
24. Tedroff K, Granath F, Forssberg H, Haglund-Akerlind Y. Long-term effects of botulinum toxin a in children with cerebral palsy. Dev Med Child Neurol. 2009;51(2):120–7. https://doi.org/10.1111/j.1469-8749.2008.03189.x.
25. Bell KJ, Ounpuu S, DeLuca PA, Romness MJ. Natural progression of gait in children with cerebral palsy. J Pediatr Orthop. 2002;22(5):677–82.
26. Johnson DC, Damiano DL, Abel MF. The evolution of gait in childhood and adolescent cerebral palsy. J Pediatr Orthop. 1997;17(3):392–6.
27. Barber LA, Read F, Lovatt Stern J, Lichtwark G, Boyd RN. Medial gastrocnemius muscle volume in ambulant children with unilateral and bilateral cerebral palsy aged 2 to 9 years. Dev Med Child Neurol. 2016;58(11):1146–52. https://doi.org/10.1111/dmcn.13132.
28. Barber LEE, Hastings-Ison T, Baker R, Barrett ROD, Lichtwark G. Medial gastrocnemius muscle volume and fascicle length in children aged 2 to 5 years with cerebral palsy. Dev Med Child Neurol. 2011;53(6):543–8. https://doi.org/10.1111/j.1469-8749.2011.03913.x.
29. Handsfield GG, Meyer CH, Abel MF, Blemker SS. Heterogeneity of muscle sizes in the lower limbs of children with cerebral palsy. Muscle Nerve. 2016;53(6):933–45. https://doi.org/10.1002/mus.24972.
30. Noble JJ, Fry NR, Lewis AP, Keevil SF, Gough M, Shortland AP. Lower limb muscle volumes in bilateral spastic cerebral palsy. Brain Dev. 2014;36(4):294–300. https://doi.org/10.1016/j.braindev.2013.05.008.
31. Herskind A, Ritterband-Rosenbaum A, Willerslev-Olsen M, Lorentzen J, Hanson L, Lichtwark G, Nielsen JB. Muscle growth is reduced in 15-month-old children with cerebral palsy. Dev Med Child Neurol. 2016;58(5):485–91. https://doi.org/10.1111/dmcn.12950.
32. Oeffinger D, Conaway M, Stevenson R, Hall J, Shapiro R, Tylkowski C. Tibial length growth curves for ambulatory children and adolescents with cerebral palsy. Dev Med Child Neurol. 2010;52(9):e195–201. https://doi.org/10.1111/j.1469-8749.2010.03711.x.
33. Bobroff ED, Chambers HG, Sartoris DJ, Wyatt MP, Sutherland DH. Femoral anteversion and neck-shaft angle in children with cerebral palsy. Clin Orthop Relat Res. 1999;364:194–204.
34. Graham HK, Rosenbaum P, Paneth N, Dan B, Lin JP, Damiano DL, Becher JG, Gaebler-Spira D, Colver A, Reddihough DS, Crompton KE, Lieber RL. Cerebral palsy. Nat Rev Dis Primers. 2016;2:15082. https://doi.org/10.1038/nrdp.2015.82.

35. Rethlefsen SA, Healy BS, Wren TA, Skaggs DL, Kay RM. Causes of intoeing gait in children with cerebral palsy. J Bone Joint Surg Am. 2006;88(10):2175–80. https://doi.org/10.2106/jbjs.e.01280.
36. Graham HK, Selber P. Musculoskeletal aspects of cerebral palsy. J Bone Joint Surg Br. 2003;85-B(2):157–66. https://doi.org/10.1302/0301-620x.85b2.14066.
37. Thomason P, Rodda J, Sangeux M, Selber P, Kerr G. Management of children with ambulatory cerebral palsy: an evidence-based review. Commentary by Hugh Williamson gait laboratory staff. J Pediatr Orthop. 2012;32(Suppl 2):S182–6. https://doi.org/10.1097/BPO.0b013e31825b6136.
38. Lieber RL, Fridén J. Spasticity causes a fundamental rearrangement of muscle-joint interaction. Muscle Nerve. 2002;25(2):265–70.
39. Pontén E, Gantelius S, Lieber RL. Intraoperative muscle measurements reveal a relationship between contracture formation and muscle remodeling. Muscle Nerve. 2007;36(1):47–54. https://doi.org/10.1002/mus.20780.
40. Mathewson MA, Ward SR, Chambers HG, Lieber RL. High resolution muscle measurements provide insights into equinus contractures in patients with cerebral palsy. J Orthop Res. 2015;33(1):33–9. https://doi.org/10.1002/jor.22728.
41. Smith LR, Lee KS, Ward SR, Chambers HG, Lieber RL. Hamstring contractures in children with spastic cerebral palsy result from a stiffer extracellular matrix and increased in vivo sarcomere length. J Physiol. 2011;589(Pt 10):2625–39. https://doi.org/10.1113/jphysiol.2010.203364.
42. Smith LR, Chambers HG, Subramaniam S, Lieber RL. Transcriptional abnormalities of hamstring muscle contractures in children with cerebral palsy. PLoS One. 2012;7(8):e40686. https://doi.org/10.1371/journal.pone.0040686.
43. Smith LR, Pontén E, Hedström Y, Ward SR, Chambers HG, Subramaniam S, Lieber RL. Novel transcriptional profile in wrist muscles from cerebral palsy patients. BMC Med Genet. 2009;2:44. https://doi.org/10.1186/1755-8794-2-44.
44. Schiaffino S, Rossi AC, Smerdu V, Leinwand LA, Reggiani C. Developmental myosins: expression patterns and functional significance. Skeletal Muscle. 2015;5(1):22. https://doi.org/10.1186/s13395-015-0046-6.
45. Gillies AR, Lieber RL. Structure and function of the skeletal muscle extracellular matrix. Muscle Nerve. 2011;44(3):318–31. https://doi.org/10.1002/mus.22094.
46. Pingel J, Suhr F. Are mechanically sensitive regulators involved in the function and (patho) physiology of cerebral palsy-related contractures? J Muscle Res Cell Motil. 2017;38(3):317–30. https://doi.org/10.1007/s10974-017-9489-1.
47. de Bruin M, Smeulders MJ, Kreulen M, Huijing PA, Jaspers RT. Intramuscular connective tissue differences in spastic and control muscle: a mechanical and histological study. PLoS One. 2014;9(6):e101038. https://doi.org/10.1371/journal.pone.0101038.
48. Booth CM, Cortina-Borja MJF, Theologis TN. Collagen accumulation in muscles of children with cerebral palsy and correlation with severity of spasticity. Dev Med Child Neurol. 2001;43(5):314–20. https://doi.org/10.1111/j.1469-8749.2001.tb00211.x.
49. Von Walden F, Gantelius S, Liu C, Borgstrom H, Bjork L, Gremark O, Stal P, Nader GA, Ponte NE. Muscle contractures in patients with cerebral palsy and acquired brain injury are associated with extracellular matrix expansion, pro-inflammatory gene expression, and reduced rRNA synthesis. Muscle Nerve. 2018;58(2):277–85. https://doi.org/10.1002/mus.26130.
50. Meyer GA, Lieber RL. Elucidation of extracellular matrix mechanics from muscle fibers and fiber bundles. J Biomech. 2011;44(4):771–3. https://doi.org/10.1016/j.jbiomech.2010.10.044.
51. Lieber RL, Runesson E, Einarsson F, Friden J. Inferior mechanical properties of spastic muscle bundles due to hypertrophic but compromised extracellular matrix material. Muscle Nerve. 2003;28(4):464–71. https://doi.org/10.1002/mus.10446.
52. Yin H, Price F, Rudnicki MA. Satellite cells and the muscle stem cell niche. Physiol Rev. 2013;93(1):23–67. https://doi.org/10.1152/physrev.00043.2011.
53. Mauro A. Satellite cell of skeletal muscle fibers. J Biophys Biochem Cytol. 1961;9(2):493–5. https://doi.org/10.1083/jcb.9.2.493.

54. Moss FP, Leblond CP. Satellite cells as the source of nuclei in muscles of growing rats. Anat Rec. 1971;170(4):421–35. https://doi.org/10.1002/ar.1091700405.
55. Weissman IL. Stem cells: units of development, units of regeneration, and units in evolution. Cell. 2000;100(1):157–68. https://doi.org/10.1016/S0092-8674(00)81692-X.
56. Seale P, Sabourin LA, Girgis-Gabardo A, Mansouri A, Gruss P, Rudnicki MA. Pax7 is required for the specification of myogenic satellite cells. Cell. 2000;102(6):777–86.
57. Collins CA, Olsen I, Zammit PS, Heslop L, Petrie A, Partridge TA, Morgan JE. Stem cell function, self-renewal, and behavioral heterogeneity of cells from the adult muscle satellite cell niche. Cell. 2005;122(2):289–301. https://doi.org/10.1016/j.cell.2005.05.010.
58. Halevy O, Piestun Y, Allouh MZ, Rosser BWC, Rinkevich Y, Reshef R, Rozenboim I, Wleklinski-Lee M, Yablonka-Reuveni Z. Pattern of Pax7 expression during myogenesis in the posthatch chicken establishes a model for satellite cell differentiation and renewal. Dev Dyn. 2004;231(3):489–502. https://doi.org/10.1002/dvdy.20151.
59. Zammit PS, Golding JP, Nagata Y, Hudon V, Partridge TA, Beauchamp JR. Muscle satellite cells adopt divergent fates: a mechanism for self-renewal? J Cell Biol. 2004;166(3):347–57. https://doi.org/10.1083/jcb.200312007.
60. Kuang S, Gillespie MA, Rudnicki MA. Niche regulation of muscle satellite cell self-renewal and differentiation. Cell Stem Cell. 2008;2(1):22–31. https://doi.org/10.1016/j.stem.2007.12.012.
61. Lepper C, Conway SJ, Fan CM. Adult satellite cells and embryonic muscle progenitors have distinct genetic requirements. Nature. 2009;460(7255):627–31. https://doi.org/10.1038/nature08209.
62. Oustanina S, Hause G, Braun T. Pax7 directs postnatal renewal and propagation of myogenic satellite cells but not their specification. EMBO J. 2004;23(16):3430–9.
63. Günther S, Kim J, Kostin S, Lepper C, Fan C-M, Braun T. Myf5-positive satellite cells contribute to Pax7-dependent long-term maintenance of adult muscle stem cells. Cell Stem Cell. 2013;13(5):590–601.
64. Lepper C, Partridge TA, Fan CM. An absolute requirement for Pax7-positive satellite cells in acute injury-induced skeletal muscle regeneration. Development. 2011;138(17):3639–46. https://doi.org/10.1242/dev.067595.
65. Sambasivan R, Yao R, Kissenpfennig A, Van Wittenberghe L, Paldi A, Gayraud-Morel B, Guenou H, Malissen B, Tajbakhsh S, Galy A. Pax7-expressing satellite cells are indispensable for adult skeletal muscle regeneration. Development. 2011;138(17):3647–56. https://doi.org/10.1242/dev.067587.
66. von Maltzahn J, Jones AE, Parks RJ, Rudnicki MA. Pax7 is critical for the normal function of satellite cells in adult skeletal muscle. Proc Natl Acad Sci USA. 2013;110(41):16474–9. https://doi.org/10.1073/pnas.1307680110.
67. Keefe AC, Lawson JA, Flygare SD, Fox ZD, Colasanto MP, Mathew SJ, Yandell M, Kardon G. Muscle stem cells contribute to myofibres in sedentary adult mice. Nat Commun. 2015;6:7087. https://doi.org/10.1038/ncomms8087.
68. Pawlikowski B, Pulliam C, Betta ND, Kardon G, Olwin BB. Pervasive satellite cell contribution to uninjured adult muscle fibers. Skeletal Muscle. 2015;5(1):1–13. https://doi.org/10.1186/s13395-015-0067-1.
69. Smith LR, Chambers HG, Lieber RL. Reduced satellite cell population may lead to contractures in children with cerebral palsy. Dev Med Child Neurol. 2013;55(3):264–70. https://doi.org/10.1111/dmcn.12027.
70. Dayanidhi S, Dykstra PB, Lyubasyuk V, McKay BR, Chambers HG, Lieber RL. Reduced satellite cell number in situ in muscular contractures from children with cerebral palsy. J Orthop Res. 2015;33(7):1039–45. https://doi.org/10.1002/jor.22860.
71. Bentzinger CF, Wang YX, Dumont NA, Rudnicki MA. Cellular dynamics in the muscle satellite cell niche. EMBO Rep. 2013;14(12):1062–72.
72. Murphy MM, Lawson JA, Mathew SJ, Hutcheson DA, Kardon G. Satellite cells, connective tissue fibroblasts and their interactions are crucial for muscle regeneration. Development. 2011;138(17):3625–37. https://doi.org/10.1242/dev.064162.

73. Fry CS, Lee JD, Jackson JR, Kirby TJ, Stasko SA, Liu H, Dupont-Versteegden EE, McCarthy JJ, Peterson CA. Regulation of the muscle fiber microenvironment by activated satellite cells during hypertrophy. FASEB J. 2014;28(4):1654–65. https://doi.org/10.1096/fj.13-239426.
74. Fry CS, Lee JD, Mula J, Kirby TJ, Jackson JR, Liu F, Yang L, Mendias CL, Dupont-Versteegden EE, McCarthy JJ, Peterson CA. Inducible depletion of satellite cells in adult, sedentary mice impairs muscle regenerative capacity without affecting sarcopenia. Nat Med. 2015;21(1):76–80. https://doi.org/10.1038/nm.3710.
75. Nishimura T, Nakamura K, Kishioka Y, Kato-Mori Y, Wakamatsu J, Hattori A. Inhibition of matrix metalloproteinases suppresses the migration of skeletal muscle cells. J Muscle Res Cell Motil. 2008;29(1):37–44. https://doi.org/10.1007/s10974-008-9140-2.
76. Pallafacchina G, Francois S, Regnault B, Czarny B, Dive V, Cumano A, Montarras D, Buckingham M. An adult tissue-specific stem cell in its niche: a gene profiling analysis of in vivo quiescent and activated muscle satellite cells. Stem Cell Res. 2010;4(2):77–91. https://doi.org/10.1016/j.scr.2009.10.003.
77. Pingel J, Bartels EM, Nielsen JB. New perspectives on the development of muscle contractures following central motor lesions. J Physiol. 2017;595(4):1027–38. https://doi.org/10.1113/jp272767.
78. Kinney MC, Dayanidhi S, Dykstra PB, McCarthy JJ, Peterson CA, Lieber RL. Reduced skeletal muscle satellite cell number alters muscle morphology after chronic stretch but allows limited serial sarcomere addition. Muscle Nerve. 2016;55(3):384–92. https://doi.org/10.1002/mus.25227.
79. Domenighetti AA, Mathewson MA, Pichika R, Sibley LA, Zhao L, Chambers HG, Lieber RL. Loss of myogenic potential and fusion capacity of muscle stem cells isolated from contractured muscle in children with cerebral palsy. Am J Physiol Cell Physiol. 2018;315(2):C247–c257. https://doi.org/10.1152/ajpcell.00351.2017.
80. Crowgey EL, Marsh AG, Robinson KG, Yeager SK, Akins RE. Epigenetic machine learning: utilizing DNA methylation patterns to predict spastic cerebral palsy. BMC Bioinformatics. 2018;19(1):225. https://doi.org/10.1186/s12859-018-2224-0.
81. Schiaffino S, Reggiani C. Fiber types in mammalian skeletal muscles. Physiol Rev. 2011;91(4):1447–531. https://doi.org/10.1152/physrev.00031.2010.
82. Rose J, Haskell WL, Gamble JG, Hamilton RL, Brown DA, Rinsky L. Muscle pathology and clinical measures of disability in children with cerebral palsy. J Orthop Res. 1994;12(6):758–68. https://doi.org/10.1002/jor.1100120603.
83. Pontén EM, Stål PS. Decreased capillarization and a shift to fast myosin heavy chain IIx in the biceps brachii muscle from young adults with spastic paresis. J Neurol Sci. 2007;253(1–2):25–33. https://doi.org/10.1016/j.jns.2006.11.006.
84. Zogby AM, Dayanidhi S, Chambers HG, Schenk S, Lieber RL. Skeletal muscle fiber-type specific succinate dehydrogenase activity in cerebral palsy. Muscle Nerve. 2017;55(1):122–4. https://doi.org/10.1002/mus.25379.
85. Andersen IT, Harrison A, Broholm R, Harder A, Nielsen JB, Bulow J, Pingel J. Microvascularization is not a limiting factor for exercise in adults with cerebral palsy. J Appl Physiol (1985). 2018;125(2):536–44. https://doi.org/10.1152/japplphysiol.00827.2017.
86. Duchateau J, Enoka RM. Human motor unit recordings: origins and insight into the integrated motor system. Brain Res. 2011;1409:42–61. https://doi.org/10.1016/j.brainres.2011.06.011.
87. Fuglevand AJ. Mechanical properties and neural control of human hand motor units. J Physiol. 2011;589(23):5595–602. https://doi.org/10.1113/jphysiol.2011.215236.
88. Rose J, McGill KC. Neuromuscular activation and motor-unit firing characteristics in cerebral palsy. Dev Med Child Neurol. 2005;47(5):329–36. https://doi.org/10.1111/j.1469-8749.2005.tb01144.x.
89. Robinson KG, Mendonca JL, Militar JL, Theroux MC, Dabney KW, Shah SA, Miller F, Akins RE. Disruption of basal lamina components in neuromotor synapses of children with spastic quadriplegic cerebral palsy. PLoS One. 2013;8(8):e70288. https://doi.org/10.1371/journal.pone.0070288.

90. Theroux MC, Oberman KG, Lahaye J, Boyce BA, DuHadaway D, Miller F, Akins RE. Dysmorphic neuromuscular junctions associated with motor ability in cerebral palsy. Muscle Nerve. 2005;32(5):626–32. https://doi.org/10.1002/mus.20401.
91. Valentine J, Stannage K, Fabian V, Ellis K, Reid S, Pitcher C, Elliott C. Muscle histopathology in children with spastic cerebral palsy receiving botulinum toxin type a. Muscle Nerve. 2016;53(3):407–14. https://doi.org/10.1002/mus.24763.

Mechanisms of Development of Passive Mechanical Muscle Stiffness

6

Preeti Raghavan, Antonio Stecco, Rajiv Menon, Mary K. Cowman, and Ravinder Regatte

...at each level of complexity entirely new properties appear, and the understanding of the new behaviors requires research which I think is as fundamental in its nature as any other.
– Philip W. Anderson, More is Different, Science, 1972.

- Spastic paresis due to neurologic injury results in both disruption of active force generation and increase in passive muscle forces that generate resistance to movement. However, the mechanisms of development of passive mechanical forces and their effect on active force generation are not well understood.
- This chapter considers the three-dimensional geometry of muscle, the structure and function of the extracellular matrix (ECM), and the role of intramuscular fluid in influencing the passive mechanical properties of the ECM via changes in intramuscular fluid volume, hyaluronan (HA) content, and ECM viscosity. These mechanisms form the basis of the hyaluronan hypothesis of muscle stiffness, where disruption of ECM homeostasis leads to the accumulation, biophysical alteration, and aggregation of HA in muscle.

P. Raghavan (✉)
Departments of Physical Medicine and Rehabilitation and Neurology, The Johns Hopkins University School of Medicine, Baltimore, MD, USA
e-mail: praghavan@jhmi.edu

A. Stecco
Rusk Rehabilitation, NYU Grossman School of Medicine, New York, NY, USA

R. Menon · R. Regatte
Bernard and Irene Schwartz Center for Biomedical Imaging, NYU Grossman School of Medicine, New York, NY, USA

M. K. Cowman
Tandon School of Engineering, Grossman School of Medicine, New York University, New York, NY, USA

P. Raghavan (ed.), *Spasticity and Muscle Stiffness*,
https://doi.org/10.1007/978-3-030-96900-4_6

- Both muscle unloading, due to paresis and immobility, and muscle overloading due to spastic muscle overactivity and compensatory overuse of specific muscles can trigger the accumulation of HA, increased viscoelasticity of the ECM, and muscle stiffness.
- The HA-rich matrix, in turn, controls the deposition of fibronectin and collagen and modulates the induction of myofibroblasts that are responsible for the excessive production of collagen leading to fibrosis and eventually to contracture.

Introduction

Spastic muscles are weaker, shorter, and stiffer – a key question is how do they get this way? Muscle weakness is explained by the paresis that invariably accompanies spasticity as part of the upper motor neuron syndrome. However, muscle shortening and stiffness have eluded a full explanation. The mechanisms of active muscle force generation are relatively well-described by excitation-contraction coupling, where the neural signal leads to the release of the neurotransmitter acetylcholine from the motor neuron terminal, which initiates the action potential and its spread along the sarcolemma of the sarcomeres (the basic functional unit of a muscle fiber) releasing calcium, which in turn facilitates the cross-bridge interactions between actin and myosin filaments that conclude with the release and reuptake of calcium by the sarcoplasmic reticulum, and the cycle repeats [1]. The active muscle force generated depends on the level of activation of each muscle fiber, as well as its length, and the velocity of contraction. The relationship between sarcomere length and active force generation is thought to reflect the degree of overlap between the actin and myosin filaments. At longer and shorter sarcomere lengths, the binding of actin and myosin is not complete leading to reduced force generation.

Even in the absence of any active force generation, the intracellular and extracellular noncontractile elastic elements in muscle generate passive forces. When a muscle is stretched, resistance from these noncontractile elements increases the passive force [2], and even small changes in muscle length have large implications for active force generation [3]. However, the precise mechanisms underlying passive mechanical properties of whole skeletal muscles are not well understood [4]. It was proposed that passive muscle stiffness may arise from a change in the configuration of the giant intracellular protein titin, also known as connectin, which forms elastic links between the ends of the thick filaments and the ends of the sarcomere (Z disks) [5], especially in shortened muscles. However, as reviewed in Chap. 5, subsequent studies found that the sarcomere is *lengthened* in patients with shortened whole muscle due to contracture [6, 7], and that the titin isoform and passive mechanics of single muscle fibers are not significantly different in spastic muscles, even though the muscle fascicles are stiffer [8]. This suggests that passive stiffness may arise from alterations in the extracellular matrix (ECM) of the muscle rather than from alterations in single muscle fibers. The structure and function of the ECM in muscle and its role in passive force development is complex. It has been found that the passive mechanical properties of muscle scale nonlinearly with size, i.e., small muscle fiber bundles are stiffer than single muscle cells, and larger fascicles and whole muscles are at least an order of magnitude stiffer [4, 9, 10], likely due to greater amounts of ECM. These findings are extremely relevant to individuals with spasticity and necessitate an understanding of the three-dimensional geometry of muscle and its effect on active and passive muscle force generation.

Three-dimensional Muscle Geometry and its Effect on Active and Passive Force Generation

The Architecture of Muscle Affects its Force Generating Capacity

Skeletal muscle is often thought of as a linear force generator, where the muscle fibers are connected end-to-end, i.e., between the origin and insertion of a muscle defining its line of action. However, there are several different muscle architecture types including parallel, pennate, and hydrostats. The vast majority of limb muscles have pennate architecture [11]. In pennate muscles, the fibers are oriented at an angle to the muscle's line of action; the "pennation angle" is the angle between the fiber orientation and the muscle's line of action. Hence, the direction in which the fibers generate force is not the same as the direction of the whole muscle's action. The muscle fibers also rotate as they shorten, becoming more oblique such that the fraction of force directed along the muscle's line of action decreases throughout a contraction. Fiber rotation decreases a muscle's output force but increases output velocity by allowing the muscle to function at a higher gear ratio (muscle velocity/fiber velocity). The magnitude of fiber rotation, and therefore gear ratio, depends on how the muscle changes shape in the dimensions orthogonal to the muscle's line of action. The gear ratio is not fixed for a given muscle but decreases significantly with the force of contraction, where dynamic muscle shape changes promote fiber rotation at low forces and resist fiber rotation at high forces [12–14]. Pennate architecture also allows muscle fibers to be packed such that there is a larger cross-sectional area of muscle for a given volume [15]. A muscle with a larger cross-sectional area can generate higher force per unit muscle compared to a muscle with parallel arrangement of fibers [16]. Thus, muscle force production varies depending on various parameters such as muscle length, fiber length, pennation angle, gearing, and its physiological cross-sectional area.

The ECM Transmits Force Laterally and Facilitates Muscle Shape Changes

The broad organization of a muscle and its ECM is as follows: each muscle fiber is surrounded by endomysium, the muscle fiber bundles or fascicles are surrounded by perimysium, and the thick outer layer, the epimysium, surrounds the whole muscle and is continuous with the tendon. The endomysium, perimysium, and epimysium collectively form the ECM and are composed of collagens and elastic fibers embedded in a viscoelastic gel of proteoglycans, glycosaminoglycans (GAGs) such as hyaluronan, and assorted glycoproteins, which interact by entanglement, cross-linking, and charge-dependent interactions. When the myofibrillar proteins and proteoglycans are removed, the honeycombed three-dimensional network of the connective tissue can be seen (Fig. 6.1) [17–19]. Given that most muscle fibers do not span the entire length of the fascicle, or the whole muscle, the contractile forces generated by these muscle fibers can only be transmitted laterally via the endomysium by translaminar shear [20, 21]. In fact, force is transmitted laterally from contractile proteins to endomysial collagen fibrils across the fiber membranes via transverse filaments known as costameres, which mark sites of attachment between myofibrils and the sarcolemma [22–24]. The endomysium itself is a reticular fibrous network of quasi-randomly orientated wavy collagen fibers embedded in a proteoglycan matrix that forms a continuum between the basement membranes of two adjacent muscle fibers. When a muscle fiber contracts or is stretched, the preferred orientation of the collagen fibers in the endomysium changes but remains wavy and relatively compliant under tension at all sarcomere lengths. The change in collagen fibril orientation accounts for the nonlinear increase in passive resistance with increasing sarcomere length, and leads to translaminar shear through the endomysium and perimysium during lateral force transmission [19, 25]. The perimysium and epimysium define slip planes between muscle fascicles and whole muscles, and enable the fascicles and muscles to slide past each other allowing large shear displacements and shape changes in the whole muscle [26]. The shear forces across adjacent muscle fibers, muscle bundles, and whole muscles are strongly determined

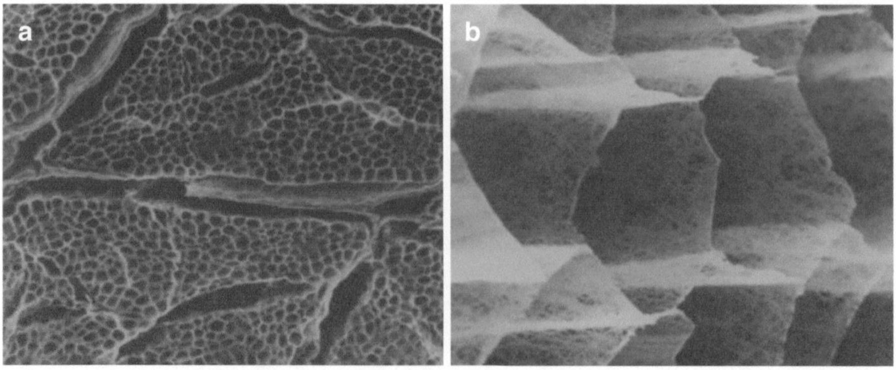

Fig. 6.1 Structure of intramuscular connective tissue. (**a**) Scanning electron micrographs (SCM) of muscle after NaOH treatment to remove the myofibrillar proteins and proteoglycans at low magnification (×100) showing the honeycombed endomysial connective tissue within fascicles separated by the thick perimysial connective tissue. (**b**) Higher magnification (×3200) SCM view of the endomysial network separating (extracted) individual muscle cells. The planar feltwork of collagen fibrils in the endomysial reticular layer is clearly seen. (From Purslow PP (1994), with permission)

by the composition and viscoelastic properties of the proteoglycan matrix of the ECM (see below).

The Three-dimensional Nature of Muscle Contraction

Until recently, only the linear interaction of the actin and myosin filaments within sarcomeres was accounted for in force generation. However, the actin and myosin filaments are arranged in a hexagonal array, known as the filament lattice, within the sarcomere. It is now recognized that changes in the transverse or radial distance between the actin and myosin filaments (i.e., lattice spacing, Fig. 6.2) can also significantly influence the muscle force generated [27, 28]. The decline in muscle force or tension at longer and shorter lengths than optimal has previously been attributed solely to changes in actin-myosin overlap in the longitudinal or axial dimension [29]. However, as a muscle shortens longitudinally, it also swells radially, changing lattice spacing. It has been found that lattice spacing may actually explain 20–50% of the length-dependent change in force in the radial dimension [28]. Modeling muscle three-dimensionally to generate both axial and radial forces suggests that

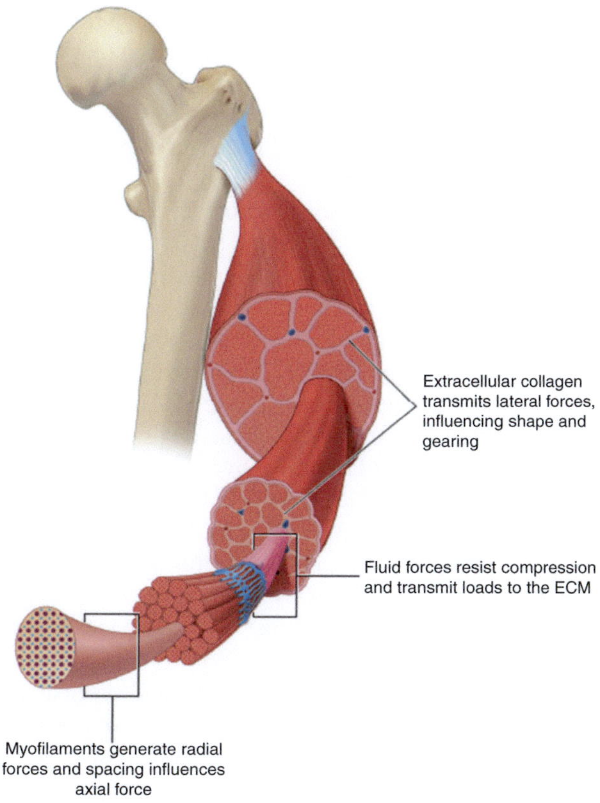

Fig. 6.2 Schematic diagram showing the various structures that influence force transmission at different levels of organization of the muscle, in directions both along the line of action of the muscle and orthogonal to it. (From Roberts TJ (2019), with permission)

the radial forces generated are of the same order of magnitude as the axial forces, but that radial forces and axial forces vary differently with changes in sarcomere length – the magnitude of the radial force is 2.4 times greater than the axial force at extremely short sarcomere lengths, and 0.9 times that of the axial force at the longest sarcomere lengths [30].

A consideration of the three-dimensional nature of muscle contraction (see [31] for review) suggests that the structure and composition of the ECM [32, 33], and intracellular and extracellular fluids [34, 35], also influence active and passive forces in the muscle through their effects on muscle architecture, radial and axial force generation, and lateral force transmission (Fig. 6.2) [36, 37]. The ECM acts as a pathway for lateral force transmission across myofibrils via the endomysium [38], across multiple heads of the same muscle via the perimysium [39], and also across adjacent synergistic and antagonistic muscles via the epimysium and the intermuscular fascia [40–42]. The composition of the ECM is particularly important in the generation of passive muscle tension in mammalian muscles [43, 44]. As the proportion of ECM in muscle increases, the thickened ECM acts as a splint or sleeve and resists the radial expansion of the muscle, which in turn restricts muscle shortening in the axial dimension as well [45]. Transverse compression of a muscle with a load has a similar effect in limiting radial expansion and reducing the force generated by the muscle [46, 47]. Interestingly, release of fascial compartment boundaries also reduces force output [48], suggesting that restoring the health of the ECM may be critically important to preserve force output.

Effect of Fluid-ECM Interactions on Muscle Mechanics

Role of Intramuscular Fluid on the Properties of the ECM

Forces transmitted by fluid within muscle have been shown to be important in the three-dimensional dynamics of muscle contraction. Extracellular water in muscle regulates ion concentrations and pH, which affect muscle contraction and force development during exercise [49]. Activity moves fluid from blood plasma into muscle due to increased hydrostatic [50, 51] and osmotic forces [52, 53]. At the onset of muscle activity, the hydrostatic pressure gradient from the vascular toward the interstitial space of muscle moves fluid into the muscle [54, 55]. Muscular activity increases the osmotic pressure in the interstitial space due to the accumulation of exercise-related metabolites [52, 56, 57], which is proportional to the intensity of muscle action [58]. This leads to a further reduction in plasma volume, which is only partially made up for by reflex decrease of capillary pressure and increased hydrostatic pressure toward the vascular space, increased plasma osmolality, and some lymphatic return [59, 60]. With prolonged submaximal exercise, lactate is removed from active muscle to the vascular space at a higher rate leading to further changes in osmotic pressure gradients [61, 62]. Overall, a *net increase* in activity-induced intramuscular fluid volume has been observed after different kinds of activities such as short-term high-intensity exercise [63–66], and prolonged isometric contraction [67]. Furthermore, the accumulation of metabolites within muscle cells is related to the fiber type distribution in the muscle, where the increase is greater in fast-twitch type 2 fibers [68].

The intramuscular fluid pressure developed during active muscle contraction is estimated to be proportional to the developed muscle force, and influences muscle shape as it shortens longitudinally and swells radially [69–71]. Studies on isolated muscles have demonstrated that increased muscle fluid volume leads to an increase in passive muscle tension [35]. The passive tension at a given length changes in proportion to the volume change, and a measurable change in force can be observed with volume changes as small as 5% in isolated muscles [72]. The changes in muscle volume may also influence active contractile force by limiting radial transmission of muscle force [73]. Passive forces contribute substantially to normal movement, such as walking, and biarticular muscles play a role in passively transferring energy across joints [74]. The passive force contributions occur at the end ranges of joint motions (i.e., peak hip extension, peak knee extension, and peak ankle dorsiflexion) and hence increased passive resistance can compromise the overall active and passive range of motion [74]. Thus, intramuscular fluid can increase compression of contractile muscle tissue, reduce radial transmission of muscle force, increase passive tension in muscle, and reduce overall range of motion.

Intramuscular Fluid Affects the Viscosity of the Ground Substance of the ECM

The ECM is highly dynamic, and its composition is balanced by continuous production, degradation, and remodeling of its components to maintain homeostasis. The ECM regulates the biomechanical properties of tissues, maintains the structural integrity of muscles, and regulates cell growth and tissue function in health and disease [75–77]. GAGs are key components of the ECM, as they are responsible for most of its physical properties, and they modulate cellular behavior (see below). Hyaluronan (hyaluronic acid, HA), traditionally regarded as a space-filling ground substance is the most abundant GAG in the ECM, found in the endomysium, perimysium, and epimysium of muscle [78, 79], as well as in the loose connective tissue or fascia surrounding muscle [80, 81]. HA is the only nonsulfated GAG, composed of a repeating disaccharide of glucuronic acid and N-acetyl glucosamine, that forms long chains or polymers assuming molecular weights of the order of 10^5 to 10^7 Da and an extended length of 0.25–25 μm [82]. It is synthesized by HA synthases (HAS 1-3) located on the plasma membrane, and HA molecules of different molecular weights are extruded from the cytoplasm to the ECM through the HAS pores that link the intracellular with the extracellular space (Fig. 6.3) [83]. The chemical structure of HA, in particular the presence of -OH groups, makes it highly hydrophilic enabling the molecule to retain water and swell which makes it an ideal space-filling molecule. Under physiological conditions, molecules of high molecular weight HA start to entangle at concentrations of less than 1 g/l and assume an expanded random coil structure surrounded by

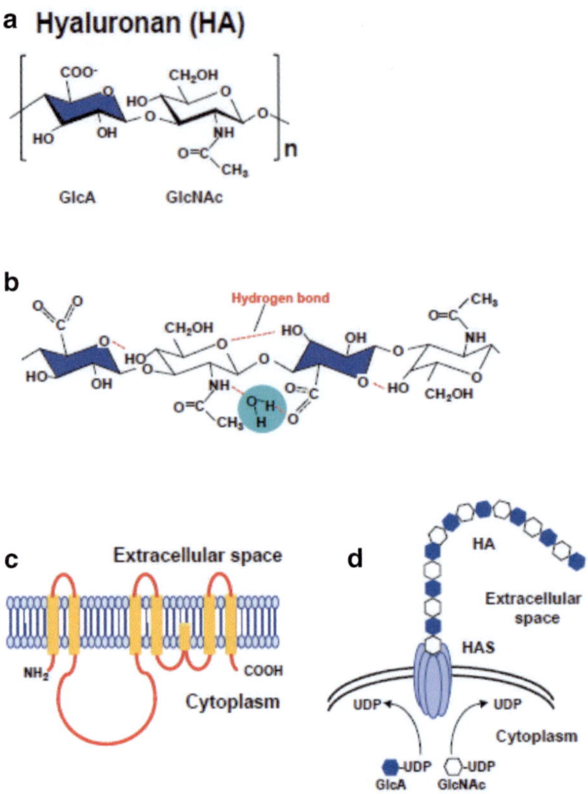

Fig. 6.3 Structure and synthesis of hyaluronan (HA). (**a**) Molecular structure of a HA disaccharide unit. HA is a negatively charged polysaccharide composed of repeating disaccharide units of glucuronic acid (GlcA; blue) and N-acetylglucosamine (GlcNAc). (**b**) Secondary structure of a HA tetrasaccharide with water. Hydrogen bonds are represented by red dashed lines. (**c**) Predicted structure of mammalian HAS. HAS enzymes contain multiple membrane-spanning regions at both the amino and carboxyl terminus and catalytic sites at the central part of the molecule. (**d**) Schematic illustration of HA synthesis and secretion. HAS enzymes catalyze the alternative addition of UDP-GlcA and UDP-GlcNAc to the nascent HA chain and extrude it through the plasma membrane. (From Kobayashi T (2020), with permission)

water molecules, which occupies a very large volume. Most of the volume of high molecular weight HA is water, which is not bound by the polymer. The polymer shape is constantly changing, but the water still contributes to the effective size of each molecule because of its frictional interaction with closely spaced polymer segments. The time-average shape of HA can be described as a sphere, with greatest density of chain segments near the center. Furthermore, the effective sphere-like volume of a wormlike HA chain grows exponentially as the molecular weight of HA increases, accounting for its unique hydrodynamic properties which affect tissue hydration, viscosity, and physical stiffness [84].

Muscle Hydration, Lubrication, Viscoelasticity, and ECM Stiffness

The production and degradation of HA, its hydrodynamic properties, and distribution throughout the ECM significantly affect intramuscular fluid dynamics, ECM viscoelasticity, and the passive resistance of the ECM. As noted above, as the concentration and molecular weight of HA increases, it entrains more water within its hydrodynamic volume, and the viscosity of the solution increases exponentially (a 10 mg/ml solution of 1.5×10^6 Da HA has a viscosity 5000× that of water) due to macromolecular crowding of the polymer (Fig. 6.4) [85, 86]. Viscosity is the resistance to flow of a liquid. Under shear stress, the viscosity of HA drops rapidly while maintaining elasticity, making it an ideal biological lubricant [87]. However, the molecular weight and viscosity of HA solutions affects the lubrication of tissues. For example, at the cartilage-cartilage interface, the relative effectiveness of friction reduction (especially static friction, the resistance to start up motion) is dependent on the molecular weight of HA: the higher the molecular weight, the lower the friction [88]. This is thought to be due to a "viscous boundary layer" of HA at the surface of cartilage that facilitates low-velocity high-load movements [89]. In contrast, for high-velocity low-load movements, such as in the endomysium and perimysium of muscle, the thickness of the HA-containing boundary is large compared with the diameter of the molecules [79]. Here friction would be predicted to increase with increased HA concentration and viscosity, negatively affecting lubrication, i.e., the

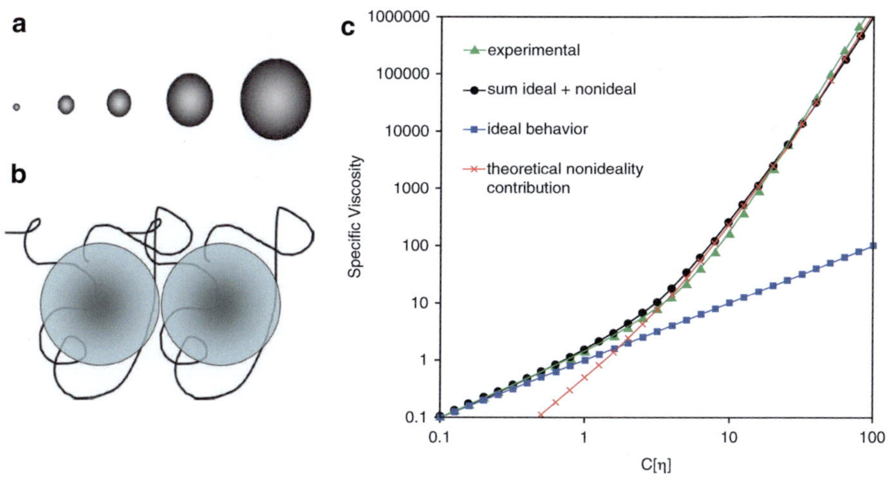

Fig. 6.4 Hydrodynamic properties and viscosity of hyaluronan (HA). (**a**) HA chains of increasing molecular weight (from left to right) 0.1, 0.5, 1, 3 and 6 million have hydrodynamic diameters of approximately 50, 140, 210, 400 and 600 nm, respectively in physiological saline solution. (**b**) The effective hydrodynamic domain of each chain is modeled as a sphere, the volume of which is dependent on the molecular weight to the 1.8 power. (**c**) Experimental data for HA in physiological saline shows a marked increase in viscosity with increasing concentration and intrinsic viscosity, as expected for nonideal solutions. (Adapted from Cowman MK (2015), with permission)

higher the molecular weight, the greater the friction [90]. Viscoelasticity is the time-dependent resistance to loading or deformation. Hyaluronan solutions also exhibit viscoelastic behavior that is highly dependent on HA concentration, temperature, pH, and the ionic strength of the solution [91]. HA shows nonlinear viscoelastic behavior with higher concentration, temperatures, and with increased or decreased pH [92–96], implying that a muscle with higher HA concentrations, and hence higher viscoelasticity will show greater passive resistance to stretch or contraction. Thus, the concentration and rheological properties of HA in the ECM of muscle can contribute significantly to increased passive resistance during movement [97, 98].

Effect of Exercise, Immobility, and Overuse on Hyaluronan Concentration

The HA in muscle is primarily of high molecular weight (>4 million Da), whereas the HA contained in lymph is primarily of low molecular weight. Volume loading produces a preferential increase in the flux of low molecular weight HA, although the maximum daily removal of HA by lymph is <1% of the tissue content in a homeostatic state [99]. In human muscle, HA is especially abundant in the perimysium (Fig. 6.5). HA muscle concentrations show large interindividual variation at rest, with no correlation between muscle and serum HA levels in the healthy state. Exercise does not immediately change muscle HA concentration, but serum HA increases significantly and decreases rapidly to lower than resting levels by 30-min postexercise [79]. However, inducing muscle hypertrophy, for example by synergist elimination after Achilles tenectomy in mice increased the concentration of

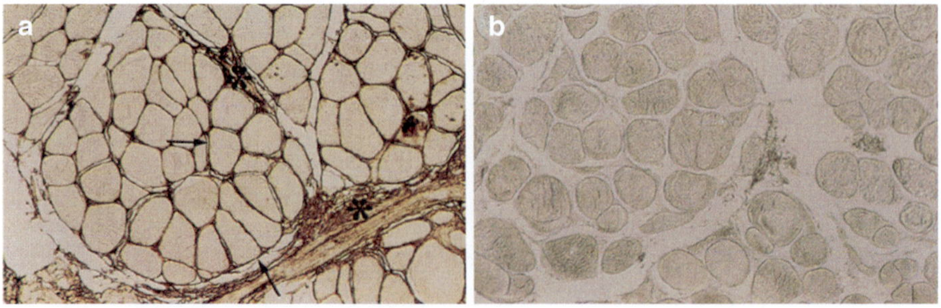

Fig. 6.5 Location of hyaluronan (HA) in human muscle. (**a**) Light micrograph of histological section of quadriceps femoris muscle obtained at surgery stained with brown staining biotinylated HA binding protein (HABP). The endomysium (arrows) and perimysium (asterisks) are rich in HA. (**b**) Control slide treated with Streptomyces hyaluronidase showed no staining, indicating that the HABP specifically reacted with HA and not with any of the other GAGs. (From Piehl-Aulin K (1991), with permission)

HA in the ECM of the compensating plantaris muscle and increased the expression of HA synthases within a variety of cell types [100]. The hypertrophic stimulus significantly increased muscle HA concentration 2.8-fold after two days, which remained significantly increased at seven days, and then decreased gradually toward control levels by 14 days (Fig. 6.6). Endogenous hyaluronidase genes, HYAL1 and HYAL2, were also highly expressed in skeletal muscle but did not change after the tenectomy. These results indicate that HA levels change dynamically in response to a hypertrophic stimulus and various cell types participate in its synthesis. Similar prior studies in rats also showed hypertrophy of the compensating muscle after synergist elimination, accompanied by large increases in the ECM, particularly thickening of the endomysium [101] and increase in the muscle's wet weight after 21 days mediated by interleukin-6 [102]; however HA was not quantified. Taken together, these studies demonstrate that muscle HA synthesis increases in response to exercise overload, and can contribute to thickening of the ECM. Interestingly, unloading of the rat soleus muscle by immobilization of the ankle joint resulted in muscle shortening and increase in muscle HA content four weeks postimmobilization compared to controls. However, thickening and disorganization of endomysial collagen fibrils only became apparent by 12 weeks postimmobilization (Fig. 6.7) [103]. Thus, disruption of HA homeostasis by both muscle overloading and unloading leads to changes in muscle HA content, and *precedes* changes in collagen fiber organization and content in the muscle ECM.

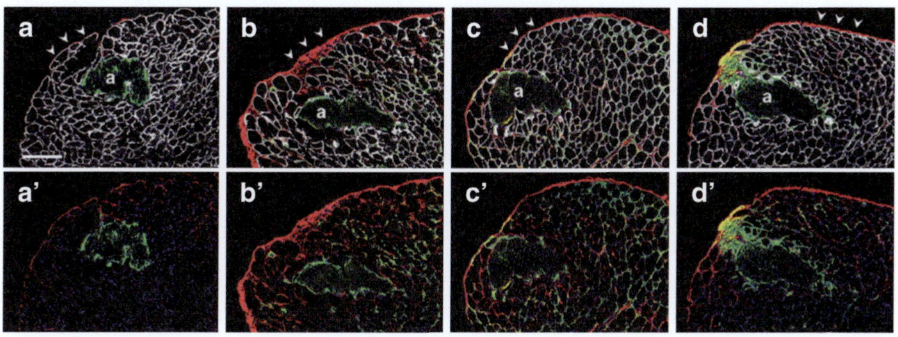

Fig. 6.6 Upregulation of hyaluronan (HA) and tenascin-C (TN-C) during compensatory hypertrophy in the mouse plantaris muscle. (**a** and **a'**) In control muscles, HA (labeled with hyaluronic acid binding protein, red) was expressed at low levels and TN-C (green) was restricted to the aponeurosis (a). (**b** and **b'**) Two days after Achilles tenectomy, the epimysium became enriched with HA (arrowheads), and both HA and TN-C appeared to infiltrate the basal lamina surrounding individual myofibers (white laminin). (**c** and **c'**) HA and TN-C were ubiquitous within the interstitial space after seven days. (**d** and **d'**) By 14 days, HA and TN-C expression had decreased within the muscle body, whereas the epimysium was still strongly labeled for HA compared with the control (**a**). Bar 200 μm; x 10. (Modified from Calve S (2012), with permission)

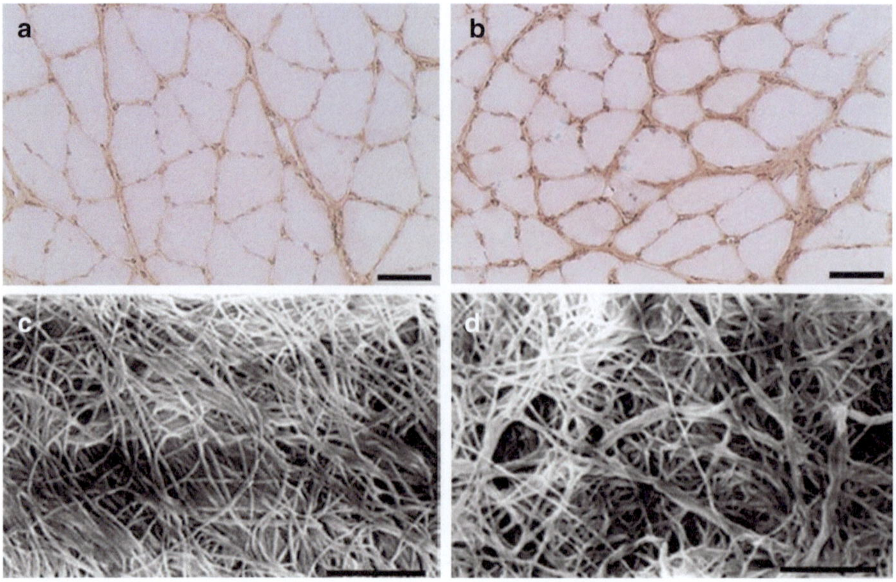

Fig. 6.7 Upregulation of hyaluronan (HA) and thickening of soleus muscle endomysia after immobilization of a rat ankle joint. (**a**) Control muscles, HA (labeled with hyaluronic acid binding protein, brown) was expressed at low levels. (**b**) Four weeks after immobilization the endomysium and perimysium are strongly labeled for HA compared with the control; bar 50 µm. (**c**) Scanning electron micrographs (SCM) of soleus muscle endomysia four weeks after immobilization. (**d**) SCM of soleus muscle endomysia 12 weeks after immobilization; bar 1 µm. (Modified from Okita M (2004), with permission)

The Hyaluronan Hypothesis of Muscle Stiffness: its Role in Spasticity, Fibrosis, and Contracture

The Hyaluronan Hypothesis of Muscle Stiffness

The hyaluronan hypothesis of muscle stiffness postulated that the excessive deposition of HA in the ECM of muscle contributes to the development of muscle stiffness by dramatically altering its viscosity [104, 105]. As alluded to earlier in this chapter, HA is a high molecular weight GAG in the ECM, where it serves as a lubricant, allowing contracting muscle fibers to glide past each other and facilitate force transmission [79, 106]. The hyaluronan hypothesis is based on several findings. First, paresis and immobility after stroke lead to rapid muscle atrophy [107]. Second, immobility results in a relative increase in the proportion of the ECM which is initially composed of space-filling HA and subsequently results in the deposition of collagen as shown in animal models [103]. Third, at high concentrations, hyaluronan and protein-crosslinked assemblies of HA aggregate [108], and interact with water molecules to dramatically increase the viscoelasticity of the ECM [90]. These large, aggregated HA molecules cannot be cleared from the muscle particularly when mobility is reduced. Thus, hyperviscous HA in the ECM can increase the passive stiffness of the ECM, and reduce lubrication and gliding during force transmission causing myofibers, muscle fascicles, and whole muscles to be stuck together. Finally, as discussed below, hyperreflexia and "muscle overactivity" in patients with spasticity, as well as compensatory muscle overuse can trigger excessive production of HA by mechanically overloading specific muscles.

Evidence for the hyaluronan hypothesis is obtained from clinical data which showed that treatment with the enzyme hyaluronidase, which hydrolyzes high molecular weight HA into smaller fragments, led to a dramatic reduction in resistance to passive motion measured using the Modified Ashworth Scale, and increased passive and active range of motion [104] (see Chap. 13). In addition, T1 rho (T1ρ) muscle MRI which images intramuscular GAG content showed increased T1ρ relaxation times in patients with poststroke muscle stiffness, and a reduction to more normal levels after treatment with the enzyme hyaluronidase (Fig. 6.8) [109]. A more recent study with biexponential T1ρ muscle MRI quantified the structure of

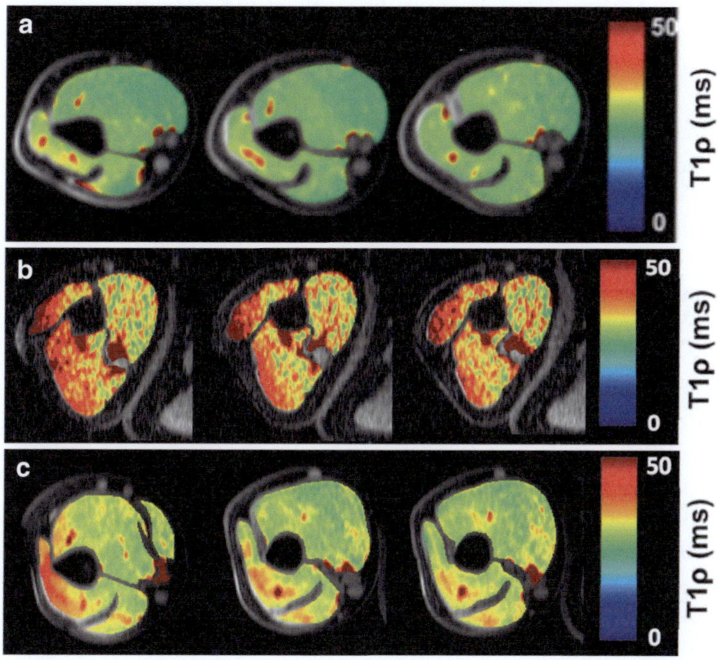

Fig. 6.8 Imaging hyaluronan (HA) in post stroke muscle stiffness using T1ρ muscle MRI. (**a**) T1ρ maps of representative slices overlaid over anatomy in a control subject. (**b**) T1ρ maps of three representative slices overlaid over anatomy in a patient with poststroke muscle stiffness prior to hyaluronidase injection treatment. (**c**) T1ρ maps of the same patient in (b) at approximately similar slice locations following hyaluronidase injection treatment. Note the difference in shape of the muscle before and after the injections. (Modified from Menon R (2019), with permission)

HA in relation to its association with water molecules, and showed that the accumulated HA in stiff muscles traps intramuscular free water, which is released after treatment with hyaluronidase [110]. The affinity of HA for water in stiff muscles can also be observed as a hypoechoic signal on gray scale ultrasound imaging [111]. Additionally, the demonstration of increased muscle viscosity in spastic muscles of stroke survivors using ultrasound shear wave velocity measurements and muscle modeling [112–114] also supports the hyaluronan hypothesis.

Spasticity Versus Muscle Stiffness

The hyperreflexia associated with spasticity became synonymous with "muscle overactivity" with the availability of botulinum toxin injections for focal treatment of muscle overactivity [115, 116], as explained in Chap. 1. Muscle overactivity then became undifferentiated from hypertonia and muscle stiffness, although it has been recognized that paralysis, muscle shortening, and muscle overactivity are three separate disabling factors in patients with spasticity that may need to be treated differently [117] (see also Chaps. 2 and 3). It has been suggested that paresis leads to muscle shortening via nonreflex (i.e., non-neural) increases in passive resistance to movement or stretch, which may increase the sensitivity to stretch and hence produce muscle overactivity via reflex mechanisms [118, 119]. However, the pathophysiologic basis of non-neural muscle shortening and its relationship to neural reflex mechanisms and muscle overactivity has been difficult to elucidate. The finding above that muscle unloading from paresis and immobility leads to an increase in HA in muscle ECM [103], which increases its viscosity and intrinsic stiffness, suggests that HA may be the missing link that connects paresis, muscle shortening, and spasticity [105].

Muscle stretch is sensed by muscle spindle receptors which reside within the HA-rich perimysium of the muscle. The muscle spindles are fusiform structures consisting of a bundle of intrafusal fibers, classified as nuclear bag and chain fibers, enclosed in a connective tissue capsule. The muscle spindle capsule consists of two distinct portions, the inner and the outer capsule [120]. The inner capsule encloses the intrafusal fibers within an innermost axial space, whereas the outer capsule is multilayered and encloses a fluid-filled space in the equatorial region of the spindle called the periaxial space. HA is abundant in the axial and periaxial spaces of the muscle spindles, in all layers of the spindle capsule, as well as in the endoneurium and in the space in between individual axons in the perimysium (Fig. 6.9) [121]. The presence of HA in the periaxial fluid has been shown to be responsible for the transcapsular potential which increases the sensitivity of the sensory endings to mechanical stimuli [122]. Alteration in the viscosity of the HA solution in the muscle spindle can thus increase the sensitivity of the muscle spindle to stretch based on models of mechanosensation [123]. Furthermore, a muscle that is in a shortened position shows increased sensitivity to stretch [124]. Taken together, paresis and immobility can lead to HA accumulation in the ECM of muscle which may increase the stretch-sensitivity of the muscle spindle particularly in shortened paretic muscles. This along with the excitatory-inhibitory imbalance in the spinal cord

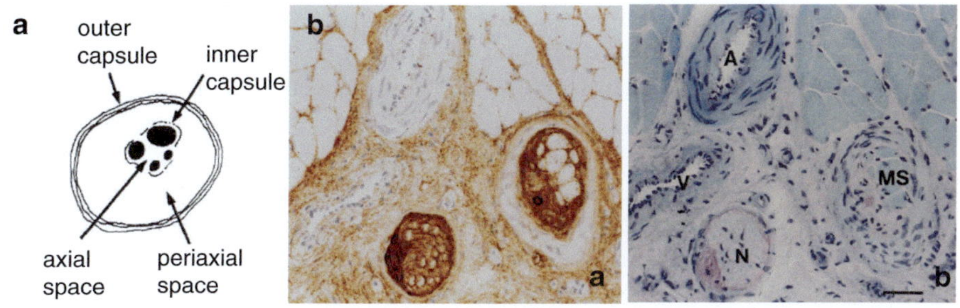

Fig. 6.9 Muscle spindle structure, location and hyaluronan (HA) content. (**a**) Schematic drawing of the structure of the muscle spindle in the equatorial region. The intrafusal fibers are shown in the axial spaces within the inner capsule. (**b**) Serial cross-sections of human lumbrical muscle stained with brown staining biotinylated HA binding protein (HABP) (**a**) and toluidine blue (**b**) showing a neurovascular bundle (*A* artery, *V* vein, *N* nerve) and a muscle spindle (*MS*). Notice the strong HABP staining in (**a**) that fills the capsular space of the muscle spindle and surrounds the nerve fibres in the perimysium; bar 50 μm. (Modified from Pedroso-Domellof F (1998), with permission)

interneuronal network after upper motor neuron lesions (see Chap. 1), may further potentiate stretch reflex hyperexcitability that is characteristic of spastic muscles. The finding that muscle overloading (due to compensatory overuse of specific muscles and potentially reflex overactivity) increases HA synthesis [100], suggests that the excessive HA can further increase the viscosity and intrinsic stiffness of the ECM and contribute to stiffness of the whole muscle. Thus, HA accumulation may be central to both the non-neural and neural mechanisms that produce increased resistance to passive joint motion in patients with spasticity demonstrated in Chap. 4.

Role of Hyaluronan in the Progression to Fibrosis and Contracture

As discussed in Chap. 5, the thickness and collagen content of the ECM in the endomysium, perimysium, and epimysium are increased in chronically spastic muscles that are contractured [125]. Therefore, increased collagen content has been associated with muscle stiffness in patients with spasticity. If this is the case, muscles with higher collagen content and disorganization would be expected to be stiffer. Interestingly, surgical samples of spastic muscle bundles showed significantly lower passive mechanical stiffness when compared with nonspastic muscle bundles [126]. Thus, recent studies do not support a role for increased content and disorganization of collagen in the development of passive muscle stiffness [127, 128]. In contrast, the viscoelastic properties of spastic muscles of stroke survivors under passive conditions were shown to be significantly altered using ultrasound shear wave velocity measurements, which were used in pure elastic and viscoelastic (Voigt) muscle models [112–114]. The effect of stroke was mainly evident in the viscous parameter, and the differences between stroke-affected and nonaffected muscles were more evident at large joint angles, suggesting that the increase in passive muscle stiffness poststroke was largely due to an increase in muscle viscosity.

The viscoelasticity or stiffness of the ECM has important implications for cell–ECM adhesion, cell spreading, migration, differentiation, and even organoid formation [129–131]. The molecular weight of HA is associated with different biological functions: low molecular weight HA is usually associated with proinflammatory response, proangiogenic activity, and migration and proliferation of cells, whereas high molecular weight HA is linked to cellular differentiation and anti-inflammatory effects. HA binding receptors include specific cell-surface receptors such as CD44 and RHAMM (receptor for hyaluronic-acid-mediated motility), as well as hyaluronan receptor for endocytosis (HARE), hyaluronan-binding protein 1 (HABP1), and lymphatic vessel endothelial receptor for hyaluronan 1 (LYVE1). HA interacts with cell surfaces in at least two ways — it can bind to cell-surface receptors to induce the transduction of a range of intracellular signals, either directly or by activating other receptors, and/or it can be retained at the cell surface by sustained transmembrane interactions with its synthases. Either means of retention can generate a voluminous pericellular matrix, or "coat" that incorporates several other HA-binding molecules. This "provisional matrix" provides a hydrated environment in which HA functions as a microenvironmental cue that regulates cell behavior [132]. HA in the pericellular matrix controls the deposition of fibronectin and collagen and modulates the induction of myofibroblasts [133], which are a specialized form of fibroblast responsible for the excessive production of collagen leading to fibrosis and tissue destruction in multiple diseases [134–136].

The differentiation of fibroblasts to myofibroblasts is primarily driven by mechanical tension, and cytokines such as TGF-β, and fibronectin [137, 138]. Several studies have shown that HA is intimately connected with the maintenance of the myofibroblast phenotype [139–145]. Removal of cell-surface HA is known to destabilize focal adhesions involved in cell attachment [146], suggesting that HA in the cross-linked pericellular matrix may cooperate with focal adhesions to provide the mechanical tension needed to maintain the myofibroblast phenotype. Association of HA with the cell-surface receptor CD44 influences the positioning of TGF-β receptors which can have an impact on TGF-β signaling [147], and blocking the synthesis of HA in fibroblasts inhibits the fibroblast-to-myofibroblast conversion [144]. HA also interacts with the fibrillar collagens in the ECM to modulate the mechanical properties of collagen and alter the contractile forces that can be generated by the cells [148]. In fact, the addition of HA to a collagen preparation with a slow rate of fibril formation led to an acceleration in fibril formation, and injection of the collagen solution into tissue promoted the migration of fibroblast-like cells into the region occupied by the injected collagen [149]. Overexpression of HA synthases has also been shown to regulate the invasiveness of fibroblasts, promote fibrosis, and control fibroblast senescence in a lung model of fibrosis [150, 151]. These studies suggest that targeting HA accumulation or synthesis could be an effective therapeutic approach to prevent fibrosis (Fig. 6.10). However, one study suggested that removal of HA may increase the expression and accumulation of collagen I and fibronectin [133], which may point to the balance of HA necessary for tissue homeostasis – both too little and too much may signal a tipping point

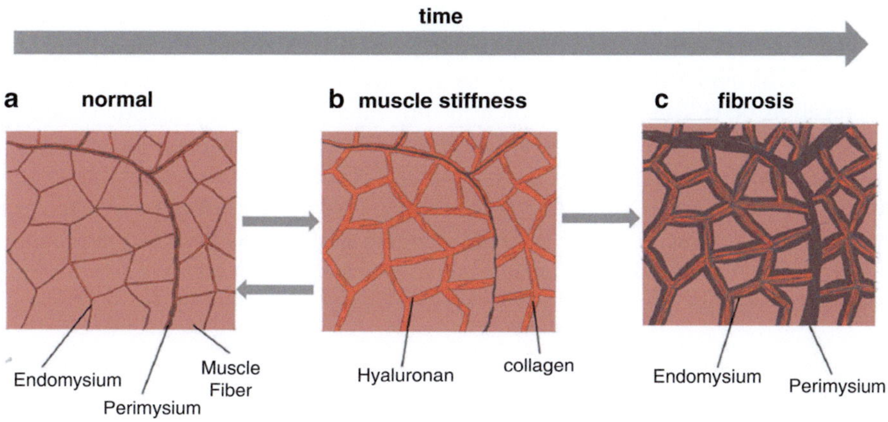

Fig. 6.10 Schematic model for evolution of muscle stiffness to fibrosis and contracture. (**a**) Cross-section of a normal skeletal muscle. (**b**) Development of muscle stiffness due to the accumulation of hyaluronan (HA) in the extracellular space, which increases the viscosity of the ECM, and causes the muscle fibers to stick together. (**c**) Continued HA accumulation initiates fibrosis leading to the replacement of HA by collagen, thickened endomysium and perimysium, and further muscle fiber atrophy. Note that whereas fibrosis is irreversible, muscle stiffness may be reversible, representing a potential therapeutic target. (Modified from Menon R (2019), with permission)

toward fibrosis. Despite the gaps in a complete mechanistic understanding of fibrosis, increased levels of HA have been shown to precede fibrosis in several organs [152–156]. Fibrosis is the end stage of many different diseases and often results from a chronic inflammatory insult, although remodeling of the ECM toward a fibrotic phenotype does not have to involve an inflammatory component [157–159]. Processes that result in muscle fibrosis include chronic inflammation [160], denervation [161], neurotoxin injection [162, 163], and direct trauma [161, 164, 165]. Muscle contractures that occur secondary to cerebral palsy, stroke and other chronic neurological conditions, and muscular diseases are due to fibrosis [126, 166, 167], and surgical approaches are used to release these contractures. However, there is no current therapy for recovery from fibrosis.

Conclusion

Spastic paresis due to neurologic injury from an upper motor neuron lesion results in both disruption of active force generation and excessive increase in passive muscle forces that generate resistance to movement. The three-dimensional geometry of muscle, the structure and function of the extracellular matrix (ECM), and changes in intramuscular fluid volume, hyaluronan (HA) content, and ECM viscosity influence the development of passive mechanical stiffness and form the basis for understanding the hyaluronan hypothesis of muscle stiffness. Both muscle unloading, due to paresis and immobility, and muscle overloading due to spastic muscle overactivity and compensatory overuse of specific muscles in individuals with spasticity can disrupt ECM homeostasis leading to the accumulation, biophysical alteration, and aggregation of HA in muscle, which in turn increases the viscoelasticity of the ECM, and leads to muscle stiffness. The HA-rich matrix in turn controls the deposition of fibronectin and collagen and modulates the induction of myofibroblasts that are responsible for the excessive production of collagen leading to fibrosis and eventually to contracture. A better understanding of the role of HA in the progression to fibrosis in muscle could lead to the prevention of contractures and the consequent disability.

References

1. Shishmarev D. Excitation-contraction coupling in skeletal muscle: recent progress and unanswered questions. Biophys Rev. 2020;12(1):143–53.
2. Hill AV. The mechanics of active muscle. Proc R Soc Lond B Biol Sci. 1953;141(902):104–17.
3. Lieber RL, Murray WM, Clark DL, Hentz VR, Friden J. Biomechanical properties of the brachioradialis muscle: implications for surgical tendon transfer. J Hand Surg Am. 2005;30(2):273–82.
4. Lieber RL, Binder-Markey BI. Biochemical and structural basis of the passive mechanical properties of whole skeletal muscle. J Physiol. 2021;599:3809.
5. Wang K, McCarter R, Wright J, Beverly J, Ramirez-Mitchell R. Regulation of skeletal muscle stiffness and elasticity by titin isoforms: a test of the segmental extension model of resting tension. Proc Natl Acad Sci U S A. 1991;88(16):7101–5.
6. Lieber RL, Ponten E, Burkholder TJ, Friden J. Sarcomere length changes after flexor carpi ulnaris to extensor digitorum communis tendon transfer. J Hand Surg Am. 1996;21(4):612–8.
7. Lieber RL, Friden J. Intraoperative measurement and biomechanical modeling of the flexor carpi ulnaris-to-extensor carpi radialis longus tendon transfer. J Biomech Eng. 1997;119(4):386–91.
8. Smith LR, Lee KS, Ward SR, Chambers HG, Lieber RL. Hamstring contractures in children with spastic cerebral palsy result from a stiffer extracellular matrix and increased in vivo sarcomere length. J Physiol. 2011;589(Pt 10):2625–39.
9. Ward SR, Winters TM, O'Connor SM, Lieber RL. Non-linear scaling of passive mechanical properties in fibers, bundles, fascicles and whole rabbit muscles. Front Physiol. 2020;11:211.
10. Smith LR, Fowler-Gerace LH, Lieber RL. Muscle extracellular matrix applies a transverse stress on fibers with axial strain. J Biomech. 2011;44(8):1618–20.
11. Ward SR, Eng CM, Smallwood LH, Lieber RL. Are current measurements of lower extremity muscle architecture accurate? Clin Orthop Relat Res. 2009;467(4):1074–82.
12. Azizi E, Brainerd EL, Roberts TJ. Variable gearing in pennate muscles. Proc Natl Acad Sci U S A. 2008;105(5):1745–50.
13. Holt NC, Danos N, Roberts TJ, Azizi E. Stuck in gear: age-related loss of variable gearing in skeletal muscle. J Exp Biol. 2016;219(Pt 7):998–1003.
14. Eng CM, Azizi E, Roberts TJ. Structural determinants of muscle gearing during dynamic contractions. Integr Comp Biol. 2018;58(2):207–18.
15. Gans C. Fiber architecture and muscle function. Exerc Sport Sci Rev. 1982;10:160–207.
16. Aagaard P, Andersen JL, Dyhre-Poulsen P, Leffers AM, Wagner A, Magnusson SP, et al. A mechanism for increased contractile strength of human pennate muscle in response to strength training: changes in muscle architecture. J Physiol. 2001;534(Pt. 2):613–23.

17. Purslow PP, Delage JP. General anatomy of the muscle fasciae. In: Fascia: the tensional network of the human body. London: Churchill Livingstone; 2012. p. 5–10.
18. Purslow PP. The structure and role of intramuscular connective tissue in muscle function. Front Physiol. 2020;11:495.
19. Purslow PP, Trotter JA. The morphology and mechanical properties of endomysium in series-fibred muscles: variations with muscle length. J Muscle Res Cell Motil. 1994;15(3):299–308.
20. Trotter JA. Functional morphology of force transmission in skeletal muscle. A brief review. Acta Anat (Basel). 1993;146(4):205–22.
21. Trotter JA, Purslow PP. Functional morphology of the endomysium in series fibered muscles. J Morphol. 1992;212(2):109–22.
22. Pardo JV, Siliciano JD, Craig SW. A vinculin-containing cortical lattice in skeletal muscle: transverse lattice elements ("costameres") mark sites of attachment between myofibrils and sarcolemma. Proc Natl Acad Sci U S A. 1983;80(4):1008–12.
23. Ervasti JM. Costameres: the Achilles' heel of Herculean muscle. J Biol Chem. 2003;278(16):13591–4.
24. Ramaswamy KS, Palmer ML, van der Meulen JH, Renoux A, Kostrominova TY, Michele DE, et al. Lateral transmission of force is impaired in skeletal muscles of dystrophic mice and very old rats. J Physiol. 2011;589(Pt 5):1195–208.
25. Passerieux E, Rossignol R, Letellier T, Delage JP. Physical continuity of the perimysium from myofibers to tendons: involvement in lateral force transmission in skeletal muscle. J Struct Biol. 2007;159(1):19–28.
26. Purslow PP. Muscle fascia and force transmission. J Bodyw Mov Ther. 2010;14(4):411–7.
27. Millman BM. The filament lattice of striated muscle. Physiol Rev. 1998;78(2):359–91.
28. Williams CD, Salcedo MK, Irving TC, Regnier M, Daniel TL. The length-tension curve in muscle depends on lattice spacing. Proc Biol Sci. 2013;280(1766):20130697.
29. Gordon AM, Huxley AF, Julian FJ. The variation in isometric tension with sarcomere length in vertebrate muscle fibres. J Physiol. 1966;184(1):170–92.
30. Williams CD, Regnier M, Daniel TL. Elastic energy storage and radial forces in the myofilament lattice depend on sarcomere length. PLoS Comput Biol. 2012;8(11):e1002770.
31. Roberts TJ, Eng CM, Sleboda DA, Holt NC, Brainerd EL, Stover KK, et al. The multiscale, three-dimensional nature of skeletal muscle contraction. Physiology (Bethesda). 2019;34(6):402–8.
32. Borg TK, Caulfield JB. Morphology of connective tissue in skeletal muscle. Tissue Cell. 1980;12(1):197–207.
33. Gillies AR, Lieber RL. Structure and function of the skeletal muscle extracellular matrix. Muscle Nerve. 2011;44(3):318–31.
34. Gindre J, Takaza M, Moerman KM, Simms CK. A structural model of passive skeletal muscle shows two reinforcement processes in resisting deformation. J Mech Behav Biomed Mater. 2013;22:84–94.
35. Sleboda DA, Roberts TJ. Incompressible fluid plays a mechanical role in the development of passive muscle tension. Biol Lett. 2017;13(1):20160630.
36. Blemker SS, Pinsky PM, Delp SL. A 3D model of muscle reveals the causes of nonuniform strains in the biceps brachii. J Biomech. 2005;38(4):657–65.
37. Sinha U, Sinha S, Hodgson JA, Edgerton RV. Human soleus muscle architecture at different ankle joint angles from magnetic resonance diffusion tensor imaging. J Appl Physiol (1985). 2011;110(3):807–19.
38. Street SF. Lateral transmission of tension in frog myofibers: a myofibrillar network and transverse cytoskeletal connections are possible transmitters. J Cell Physiol. 1983;114(3):346–64.
39. Huijing PA, Baan GC, Rebel GT. Non-myotendinous force transmission in rat extensor digitorum longus muscle. J Exp Biol. 1998;201(Pt 5):683–91.
40. Huijing PA. Epimuscular myofascial force transmission: a historical review and implications for new research. International Society of Biomechanics Muybridge Award Lecture, Taipei, 2007. J Biomech. 2009;42(1):9–21.

41. Yucesoy CA, Baan G, Huijing PA. Epimuscular myofascial force transmission occurs in the rat between the deep flexor muscles and their antagonistic muscles. J Electromyogr Kinesiol. 2010;20(1):118–26.
42. Turrina A, Martinez-Gonzalez MA, Stecco C. The muscular force transmission system: role of the intramuscular connective tissue. J Bodyw Mov Ther. 2013;17(1):95–102.
43. Wood LK, Kayupov E, Gumucio JP, Mendias CL, Claflin DR, Brooks SV. Intrinsic stiffness of extracellular matrix increases with age in skeletal muscles of mice. J Appl Physiol (1985). 2014;117(4):363–9.
44. Meyer G, Lieber RL. Muscle fibers bear a larger fraction of passive muscle tension in frogs compared with mice. J Exp Biol. 2018;221(Pt 22):jeb182089.
45. Azizi E, Deslauriers AR, Holt NC, Eaton CE. Resistance to radial expansion limits muscle strain and work. Biomech Model Mechanobiol. 2017;16(5):1633–43.
46. Siebert T, Till O, Blickhan R. Work partitioning of transversally loaded muscle: experimentation and simulation. Comput Methods Biomech Biomed Engin. 2014;17(3):217–29.
47. Siebert T, Till O, Stutzig N, Gunther M, Blickhan R. Muscle force depends on the amount of transversal muscle loading. J Biomech. 2014;47(8):1822–8.
48. Ruttiman RJ, Sleboda DA, Roberts TJ. Release of fascial compartment boundaries reduces muscle force output. J Appl Physiol (1985). 2019;126(3):593–8.
49. Sjogaard G, Saltin B. Extra- and intracellular water spaces in muscles of man at rest and with dynamic exercise. Am J Phys. 1982;243(3):R271–80.
50. Jacobsson S, Kjellmer I. Accumulation of fluid in exercising skeletal muscle. Acta Physiol Scand. 1964;60:286–92.
51. Kjellmer I. The effect of exercise on the vascular bed of skeletal muscle. Acta Physiol Scand. 1964;62:18–30.
52. Lundvall J. Tissue hyperosmolality as a mediator of vasodilatation and transcapillary fluid flux in exercising skeletal muscle. Acta Physiol Scand Suppl. 1972;379:1–142.
53. Lundvall J, Mellander S, Westling H, White T. Fluid transfer between blood and tissues during exercise. Acta Physiol Scand. 1972;85(2):258–69.
54. Folkow B, Haglund U, Jodal M, Lundgren O. Blood flow in the calf muscle of man during heavy rhythmic exercise. Acta Physiol Scand. 1971;81(2):157–63.
55. Nicolaides AN, Zukowski AJ. The value of dynamic venous pressure measurements. World J Surg. 1986;10(6):919–24.
56. Meyer RA, Prior BM. Functional magnetic resonance imaging of muscle. Exerc Sport Sci Rev. 2000;28(2):89–92.
57. Bjornberg J. Forces involved in transcapillary fluid movement in exercising cat skeletal muscle. Acta Physiol Scand. 1990;140(2):221–36.
58. Jenner G, Foley JM, Cooper TG, Potchen EJ, Meyer RA. Changes in magnetic resonance images of muscle depend on exercise intensity and duration, not work. J Appl Physiol (1985). 1994;76(5):2119–24.
59. Senay LC Jr, Pivarnik JM. Fluid shifts during exercise. Exerc Sport Sci Rev. 1985;13:335–87.
60. Greenleaf JE, Convertino VA, Stremel RW, Bernauer EM, Adams WC, Vignau SR, et al. Plasma [Na+], [Ca2+], and volume shifts and thermoregulation during exercise in man. J Appl Physiol Respir Environ Exerc Physiol. 1977;43(6):1026–32.
61. Gladden LB. Muscle as a consumer of lactate. Med Sci Sports Exerc. 2000;32(4):764–71.
62. Stallknecht B, Vissing J, Galbo H. Lactate production and clearance in exercise. Effects of training. A mini-review. Scand J Med Sci Sports. 1998;8(3):127–31.
63. Willwacher S, Sleboda DA, Mahlich D, Bruggemann GP, Roberts TJ, Bratke G. The time course of calf muscle fluid volume during prolonged running. Physiol Rep. 2020;8(9):e14414.
64. Ploutz-Snyder LL, Convertino VA, Dudley GA. Resistance exercise-induced fluid shifts: change in active muscle size and plasma volume. Am J Phys. 1995;269(3 Pt 2):R536–43.
65. Raja MK, Raymer GH, Moran GR, Marsh G, Thompson RT. Changes in tissue water content measured with multiple-frequency bioimpedance and metabolism measured with 31P-MRS during progressive forearm exercise. J Appl Physiol (1985). 2006;101(4):1070–5.

66. Shi J, Zheng YP, Chen X, Huang QH. Assessment of muscle fatigue using sonomyography: muscle thickness change detected from ultrasound images. Med Eng Phys. 2007; 29(4):472–9.
67. Jensen BR, Jorgensen K, Sjogaard G. The effect of prolonged isometric contractions on muscle fluid balance. Eur J Appl Physiol Occup Physiol. 1994;69(5):439–44.
68. Prior BM, Ploutz-Snyder LL, Cooper TG, Meyer RA. Fiber type and metabolic dependence of T2 increases in stimulated rat muscles. J Appl Physiol (1985). 2001;90(2):615–23.
69. Heukelom B, van der Stelt A, Diegenbach PC. A simple anatomical model of muscle, and the effects of internal pressure. Bull Math Biol. 1979;41(6):791–802.
70. Daggfeldt K. Muscle bulging reduces muscle force and limits the maximal effective muscle size. J Mech Med Biol. 2006;6:229–39.
71. Winters TM, Sepulveda GS, Cottler PS, Kaufman KR, Lieber RL, Ward SR. Correlation between isometric force and intramuscular pressure in rabbit tibialis anterior muscle with an intact anterior compartment. Muscle Nerve. 2009;40(1):79–85.
72. Sleboda DA, Wold ES, Roberts TJ. Passive muscle tension increases in proportion to intramuscular fluid volume. J Exp Biol. 2019;222(Pt 21):jeb209668.
73. Sleboda DA, Roberts TJ. Internal fluid pressure influences muscle contractile force. Proc Natl Acad Sci U S A. 2020;117(3):1772–8.
74. Whittington B, Silder A, Heiderscheit B, Thelen DG. The contribution of passive-elastic mechanisms to lower extremity joint kinetics during human walking. Gait Posture. 2008;27(4):628–34.
75. Csapo R, Gumpenberger M, Wessner B. Skeletal muscle extracellular matrix - what do we know about its composition, regulation, and physiological roles? A narrative review. Front Physiol. 2020;11:253.
76. Amorim S, Reis CA, Reis RL, Pires RA. Extracellular matrix mimics using Hyaluronan-based biomaterials. Trends Biotechnol. 2021;39(1):90–104.
77. Manou D, Caon I, Bouris P, Triantaphyllidou IE, Giaroni C, Passi A, et al. The complex interplay between extracellular matrix and cells in tissues. Methods Mol Biol. 2019;1952:1–20.
78. Laurent C, Johnson-Wells G, Hellstrom S, Engstrom-Laurent A, Wells AF. Localization of hyaluronan in various muscular tissues. A morphological study in the rat. Cell Tissue Res. 1991;263(2):201–5.
79. Piehl-Aulin K, Laurent C, Engstrom-Laurent A, Hellstrom S, Henriksson J. Hyaluronan in human skeletal muscle of lower extremity: concentration, distribution, and effect of exercise. J Appl Physiol (1985). 1991;71(6):2493–8.
80. Stecco C, Stern R, Porzionato A, Macchi V, Masiero S, Stecco A, et al. Hyaluronan within fascia in the etiology of myofascial pain. Surg Radiol Anat. 2011;33(10):891–6.
81. Fede C, Angelini A, Stern R, Macchi V, Porzionato A, Ruggieri P, et al. Quantification of hyaluronan in human fasciae: variations with function and anatomical site. J Anat. 2018;233(4):552–6.
82. Laurent TC. Biochemistry of hyaluronan. Acta Otolaryngol Suppl. 1987;442:7–24.
83. Kobayashi T, Chanmee T, Itano N. Hyaluronan: metabolism and function. Biomol Ther. 2020;10(11):1525.
84. Cowman MK, Lee HG, Schwertfeger KL, McCarthy JB, Turley EA. The content and size of Hyaluronan in biological fluids and tissues. Front Immunol. 2015;6:261.
85. Cowman MK, Hernandez M, Kim JR. Macromolecular crowding in the biomatrix. In: Balazs EA, editor. Structure and function of biomatrix control of cell behavior and gene expression. Edgewater: Matrix Biology Institute; 2012. p. 45–66.
86. Hascall V, Esko JD. Hyaluronan. In: Varki A, Cummings RD, Esko JD, Stanley P, Hart GW, Aebi M, et al., editors. Essentials of Glycobiology. 3rd ed. New York: Cold Spring Harbor; 2015.
87. Cowman MK, Chen CC, Pandya M, Yuan H, Ramkishun D, LoBello J, et al. Improved agarose gel electrophoresis method and molecular mass calculation for high molecular mass hyaluronan. Anal Biochem. 2011;417(1):50–6.

88. Kwiecinski JJ, Dorosz SG, Ludwig TE, Abubacker S, Cowman MK, Schmidt TA. The effect of molecular weight on hyaluronan's cartilage boundary lubricating ability--alone and in combination with proteoglycan 4. Osteoarthr Cartil. 2011;19(11):1356–62.
89. Yakubov GE, McColl J, Bongaerts JH, Ramsden JJ. Viscous boundary lubrication of hydrophobic surfaces by mucin. Langmuir. 2009;25(4):2313–21.
90. Cowman MK, Schmidt TA, Raghavan P, Stecco A. Viscoelastic properties of Hyaluronan in physiological conditions. F1000Res. 2015;4:622.
91. Gibbs DA, Merrill EW, Smith KA, Balazs EA. Rheology of hyaluronic acid. Biopolymers. 1968;6(6):777–91.
92. Caspersen MB, Roubroeks JP, Qun L, Shan H, Fogh J, Ruidong Z, et al. Thermal degradation and stability of sodium hyaluronate in solid state. Carbohydr Polym. 2014;107:25–30.
93. Cowman MK, Matsuoka S. Experimental approaches to hyaluronan structure. Carbohydr Res. 2005;340(5):791–809.
94. Matteini P, Dei L, Carretti E, Volpi N, Goti A, Pini R. Structural behavior of highly concentrated hyaluronan. Biomacromolecules. 2009;10(6):1516–22.
95. Snetkov P, Zakharova K, Morozkina S, Olekhnovich R, Uspenskaya M. Hyaluronic acid: the influence of molecular weight on structural, physical, physico-chemical, and degradable properties of biopolymer. Polymers (Basel). 2020;12(8):1800.
96. Shimada E, Matsumura G. Viscosity and molecular weight of hyaluronic acids. J Biochem. 1975;78(3):513–7.
97. Meyer GA, McCulloch AD, Lieber RL. A nonlinear model of passive muscle viscosity. J Biomech Eng. 2011;133(9):091007.
98. Elliott DM, Robinson PS, Gimbel JA, Sarver JJ, Abboud JA, Iozzo RV, et al. Effect of altered matrix proteins on quasilinear viscoelastic properties in transgenic mouse tail tendons. Ann Biomed Eng. 2003;31(5):599–605.
99. Armstrong SE, Bell DR. Relationship between lymph and tissue hyaluronan in skin and skeletal muscle. Am J Physiol Heart Circ Physiol. 2002;283(6):H2485–94.
100. Calve S, Isaac J, Gumucio JP, Mendias CL. Hyaluronic acid, HAS1, and HAS2 are significantly upregulated during muscle hypertrophy. Am J Physiol Cell Physiol. 2012;303(5):C577–88.
101. Williams PE, Goldspink G. Connective tissue changes in surgically overloaded muscle. Cell Tissue Res. 1981;221(2):465–70.
102. White JP, Reecy JM, Washington TA, Sato S, Le ME, Davis JM, et al. Overload-induced skeletal muscle extracellular matrix remodelling and myofibre growth in mice lacking IL-6. Acta Physiol (Oxf). 2009;197(4):321–32.
103. Okita M, Yoshimura T, Nakano J, Motomura M, Eguchi K. Effects of reduced joint mobility on sarcomere length, collagen fibril arrangement in the endomysium, and hyaluronan in rat soleus muscle. J Muscle Res Cell Motil. 2004;25(2):159–66.
104. Raghavan P, Lu Y, Mirchandani M, Stecco A. Human recombinant hyaluronidase injections for upper limb muscle stiffness in individuals with cerebral injury: a case series. EBioMedicine. 2016;9:306–13.
105. Stecco A, Stecco C, Raghavan P. Peripheral mechanisms of spasticity and treatment implications. Curr Phys Med Rehabil Rep. 2014;2(2):121–7.
106. Huijing PA, Jaspers RT. Adaptation of muscle size and myofascial force transmission: a review and some new experimental results. Scand J Med Sci Sports. 2005;15(6):349–80.
107. Scherbakov N, Sandek A, Doehner W. Stroke-related sarcopenia: specific characteristics. J Am Med Dir Assoc. 2015;16(4):272–6.
108. Zhao M, Yoneda M, Ohashi Y, Kurono S, Iwata H, Ohnuki Y, et al. Evidence for the covalent binding of SHAP, heavy chains of inter-alpha-trypsin inhibitor, to hyaluronan. J Biol Chem. 1995;270(44):26657–63.
109. Menon RG, Raghavan P, Regatte RR. Quantifying muscle glycosaminoglycan levels in patients with post-stroke muscle stiffness using T1rho MRI. Sci Rep. 2019;9(1):14513.
110. Menon RG, Raghavan P, Regatte RR. Pilot study quantifying muscle glycosaminoglycan using bi-exponential T1rho mapping in patients with muscle stiffness after stroke. Sci Rep. 2021;11(1):13951.

111. Stecco A, Pirri C, Caro R, Raghavan P. Stiffness and echogenicity: development of a stiffness-echogenicity matrix for clinical problem solving. Eur J Transl Myol. 2019;29(3):8476.
112. Rasool G, Wang AB, Rymer WZ, Lee SSM. Shear waves reveal viscoelastic changes in skeletal muscles after hemispheric stroke. IEEE Trans Neural Syst Rehabil Eng. 2018;26(10):2006–14.
113. Wang AB, Perreault EJ, Royston TJ, Lee SSM. Changes in shear wave propagation within skeletal muscle during active and passive force generation. J Biomech. 2019;94:115–22.
114. Rasool G, Wang AB, Rymer WZ, Lee SS. Altered viscoelastic properties of stroke-affected muscles estimated using ultrasound shear waves - preliminary data. Annu Int Conf IEEE Eng Med Biol Soc. 2016;2016:2869–72.
115. Brin MF. Dosing, administration, and a treatment algorithm for use of botulinum toxin A for adult-onset spasticity. Spasticity Study Group. Muscle Nerve Suppl. 1997;6:S208–20.
116. Gracies JM, Elovic E, McGuire J, Simpson DM. Traditional pharmacological treatments for spasticity. Part I: local treatments. Muscle Nerve Suppl. 1997;6:S61–91.
117. Gracies JM. Pathophysiology of impairment in patients with spasticity and use of stretch as a treatment of spastic hypertonia. Phys Med Rehabil Clin N Am. 2001;12(4):747–68, vi.
118. Gracies JM. Pathophysiology of spastic paresis. II: emergence of muscle overactivity. Muscle Nerve. 2005;31(5):552–71.
119. Singer B, Dunne J, Allison G. Reflex and non-reflex elements of hypertonia in triceps surae muscles following acquired brain injury: implications for rehabilitation. Disabil Rehabil. 2001;23(17):749–57.
120. Barker D, Banks RW. The muscle spindle. In: Engel AG, Franzini-Armstrong C, editors. Myology 1. 2nd ed. New York: McGraw-Hill; 1994. p. 333–60.
121. Pedrosa-Domellof F, Hellstrom S, Thornell LE. Hyaluronan in human and rat muscle spindles. Histochem Cell Biol. 1998;110(2):179–82.
122. Fukami Y. Studies of capsule and capsular space of cat muscle spindles. J Physiol. 1986;376:281–97.
123. Song Z, Banks RW, Bewick GS. Modelling the mechanoreceptor's dynamic behaviour. J Anat. 2015;227(2):243–54.
124. Edin BB, Vallbo AB. Stretch sensitization of human muscle spindles. J Physiol. 1988;400:101–11.
125. de Bruin M, Smeulders MJ, Kreulen M, Huijing PA, Jaspers RT. Intramuscular connective tissue differences in spastic and control muscle: a mechanical and histological study. PLoS One. 2014;9(6):e101038.
126. Lieber RL, Runesson E, Einarsson F, Friden J. Inferior mechanical properties of spastic muscle bundles due to hypertrophic but compromised extracellular matrix material. Muscle Nerve. 2003;28(4):464–71.
127. Chapman MA, Pichika R, Lieber RL. Collagen crosslinking does not dictate stiffness in a transgenic mouse model of skeletal muscle fibrosis. J Biomech. 2015;48(2):375–8.
128. Smith LR, Barton ER. Collagen content does not alter the passive mechanical properties of fibrotic skeletal muscle in mdx mice. Am J Physiol Cell Physiol. 2014;306(10):C889–98.
129. Pelham RJ Jr, Wang Y. Cell locomotion and focal adhesions are regulated by substrate flexibility. Proc Natl Acad Sci U S A. 1997;94(25):13661–5.
130. Chaudhuri O, Cooper-White J, Janmey PA, Mooney DJ, Shenoy VB. Effects of extracellular matrix viscoelasticity on cellular behaviour. Nature. 2020;584(7822):535–46.
131. Toole BP. Hyaluronan: from extracellular glue to pericellular cue. Nat Rev Cancer. 2004;4(7):528–39.
132. Turley EA, Noble PW, Bourguignon LY. Signaling properties of hyaluronan receptors. J Biol Chem. 2002;277(7):4589–92.
133. Evanko SP, Potter-Perigo S, Petty LJ, Workman GA, Wight TN. Hyaluronan controls the deposition of fibronectin and collagen and modulates TGF-beta1 induction of lung Myofibroblasts. Matrix Biol. 2015;42:74–92.
134. Desmouliere A, Chaponnier C, Gabbiani G. Tissue repair, contraction, and the myofibroblast. Wound Repair Regen. 2005;13(1):7–12.

135. Hinz B, Phan SH, Thannickal VJ, Galli A, Bochaton-Piallat ML, Gabbiani G. The myofibroblast: one function, multiple origins. Am J Pathol. 2007;170(6):1807–16.
136. Hinz B, Phan SH, Thannickal VJ, Prunotto M, Desmouliere A, Varga J, et al. Recent developments in myofibroblast biology: paradigms for connective tissue remodeling. Am J Pathol. 2012;180(4):1340–55.
137. Tomasek JJ, Gabbiani G, Hinz B, Chaponnier C, Brown RA. Myofibroblasts and mechanoregulation of connective tissue remodelling. Nat Rev Mol Cell Biol. 2002;3(5):349–63.
138. Gabbiani G. The myofibroblast in wound healing and fibrocontractive diseases. J Pathol. 2003;200(4):500–3.
139. Albeiroti S, Soroosh A, de la Motte CA. Hyaluronan's role in fibrosis: a pathogenic factor or a passive player? Biomed Res Int. 2015;2015:790203.
140. Jenkins RH, Thomas GJ, Williams JD, Steadman R. Myofibroblastic differentiation leads to hyaluronan accumulation through reduced hyaluronan turnover. J Biol Chem. 2004;279(40):41453–60.
141. Meran S, Thomas D, Stephens P, Martin J, Bowen T, Phillips A, et al. Involvement of hyaluronan in regulation of fibroblast phenotype. J Biol Chem. 2007;282(35):25687–97.
142. Meran S, Thomas DW, Stephens P, Enoch S, Martin J, Steadman R, et al. Hyaluronan facilitates transforming growth factor-beta1-mediated fibroblast proliferation. J Biol Chem. 2008;283(10):6530–45.
143. Simpson RM, Meran S, Thomas D, Stephens P, Bowen T, Steadman R, et al. Age-related changes in pericellular hyaluronan organization leads to impaired dermal fibroblast to myofibroblast differentiation. Am J Pathol. 2009;175(5):1915–28.
144. Webber J, Jenkins RH, Meran S, Phillips A, Steadman R. Modulation of TGFbeta1-dependent myofibroblast differentiation by hyaluronan. Am J Pathol. 2009;175(1):148–60.
145. Webber J, Meran S, Steadman R, Phillips A. Hyaluronan orchestrates transforming growth factor-beta1-dependent maintenance of myofibroblast phenotype. J Biol Chem. 2009;284(14):9083–92.
146. Twarock S, Tammi MI, Savani RC, Fischer JW. Hyaluronan stabilizes focal adhesions, filopodia, and the proliferative phenotype in esophageal squamous carcinoma cells. J Biol Chem. 2010;285(30):23276–84.
147. Ito T, Williams JD, Fraser DJ, Phillips AO. Hyaluronan regulates transforming growth factor-beta1 receptor compartmentalization. J Biol Chem. 2004;279(24):25326–32.
148. Allison DD, Wight TN, Ripp NJ, Braun KR, Grande-Allen KJ. Endogenous overexpression of hyaluronan synthases within dynamically cultured collagen gels: implications for vascular and valvular disease. Biomaterials. 2008;29(20):2969–76.
149. Tsunenaga M, Nishiyama T, Horii I, Nakayama Y, Arai K, Hayashi T. Effect of hyaluronate on physicochemical and biological properties of collagen solution which could be used as collagen filler. Connect Tissue Res. 1992;28(1–2):113–23.
150. Li Y, Jiang D, Liang J, Meltzer EB, Gray A, Miura R, et al. Severe lung fibrosis requires an invasive fibroblast phenotype regulated by hyaluronan and CD44. J Exp Med. 2011;208(7):1459–71.
151. Li Y, Liang J, Yang T, Monterrosa Mena J, Huan C, Xie T, et al. Hyaluronan synthase 2 regulates fibroblast senescence in pulmonary fibrosis. Matrix Biol. 2016;55:35–48.
152. Bensadoun ES, Burke AK, Hogg JC, Roberts CR. Proteoglycan deposition in pulmonary fibrosis. Am J Respir Crit Care Med. 1996;154(6 Pt 1):1819–28.
153. Suresh K, Scheid E, Klotz L, Venkateswaran V, Gauldie J, Foley R. Induction of specific human cytotoxic T cells using dendritic cells transduced with an adenovector encoding rat epidermal growth factor receptor 2. Int J Oncol. 2011;39(4):907–13.
154. Chandra SR, Shenoy RK, Karthikeyan SK, Chithra P, Annapoorni CS. Two cases of a rare treatable limb girdle muscle disease. J Assoc Physicians India. 2011;59:321–5.
155. Vijaya Laxmi S, Thirupathi Reddy Y, Suresh Kuarm B, Narsimha Reddy P, Crooks PA, Rajitha B. Synthesis and evaluation of chromenyl barbiturates and thiobarbiturates as potential antitubercular agents. Bioorg Med Chem Lett. 2011;21(14):4329–31.

156. Kumar V, Murthy AK, Suresh KP. Glutathione S-transferase M1 and T1 status and the risk of laryngeal cancer: a meta-analysis. Asian Pac J Cancer Prev. 2011;12(9):2221–6.
157. Eckes B, Nischt R, Krieg T. Cell-matrix interactions in dermal repair and scarring. Fibrogenesis Tissue Repair. 2010;3:4.
158. Hardie WD, Glasser SW, Hagood JS. Emerging concepts in the pathogenesis of lung fibrosis. Am J Pathol. 2009;175(1):3–16.
159. Sivakumar P, Das AM. Fibrosis, chronic inflammation and new pathways for drug discovery. Inflamm Res. 2008;57(9):410–8.
160. Meyer GA, Lieber RL. Skeletal muscle fibrosis develops in response to desmin deletion. Am J Physiol Cell Physiol. 2012;302(11):C1609–20.
161. Lewis DM, Pardoe MJ, Webb SN. The effect of denervation on the mechanical and electrical properties of cat skeletal muscle [proceedings]. J Physiol. 1978;277:48P–9P.
162. Thacker BE, Tomiya A, Hulst JB, Suzuki KP, Bremner SN, Gastwirt RF, et al. Passive mechanical properties and related proteins change with botulinum neurotoxin A injection of normal skeletal muscle. J Orthop Res. 2012;30(3):497–502.
163. Binder-Markey BI, Dewald JPA, Murray WM. The biomechanical basis of the claw finger deformity: a computational simulation study. J Hand Surg Am. 2019;44(9):751–61.
164. Carraro U, Dalla Libera L, Catani C, Danieli-Betto D. Chronic denervation of rat diaphragm: selective maintenance of adult fast myosin heavy chains. Muscle Nerve. 1982;5(7):515–24.
165. Omer GE Jr. Evaluation and reconstruction of the forearm and hand after acute traumatic peripheral nerve injuries. J Bone Joint Surg Am. 1968;50(7):1454–78.
166. Nuckolls GH, Kinnett K, Dayanidhi S, Domenighetti AA, Duong T, Hathout Y, et al. Conference report on contractures in musculoskeletal and neurological conditions. Muscle Nerve. 2020;61(6):740–4.
167. Smith LR, Irianto J, Xia Y, Pfeifer CR, Discher DE. Constricted migration modulates stem cell differentiation. Mol Biol Cell. 2019;30(16):1985–99.

7 Symptomatic and Functional After-Effects of the Syndrome of Spastic Paresis

Nathaniel H. Mayer and Alberto Esquenazi

Chiefly, the bones serve as struts, while the muscles and ligaments act as ties – cross-braces.
– D'Arcy Wentworth Thompson, On Growth and Form, 1917.

- An upper motor neuron syndrome that leads to spastic paresis can result in important symptomatic and functional consequences.
- In the upper limb, these consequences include skin and nerve problems, problems of access to the hand, elbow crease and axilla, grasp and release dysfunction, and problems of reaching.
- Symptomatic and functional consequences in the lower limb include deformities that impact skin and footwear, inadequate limb clearance, improper foot loading, abnormal limb advancement, and inadequate single limb support during locomotion.
- A thorough understanding of these disabling consequences is necessary for planning appropriate treatment.

N. H. Mayer (✉)
Lewis Katz School of Medicine at Temple University, Philadelphia, PA, USA

Motor Control Analysis Laboratory, MossRehab, Elkins Park, PA, USA
e-mail: NMAYER@einstein.edu

A. Esquenazi
Thomas Jefferson University, Philadelphia, PA, USA

Gait and Motion Analysis Laboratory, MossRehab, Elkins Park, PA, USA
e-mail: aesquena@einstein.edu

P. Raghavan (ed.), *Spasticity and Muscle Stiffness*,
https://doi.org/10.1007/978-3-030-96900-4_7

Introduction

This chapter describes important after-effects of the upper motor neuron syndrome which leads to spastic paresis that impedes function and causes deformity and disability [1]. Spastic paresis is characterized by involuntary phenomena that position limb segments in undesired and maladaptive configurations. These include both neural changes causing involuntary muscle overactivity including spastic dystonia, spastic co-contraction, increased flexor reflex afferent activity, and associated reactions, and non-neural changes in the muscle including muscle shortening, stiffness, and contracture [2, 3]. See Chaps. 1, 2, 3, 4, 5, and 6 for explanation of the pathophysiology of these phenomena. Spastic paresis is also characterized by agonist muscle weakness and lack of selective control of movement needed to generate voluntary movement. The neural and non-neural changes superimpose creating a brew of consequential after-effects that lead to skin, nerve, and joint problems, and dysfunction in movement, mobility, and activities of daily life.

Functional Consequences in the Upper Limb

Skin and Nerve Problems

Skin Problems of the Hand, at the Elbow Crease, and in the Axilla

A common presentation in individuals with spastic paresis is a clenched fist with involuntary flexion of the fingers and thumb. The wrist is typically flexed but may be hyperextended. A clenched fist that cannot be unclenched easily leads to maceration, erosion, detritus, skin erythema and breakdown, malodor, and potentially, infection (see Figs. 7.1, 7.2, 7.3, 7.4, 7.5). Severe shortening and/or spastic dystonia involving the flexor digitorum superficialis (FDS) and flexor digitorum profundus

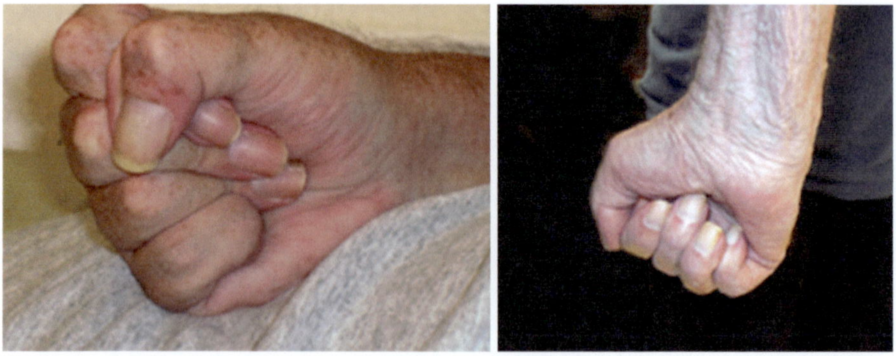

Fig. 7.1 Muscle overactivity or shortening involving the flexor digitorum superficialis (FDS) muscle results in a largely "FDS type hand" (left image), whereas overactivity or shortening involving the flexor digitorum profundus (FDP) muscle leads to an "FDP type hand" (right image). A persistently clenched fist leads to moisture retention, tissue maceration, malodor and skin breakdown

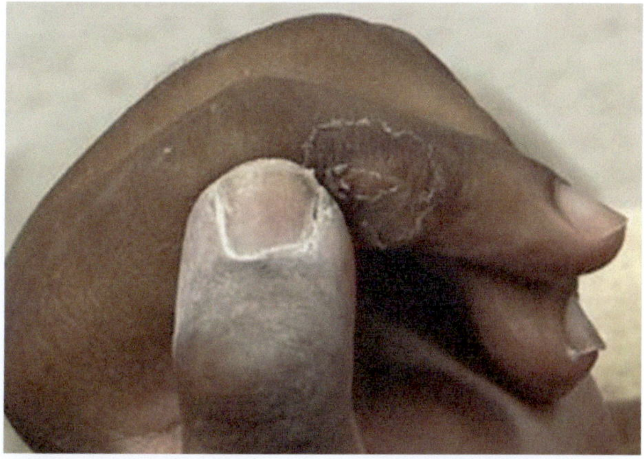

Fig. 7.2 Skin shearing and erosion due to persistent overactivity or shortening involving the flexor pollicis longus (FPL) muscle in an "FPL type thumb" is seen on the middle phalanx of the index finger

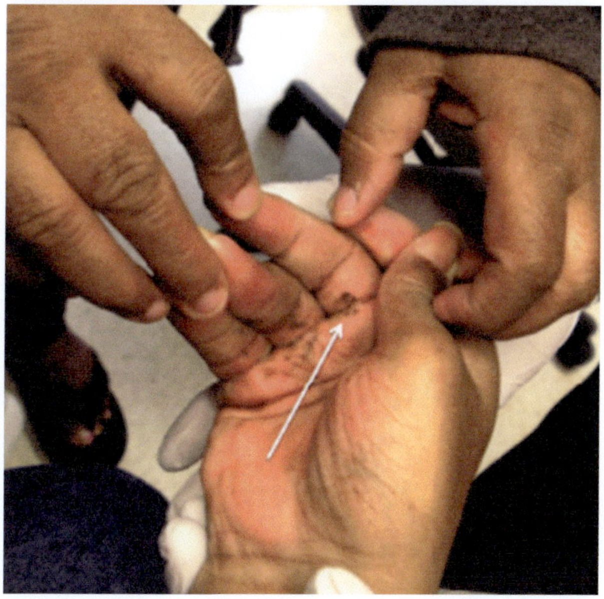

Fig. 7.3 Detritus has collected in the proximal crease of the long finger in this patient with a clenched fist

(FDP) muscles result in an "FDS hand" and an "FDP hand," respectively, as seen in Fig. 7.1. It is not unusual, however, to have mixed findings with some fingers of the FDS type and others of the FDP type. The description of the FDS hand and FDP hand can guide the selection of muscles for injection treatments. Fists that have been clenched for a long time are prone to contracture. Serial casting or serial splinting is a consideration in order to open the hand and provide access for air circulation, moisture evaporation, and elimination of malodor (see Fig. 7.6) [4]. See Chaps. 12 and 13 for local injection treatments if the muscles are not contractured. Surgical interventions such as an "STP" transfer (superficialis to profundus transfer) are a consideration when the patient is chronically affected and not expected to have

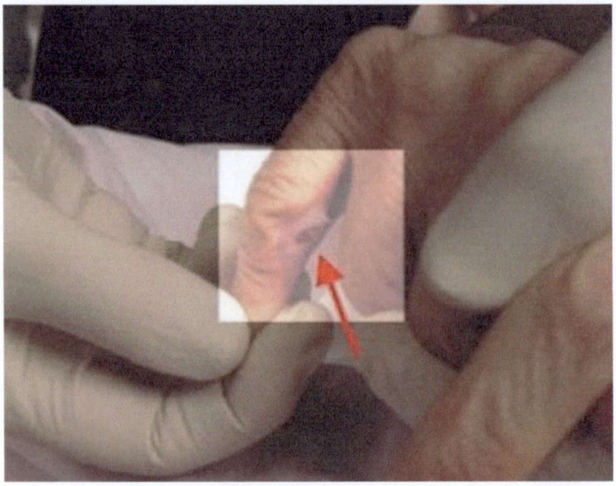

Fig. 7.4 Frank skin ulceration developed on the inner aspect of the little finger in this patient with a clenched fist

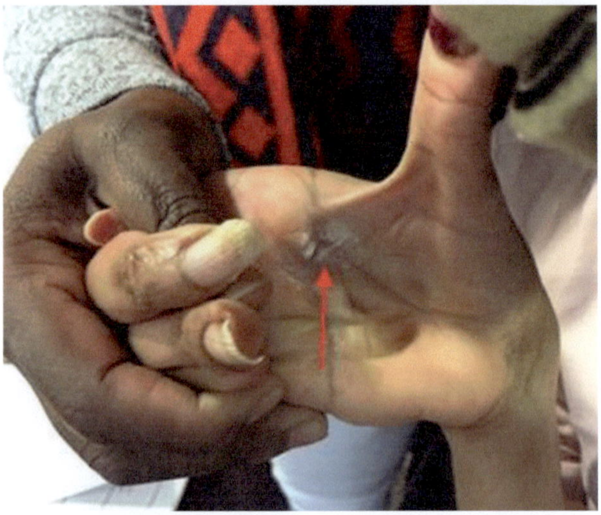

Fig. 7.5 Muscle overactivity or shortening of the flexor digitorum profundus muscle can lead to the fingernails digging into the palmar skin causing indentation and laceration

neurological recovery of voluntary finger movements [5]. An aeration splint (see Fig. 7.7) to keep the fingers away from the palm and allow air circulation through the hand is an alternative when surgery is not feasible. When volitional finger flexor movement is seen in the presence of flexor contracture, fractional lengthening may be a surgical consideration.

A flexed elbow with skin overlap can lead to moisture accumulation, irritation, erythema, and skin breakdown (see Fig. 7.8). Skin irritation and erythema can be seen in the elbow crease in the image on the right side of Fig. 7.8. The image on the left side of Fig. 7.9 shows overlapping skin of another patient with a chronically flexed elbow. Persistent flexion posturing with skin overlap led to severe ulceration and skin breakdown, seen in the image on the right side of

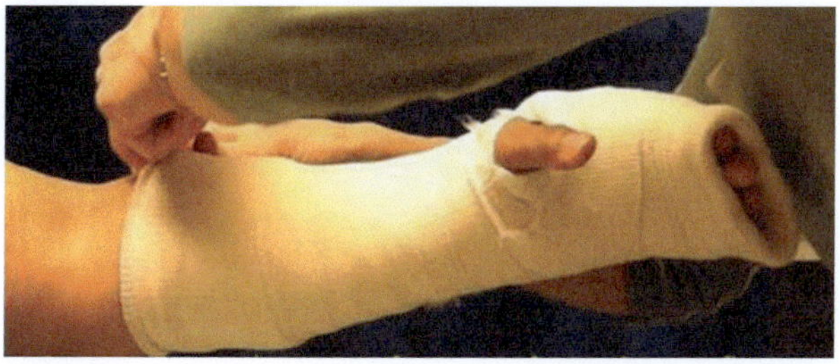

Fig. 7.6 Fists that have been clenched for a long time are prone to developing contractures. This patient is undergoing composite serial casting to stretch out the combined contracture of wrist and finger flexors with the goal of opening the hand to provide access for air circulation, moisture evaporation, and elimination of malodor

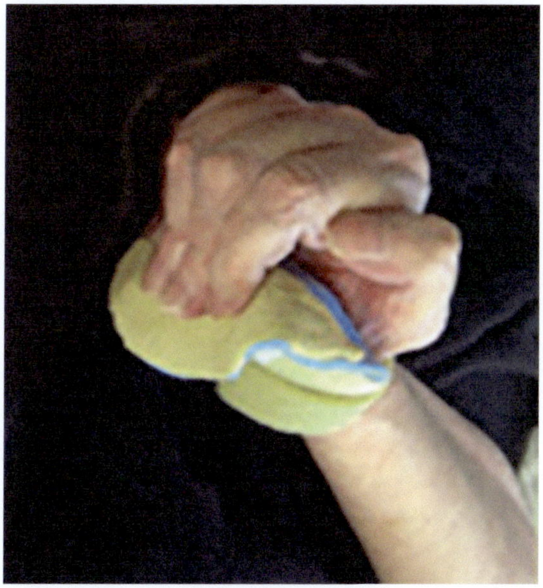

Fig. 7.7 An aeration splint has been fabricated by an occupational therapist to keep the fingers away from the palm and allow air circulation through the hand. Unlike a resting hand splint which makes full palmar contact, an aeration splint creates a tunnel to allow air to circulate across the palm

Fig. 7.9. It is important to educate families to observe skin condition when they perform passive range of motion exercises and bring the aforementioned signs to medical attention. Treatment involves releasing the shortened muscles and/or mitigating muscle overactivity prior to instituting a serial casting program. Reducing tension facilitates patient tolerance to stretching by the casting process. After completion of the casting course, a maintenance resting splint is usually provided.

An adducted shoulder can result in persistent skin overlap leading to skin irritation, maceration, and breakdown (see Figs. 7.10 and 7.11). Shortening and/or overactivity in the pectoralis major (PM), teres major (TM), latissimus dorsi (LD), and subscapularis muscles may be involved. Local treatment of skin lesions along with

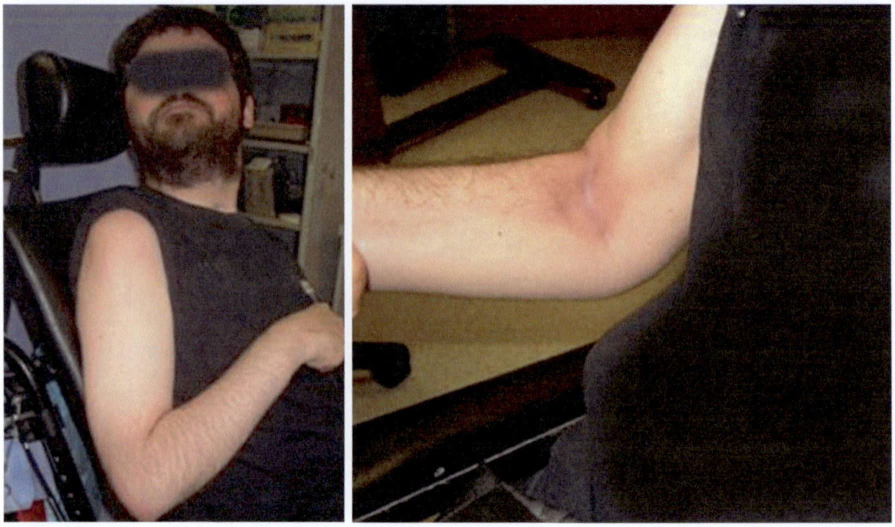

Fig. 7.8 A chronically flexed elbow seen in the left image has led to skin irritation and erythema seen in the elbow crease on the right image

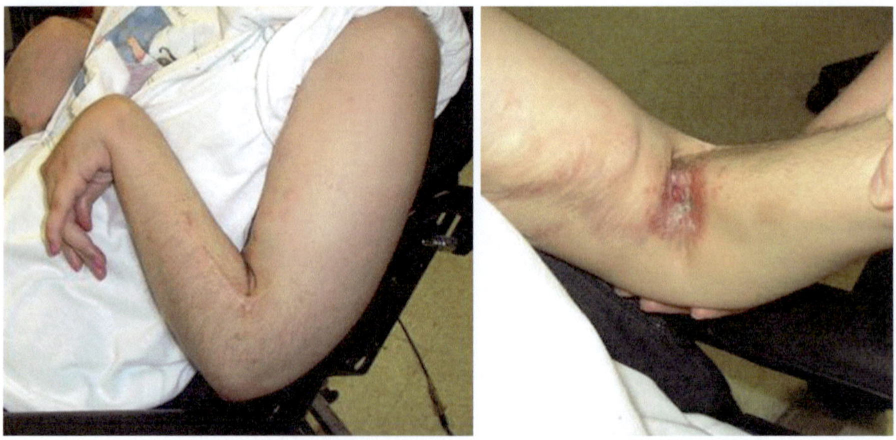

Fig. 7.9 The image on the left side shows overlapping skin in another patient with a chronically flexed elbow. Persistent flexion posturing with skin overlap led to severe skin breakdown in the elbow crease seen on the right image. In addition to the intrinsic value of doing range of motion exercises, it is important to teach families and caregivers to observe skin condition

release of muscle tension followed by vigorous passive range of motion exercises are treatment considerations. Serial casting is not a treatment consideration in this region. Ranging can be conveniently carried out when patients are showered but we also recommend that passive shoulder abduction be performed many times a day because the natural resting position of the shoulder is one of arm contact with the

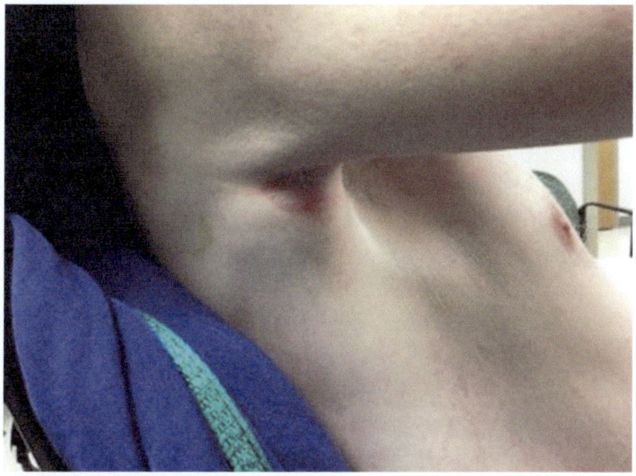

Fig. 7.10 An adducted shoulder can result in persistent skin overlap leading to skin irritation, maceration, and breakdown. Note the area of erythema at the confluence of the adductor tendons

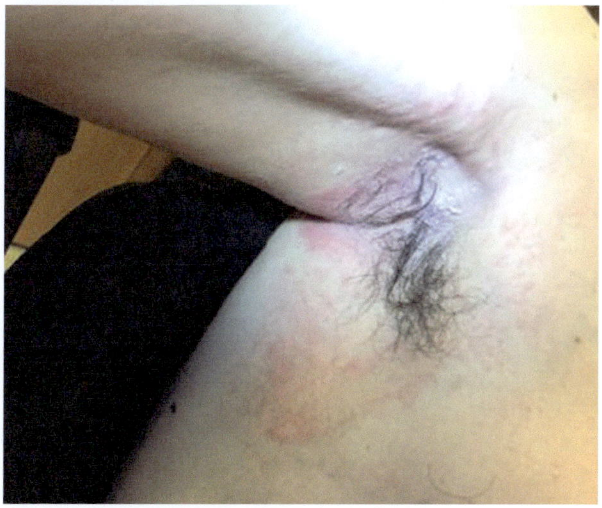

Fig. 7.11 Skin irritation due to moisture retention in the axilla is seen in this image. A persistently adducted shoulder can result from involuntary muscle overactivity or shortening of the pectoralis major, teres major, latissimus dorsi, and/or subscapularis muscles

trunk, i.e., skin overlap. When a patient is not able to actively abduct the shoulder, the ordinary rest position closes off the axilla from aeration.

Episodic Disruptive Symptoms

Sustained clonus involving the upper and lower limbs can be functionally disruptive to activities of daily living, transfers, and gait. The trigger for such episodic behavior is often unclear but some patients note that contact with a cold floor when they first get out of bed may trigger the clonus. Others recall nociceptive input or passive stretch as potential triggers. Focal chemodenervation is sometimes effective in mitigating diffuse clonus if one can identify one or more muscles that are the first to be clonic. Dantrolene sodium may help because it has been found to be effective in reducing or abolishing clonus [6, 7]. In the postsynaptic muscle membrane, the release of calcium ions, mediated by ryanodine receptors, is an essential step in muscle contraction [8]. Dantrolene depresses excitation-contraction coupling in skeletal muscles by binding to ryanodine receptor 1, thereby preventing the release of calcium ions from storage sites in the sarcoplasmic reticulum. Because tonic contractions release more calcium ions than can be inhibited by dantrolene binding, the drug is more effective in reducing low frequency (5–8 Hz) oscillations of phasic clonus than the tonic involuntary contractions that have tetanic frequencies.

Episodic flexor spasms are usually disruptive in the lower extremities, a finding that is more often seen in spinal cord pathologies [9]. Multiple spinal levels are often involved, accounting for multi-segmental involvement that typically includes muscles responsible for ankle dorsiflexion, knee flexion, and hip flexion, and may include the lower abdominal muscles as well. Oral anti-spastic agents such as baclofen or tizanidine may be used while an intrathecal baclofen system is considered for unbridled flexor spasms [10].

Associated Reactions

Physical or voluntary activity occurring in one part of the body may be accompanied by involuntary activity in another, the latter being termed an associated reaction. Associated reactions were first described by Walshe in 1923 as released postural reactions deprived of voluntary (cortical) control [11]. The involuntary movements of an affected arm during transfers and ambulation exemplify associated reactions of the upper limb. Yawning and coughing are included as associated reactions because they are considered to be semi-voluntary movements. Walshe's own words clarify the concept of associated reactions as follows:

> "… all voluntary purposive movements are accompanied by an appropriate postural adjustment of the rest of the skeletal musculature, and that in forceful movements this adjustment or adaptation is necessarily bilateral and widespread. Although carried out under voluntary control, postural adaptation is a function of reflex mechanisms situated in the brain-stem, which are not put out of action by the lesion which produces hemiplegia and abolishes voluntary control of the musculature on the affected side of the body. In these circumstances, we should still expect postural reactions to occur when forceful voluntary motor activities are carried out by the musculature of the sound half of the body. Now, however, deprived of cortical control, they would occur in exaggerated intensity and deprived of that fineness of adaptation which that control ensures. It was concluded that the associated movements of hemiplegia are phenomena of this order, appearing in the muscles of the affected side on certain voluntary movements of the normal limbs, or on such semi-voluntary movements as yawning."

Bakheit and Sawyer state that associated reactions occur in 80% of stroke patients with spastic hemiplegia and often interfere with balance and safe mobility [12]. Figures 7.12, 7.13, and 7.14 show the sequential development of activity in the biceps in a patient standing up from a chair. Figure 7.12 reveals some dystonic EMG activity of the biceps and other flexor muscles "at rest" when sitting on a chair. Figures 7.13 and 7.14 reveal increased activity in the biceps during an associated reaction as the patient completes the sequence of standing up. Associated reactions have the potential to occur frequently throughout the day and are important contributors to abnormal postures. Local injection of involved muscles is a treatment consideration.

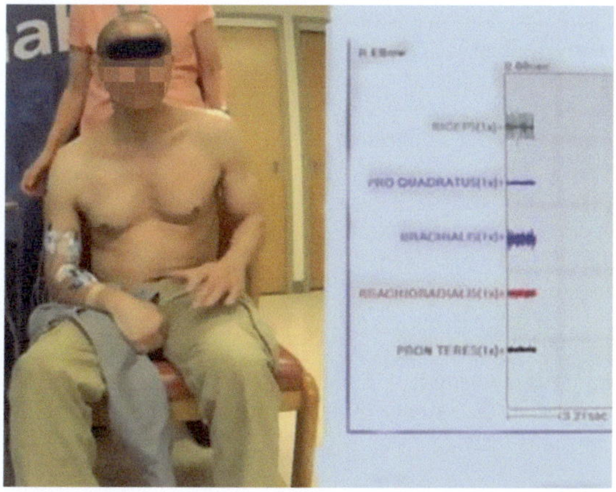

Fig. 7.12 Figures 7.12 through 7.14 show sequential development of an associated reaction during the act of standing up from a chair as reflected in biceps activity in the top trace of the EMG recording on the right side of the image. The patient, sitting quietly on a chair, has low-grade dystonic EMG activity in the biceps (green trace). Note that images were reduced in size to fit together

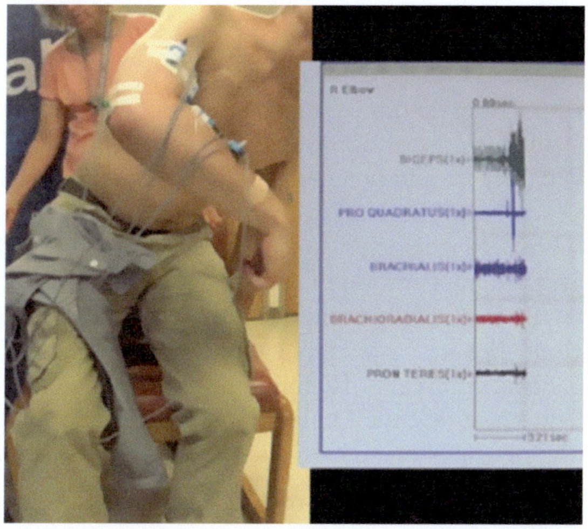

Fig. 7.13 The patient is well on his way toward standing up in this image and the EMG activity in the biceps in the top trace is seen developing more intensely than at baseline when sitting

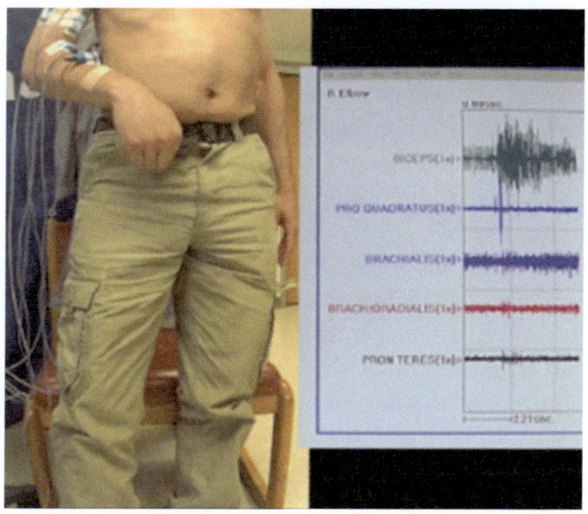

Fig. 7.14 As the person completes standing up, full activation of the biceps can be appreciated on the right side of this image in the top trace. Associated reactions occur commonly during everyday activities and are important contributors to abnormal postures

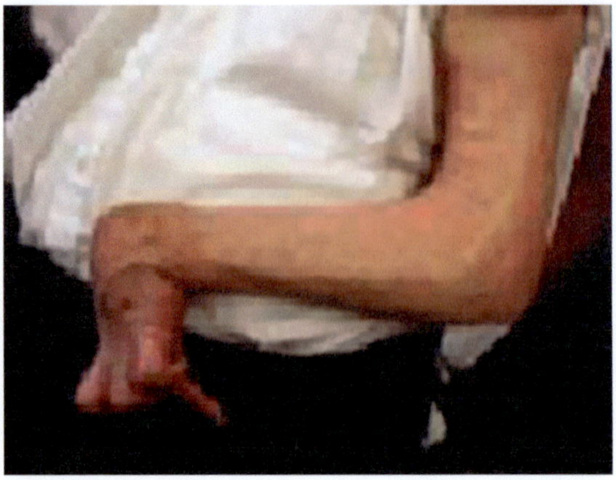

Fig. 7.15 This is a patient with left spastic hemiparesis who developed an ulnar nerve neuropathy due to chronic stretch injury around a persistently flexed elbow. A chronically flexed wrist with subluxation also led to compression of the median nerve in the carpal tunnel. Physical tissue injury is a potential after-effect in patients with spastic paresis

Physical Compression and Injury

Upper limb deformity causes a net imbalance of forces in a given direction and can result in peripheral nerve compression and injury. Figure 7.15 illustrates a patient with left spastic hemiparesis who developed an ulnar neuropathy due to chronic stretch injury around a persistently flexed elbow. A chronically flexed wrist with subluxation also led to compression of the median nerve in the carpal tunnel. Surgical intervention may be necessary in such cases. Serial casting is less successful in cases with prolonged deformity. Trauma is occasionally observed due to elbow flexor spasms that cause the hand to strike the neck, face, and chest. Some patients complain of being awakened at night by elbow flexor spasms that strike their chest or chin. Oral anti-spastic agents such as baclofen or tizanidine may be tried. Focal chemodenervation is also a consideration.

Problems of Access

Access to the Hand, Fingers, and Thumb

Access to the hand is important for object acquisition. Access can be blocked by several types of abnormal hand posturing due to shortening, stiffness, contracture, or overactivation affecting the FDS (see Fig. 7.16), FDP, and the intrinsic muscles of the hand. In addition, the thumb-in-palm configuration may involve the FPL, the flexor pollicis brevis (FPB), the adductor pollicis (AP), and the first dorsal interosseous (FDI) muscles. Mixed FDS and FDP findings for different fingers are not uncommon (see Fig. 7.17). One muscle group may also mask the effect of another. For example, the effect of finger intrinsics can be masked by the stronger contraction of the finger and thumb extrinsics. For example, examination of Fig. 7.17 reveals an "FPL type posture" of the thumb but one cannot rule out involvement of the FPB or, for that

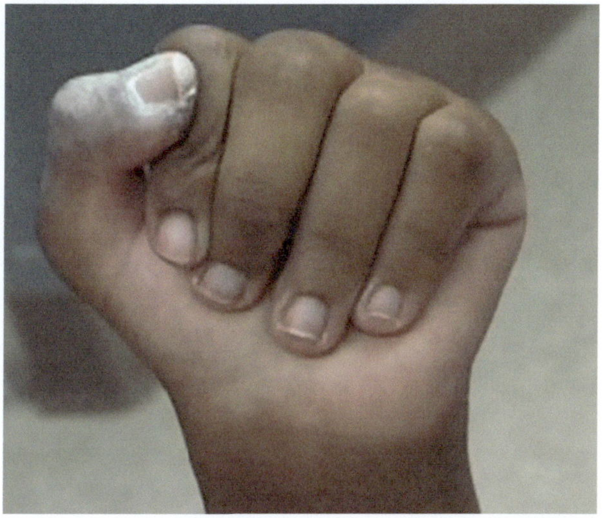

Fig. 7.16 Image of an "FDS type hand" with an "FPL type thumb-in-palm". Access to the hand is blocked by involuntary muscle overactivity or shortening affecting these muscles. *FDS* flexor digitorum superficialis, *FPL* flexor pollicis longus

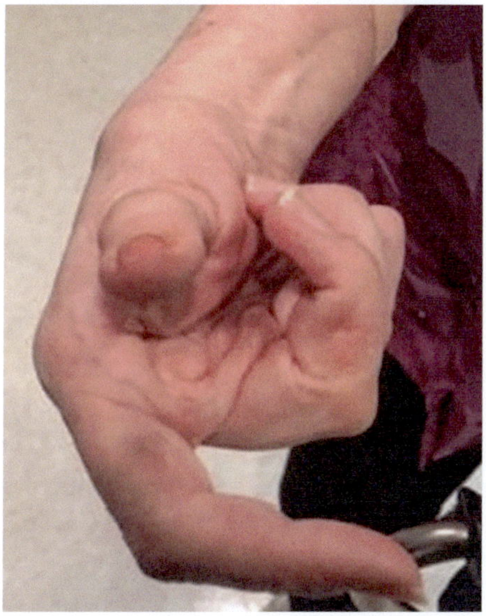

Fig. 7.17 Varied hand configurations can be seen. This figure illustrates mixed involvement of the flexor digitorum superficialis and flexor digitorum profundus muscles of different fingers. Analysis of the various finger configurations will inform the selection of muscles for treatment

matter, the intrinsics of the fingers. Dynamic polyEMG of hand muscles may be useful if there is suspicion of a combined extrinsic/intrinsic hand [13]. When extrinsic finger flexors are weakened by chemodenervation or surgical lengthening, unmasking of overactive intrinsics can result in an intrinsic plus hand (see Fig. 7.18). [An intrinsic plus hand is not common in patients with spastic paresis in our experience.]

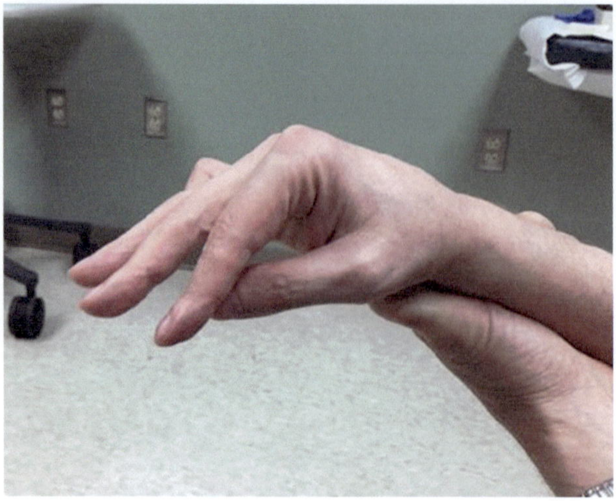

Fig. 7.18 This image shows an intrinsic plus hand involving the fingers and the thumb. The narrowed web space inlet impairs access to the hand, affecting "hand as a holder" function

Impaired access affects "hand as a holder" function. A clenched fist typically involves flexed fingers and a thumb-in-palm deformity and is a common clinical configuration in patients with spastic hemiplegia after a stroke. Sources of flexor muscle overactivity include spastic dystonia, spastic co-contraction, and associated reactions. Changes in the rheologic properties of muscle tissue including shortening, stiffness, and contracture contribute as well. An additional key finding is marked paresis or frank absence of voluntary finger extension. Nevertheless, an object can be inserted, pushed, or wriggled into a clenched fist for the functional purpose of holding. We term this motor behavior "hand as a holder" function. Treatment that reduces the degree of clenching of the fingers may allow insertion of larger sized objects into the affected hand, thus increasing its functional capacity.

The difficulty experienced by persons with a clenched fist and thumb-in-palm configurations is based on impaired or absent volitional activation of extensors and involuntary rheologic stiffness of flexor tissues along with flexor muscle overactivity. To improve access to the clenched fist, the cause must be treated and the contracture may be mitigated with serial casting or splinting [14]. Improving access to the hand by easing the intensity of a clenched fist helps make the "hand as a holder" function feasible.

Access to the Elbow Crease

Chronic elbow flexion driven by spastic dystonia, flexor spasm, and/or associated reactions often results in progressive skin overlap at the elbow, making access for washing the elbow crease difficult, leading to maceration, skin irritation and breakdown. Figure 7.19 illustrates the resting flexion posture of the elbow as well as the large degree of lost range of elbow extension. The goal of treatment is to improve

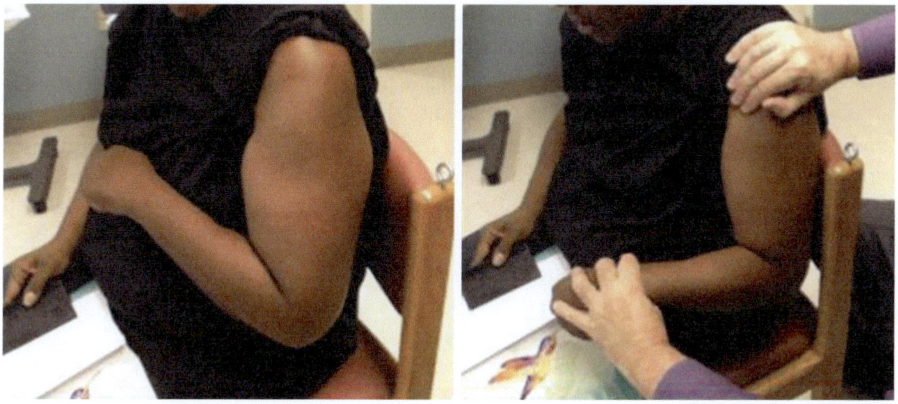

Fig. 7.19 Access for washing the elbow is made difficult by chronic elbow flexion, driven by spastic dystonia, flexor spasm, and/or associated reactions, as well as changes in the rheologic properties of muscle tissue including shortening, stiffness and contracture, leading to progressive, persistent skin overlap at the elbow. Dressing function may be affected as well

Fig. 7.20 Involuntary shoulder adduction/internal rotation often blocks access to the axilla, making washing and deodorant application difficult. Muscles that may be involved include the pectoralis major, teres major, latissimus dorsi, and subscapularis

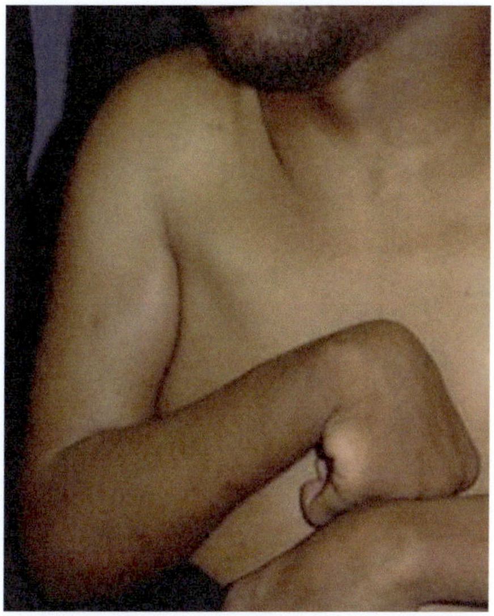

the range of motion to a point where air has access to the elbow crease at all times. Local injection to reduce the tension in the elbow flexors followed by serial casting or surgical lengthening are treatment considerations.

Access to the Axilla

Shortening and/or involuntary shoulder adduction/internal rotation often block access to the axilla, making washing and deodorant application difficult (Fig. 7.20).

Muscles that may be involved include the PM, TM, LD, and subscapularis. Phenol injection is a consideration because the PM, TM, and LD muscles are innervated by motor nerves and the clinician does not have to worry about sensory dysesthesia induced by phenol. Reasons to use phenol are the cost of the drug and saving on the amount of neurotoxin that needs to be expended for large proximal arm muscles when there may be many distal arm muscles and leg muscles that also require neurotoxin injections in the same patient. However, phenol is a neurolytic agent which can cause inflammation and fibrosis, making it difficult (after a number of injections) to find the motor nerve with electrical stimulation for future treatments [15].

Grasp and Release Dysfunction

Problems of hand opening are typically related to the triad of muscle shortening, weakness of extrinsic finger extensors, and overactivity of extrinsic finger flexors. In the polio era, paralysis of finger extensors never led to a clenched fist deformity because the finger flexors were never subjected to involuntary neural overactivity. However, spasticity by itself is also insufficient to lead to a clenched fist. Rather, other neural phenomena such as co-contraction and associated reactions occurring many times during the day along with non-neural phenomena such as muscle shortening, stiffness, and contracture due to lack of mobility summate leading to the grasp and release dysfunction.

Inadequate Hand Opening Preceding Grasp

Normally, the reach phase prior to grasp is characterized by active finger extension [16]. The fingers and thumb extend and the hand opens in proportion to the size and configurational properties of the target object. The left side of Fig. 7.21 reveals the

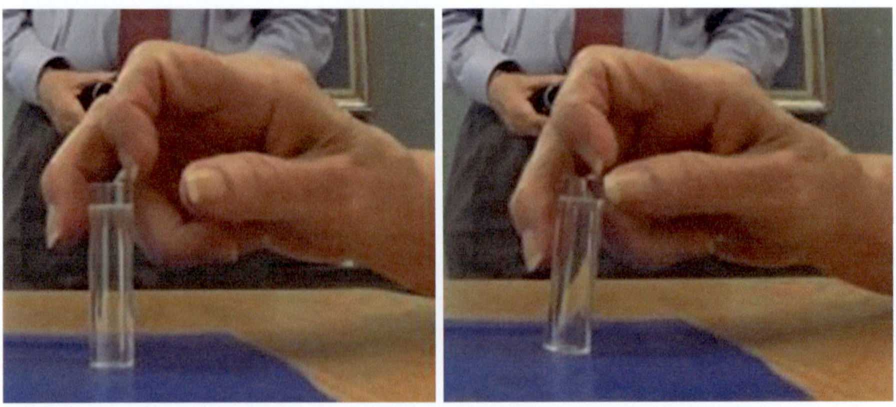

Fig. 7.21 During the pre-grasp phase of reaching, the fingers and thumb normally extend as the hand opens in proportion to the size and configuration of a target object. In this patient, the left image reveals an excessively flexed index finger during pre-grasp. The right image reveals that the index finger cannot participate in grasp of the cylinder, due to being excessively curled and past the locus of contact with the object

hand of a patient approaching a small 0.5″ diameter cylinder. Note that the index finger is excessively curled prior to grasp such that the cylinder cannot be grasped as seen on the right image of Fig. 7.21. In fact, the patient tipped the cylinder over when contact was made with the fingers and thumb (see Fig. 7.22). The motor behavior that knocked the cylinder over is analogous to the problem of lack of adequate clearance commonly seen in the lower limb of hemiparetic patients (see later in the chapter). In this case, the patient chose to retrieve the fallen cylinder using her thumb and long finger as seen in Fig. 7.23. The patient finally grasped and

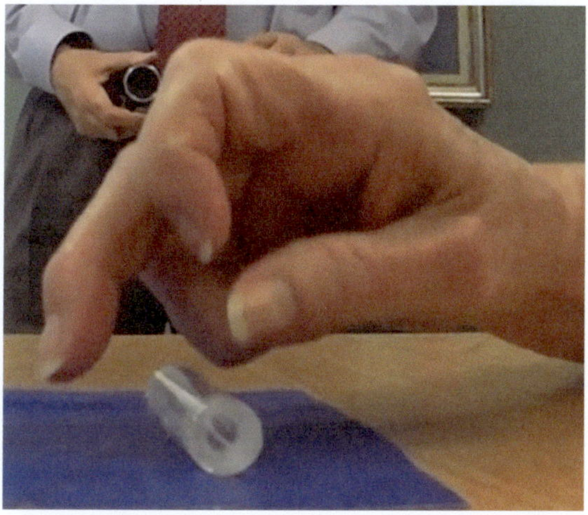

Fig. 7.22 The patient tipped the cylinder when initial contact was made with the hand

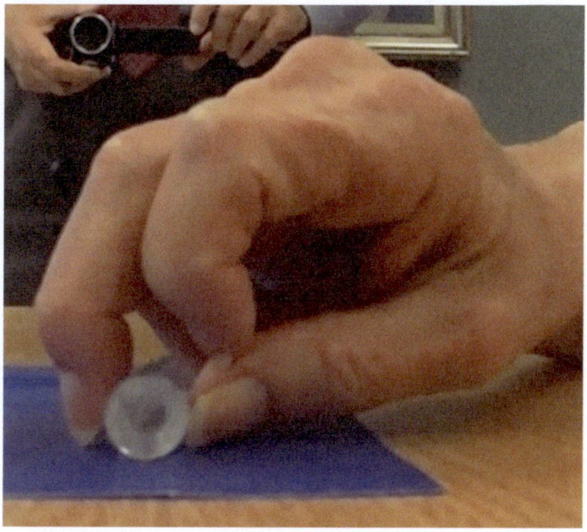

Fig. 7.23 The patient chose to retrieve the fallen cylinder using her thumb and long finger

lifted the cylinder, but the grasp appears tenuous and dysfunctional as seen in Fig. 7.24. The thumb nail rather than the thumb pad provides a partial counterforce to contact pressure with the flexed distal interphalangeal joint (DIP) joint of the long finger. The index finger is curled and makes no contact. Somewhat hidden in the photo is the middle phalanx of the ring finger which provides the other counterforce to the contact pressure of the long finger pressing on the cylinder. Objects of larger size cannot be picked up at all, as seen in Fig. 7.25.

It is clear from the figures that the FDP of the index finger is involved but the clinician has to infer the cause. Decisions about whether muscle shortening and/or overactivity are driving excessive thumb flexion and ring finger proximal interphalangeal (PIP) joint flexion need to be made. Treatment with neurotoxin is often effective in mitigating muscle overactivity but selecting muscles relevant to the

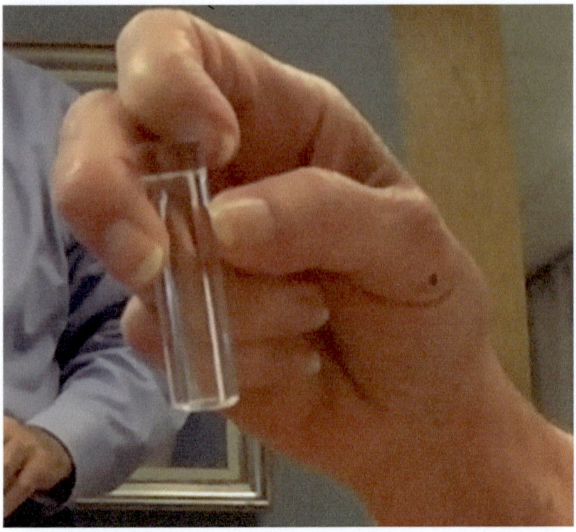

Fig. 7.24 The patient finally grasped and lifted the cylinder, but the grasp appears tenuous because the long finger compresses the cylinder against the flexed middle phalanx of the ring finger, the thumb tip rather than the pad is in contact with the cylinder, and the index finger remains excessively curled "above the fray"

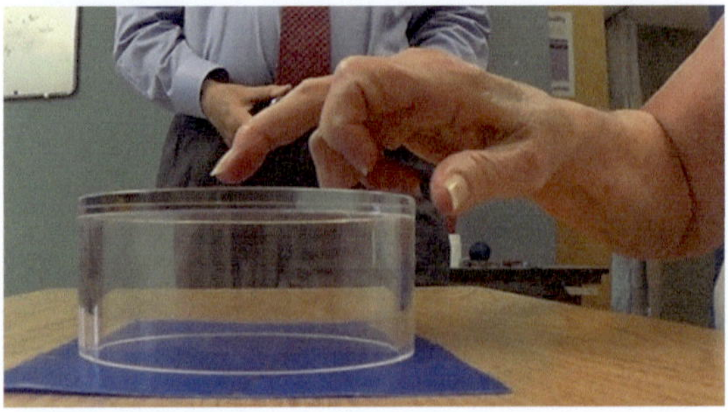

Fig. 7.25 The patient was unable to grasp a 4.5 inch diameter cylinder. Impaired access to the hand makes it difficult to pick up large diameter objects

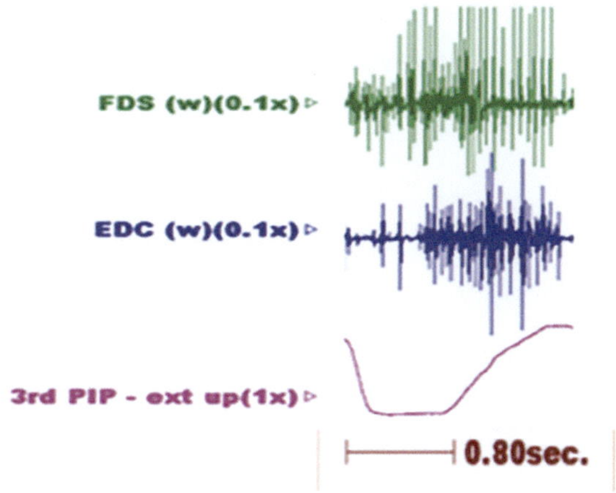

Fig. 7.26 This polyEMG record (image enlarged) reveals spastic co-contraction of the flexor digitorum superficialis (FDS, top EMG trace) during attempted finger extension by the extensor digitorum communis (EDC, middle EMG trace) that slows down finger extension of the 3rd proximal interphalangeal (PIP) joint. A patient's inability to relax involuntary overactivity of finger flexors prevents object release in many patients. Difficulty releasing is usually greater for larger sized objects than smaller ones

clinical problem is key to decision-making so as to not cause weakness. When injecting neurotoxin, consider electrical stimulation to isolate parts of the FDS and FDP muscles controlling the relevant fingers.

Inadequate Hand Opening During Release

The normal release of a handheld object is characterized by relaxation of the finger and thumb flexors followed immediately by active extension of the fingers and thumb. Patients with spastic paresis often have difficulty releasing a grasped object. Figure 7.26 reveals slowed finger extension after prior flexion due to persistent spastic co-contraction of the FDS. Difficulty releasing is usually greater for larger sized objects than for smaller ones, presumably because the larger object stretches the shortened flexors more than smaller objects. When finger extensors are very weak, the patient may let the object slip out of the hand by gravity. Weak finger extension may be aided by a spring-loaded orthosis that works as an extension assist [17].

Hyperextended Wrist and Finger Flexor Tenodesis

A hyperextended wrist produces a clenched fist by the mechanism of finger flexor tenodesis [18]. Figure 7.27 illustrates the tenodesis effect of wrist angle on finger configuration. When the wrist is flexed, the rheologic tension in the finger flexors is reduced because the finger flexors are slack. When the wrist is extended, the rheologic tension in the finger flexors is increased due to stretch of the finger flexors across the wrist. Even when there is no neural input to the finger flexors, the fingers will flex toward the palm because of rheologic tension in the finger flexors when the wrist extends. Shortening of the finger flexors, the development of stiffness, and contractures due to disuse can further exacerbate the tenodesis effect. The finger

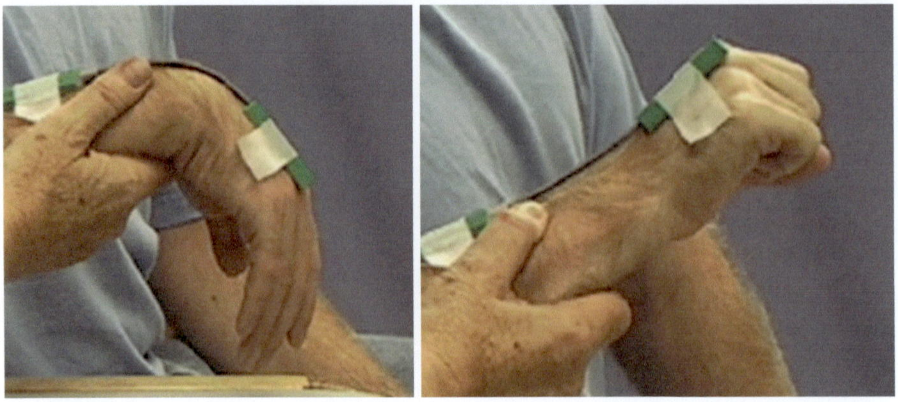

Fig. 7.27 A hyperextended wrist produces a clenched fist by the mechanism of finger flexor tenodesis. This image illustrates the tenodesis effect of wrist angle. When the wrist is flexed, rheologic tension of the finger flexors is reduced because the finger flexors are not stretched. When the wrist is extended, rheologic finger flexor tension increases due to stretch of the finger flexors across the wrist, which is exacerbated by muscle shortening, stiffness, and contracture

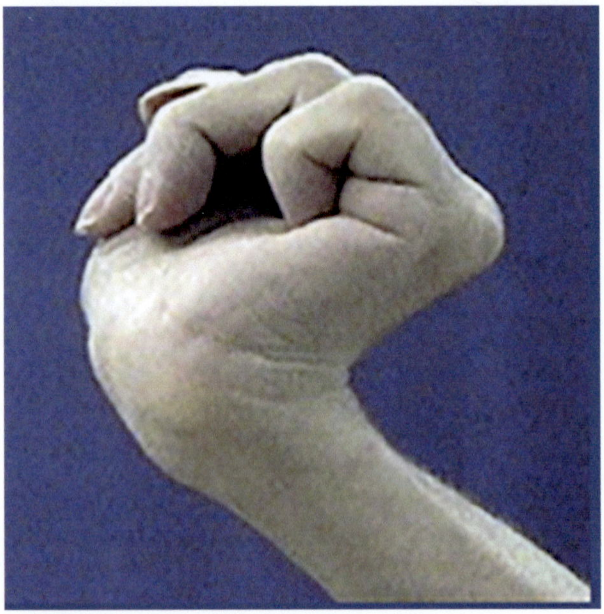

Fig. 7.28 This figure illustrates a patient with cerebral palsy whose hyperextended wrist resulted in tenodesis-driven finger flexion. Initial treatment must be aimed at restoring wrist flexion before treatment of the finger flexors

flexors may or may not be neurally overactive in such cases and, unless clinical examination is highly suggestive of spastic dystonia or a dynamic EMG study is available to ascertain FDS/FDP overactivity, weakening the finger flexors further may not be worthwhile. Figure 7.28 illustrates a patient with cerebral palsy whose hyperextended wrist resulted in tenodesis-driven finger flexion. Shortening and/or overactivity of the wrist and finger extensors may be responsible for the excessive finger flexion in this case and must be treated first to restore range of motion at the wrist.

Joint and Muscle Contractures

Contracture is often a factor that makes for difficulty with hand opening. A clinician needs to distinguish between two types of contracture: contracture of joint capsules and fixed shortening of muscle tissue. Tendons do not shorten. In actuality, other tissues such as connective tissue, vascular tissues, and nerve tissue are also subject to contracture by unremitting joint configurations. It is for this reason that a surgeon, for example, will not lengthen contractured elbow flexors all the way because strain damage to arteries, nerves, and other soft tissue is likely to occur if the joint is pulled into extension completely [19]. Lengthening is performed for "half the distance to the goal line" with the rest of the contracture worked out post-operatively by serial casting or splinting. We note that joint contractures of the fingers are unrelated to wrist position, whereas finger flexor muscle contractures are tightened by wrist extension and loosened by wrist flexion with the range of motion worsening or improving accordingly due to the tenodesis effect. The examiner keeps this in mind when distinguishing between joint and muscle contracture, noting that combined contracture of joints and muscles may frequently occur. The distinction between joint and muscle contractures is important for both conservative and surgical treatment. Neurotoxin injections do not help joint contractures. The association between immobility, accumulation and aggregation of extracellular hyaluronan in muscle, development of muscle stiffness, and contracture can explain the prevalence of finger flexion contractures [20]. Also see Chaps. 5 and 6 for non-neural changes in muscles, and Chaps. 8 and 13 for treatment of muscle shortening with pharmacologic release using hyaluronidase injections.

The Intrinsic plus Hand

When extrinsic finger flexors and extensors are very weak, the presence of voluntary intrinsic muscle activation results in an intrinsic plus hand. This is a useful hand for grasp and release but it is not a powerful hand. In addition, the web space inlet is relatively narrow so that grasp of larger sized objects may be limited.

An intrinsic plus hand (see Fig. 7.29) is sometimes seen after surgical lengthening of the extrinsic finger flexors. Figure 7.30 shows a patient who had a markedly flexed elbow, flexed wrist, clenched fist, and thumb-in-palm. Elbow flexors, wrist flexors, and extrinsic finger flexors were surgically lengthened. However, post surgery, the opposite deformities developed, namely, an extended elbow (patient couldn't flex the elbow actively), an extended, radially deviated wrist (patient could not flex the wrist actively), intrinsic plus fingers, and an intrinsic thumb. The patient could hold small objects that were placed in her hand, but she could not bring them to her body because she lacked elbow flexion. Consequently, she did not use the hand or upper limb very much. However, dressing the limb became easier because she could pull her sleeve up her straight arm more easily than up the markedly flexed elbow that she had prior to surgery. The reason for development of the opposite deformities after surgery was that prior to surgery, she actually had substantial

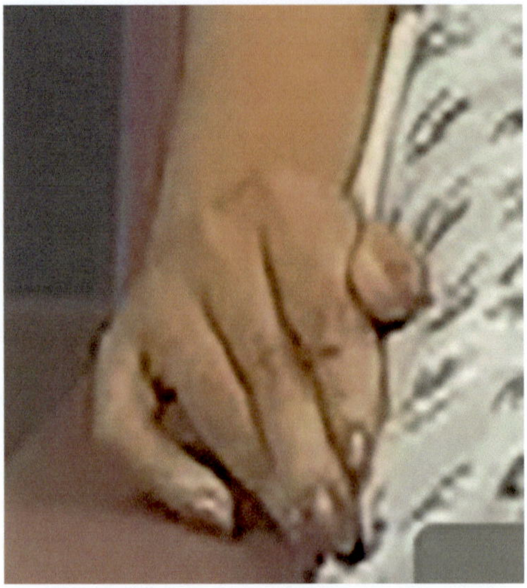

Fig. 7.29 Image of an intrinsic plus hand that developed after surgical lengthening of the extrinsic finger flexors for a clenched fist

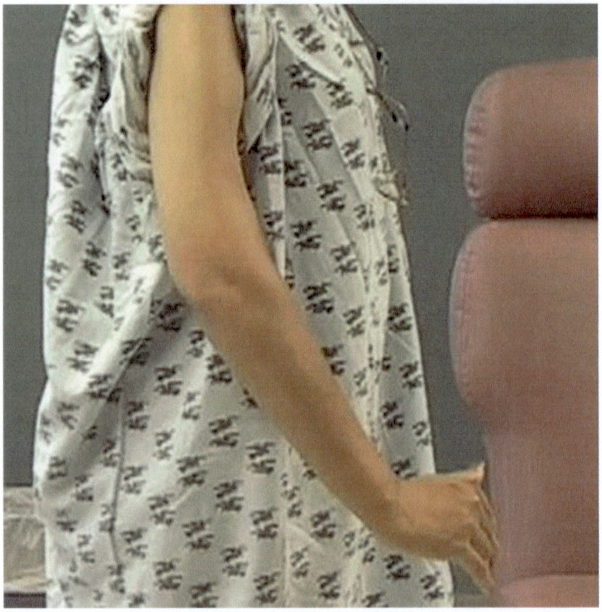

Fig. 7.30 This figure shows a patient who had a markedly flexed elbow, flexed wrist, clenched fist, and thumb-in-palm that were treated with surgical lengthening. Post surgery the patient developed opposite deformities with elbow extension, wrist extension, and an intrinsic plus hand

triceps muscle activity, wrist extensor activity, and intrinsic muscle activity. However, the neural activity of these muscle groups was masked by the much stronger activity of elbow flexors, wrist flexors, and extrinsic finger flexors. It was not anticipated that opposite deformities would occur. Nevertheless, this case serves as a cautionary tale as clinical postures reflect a net balance of forces around a joint. Weakening one muscle set of dominant forces can lead to releasing the effect of active antagonist muscles, resulting in opposite deformities. In this regard, dynamic polyEMG of agonists and antagonists around a joint may provide useful pre-operative information. Clinical postures may also represent non-neural changes in muscle that should be treated first prior to considering surgical interventions that may not lead to functional benefit.

The Flexed Thumb

The thumb is flexed by the FPL (Fig. 7.31) and FPB muscles (Fig. 7.32). The FPL is an extrinsic muscle and is subject to tenodesis tightening by wrist extension. Testing of Ashworth scores without maintaining a consistent wrist position can confuse the picture regarding which muscle is causing the thumb to flex (this is true for the finger flexors as well). Flexion of the interphalangeal (IP) joint of the thumb reflects an overactive FPL. Weakness of the extensor pollicis longus (EPL) muscle plays a negative role as well. Flexion of the IP joint of the thumb narrows the web space inlet, affecting "hand as a holder" function. An overactive FPB results in flexed metacarpophalangeal (MP) and carpometacarpal (CMC) joints, the IP joint typically being extended. The thumb ends up well into the palm, reducing access, and consequently compromising holding function (Fig. 7.32). Overactivity or shortening of the AP and FDI muscles adds to the problem.

Distinguishing between the "FPL type" deformity and the "FPB type" deformity which also involves the AP and FDI is imperative for the selection of the appropriate muscles for treatment. Thumb muscles, like other muscles elsewhere, are subject to non-neural rheologic changes, i.e., muscle shortening, stiffness, and contracture and need appropriate early treatment. Serial casting or splinting may be needed.

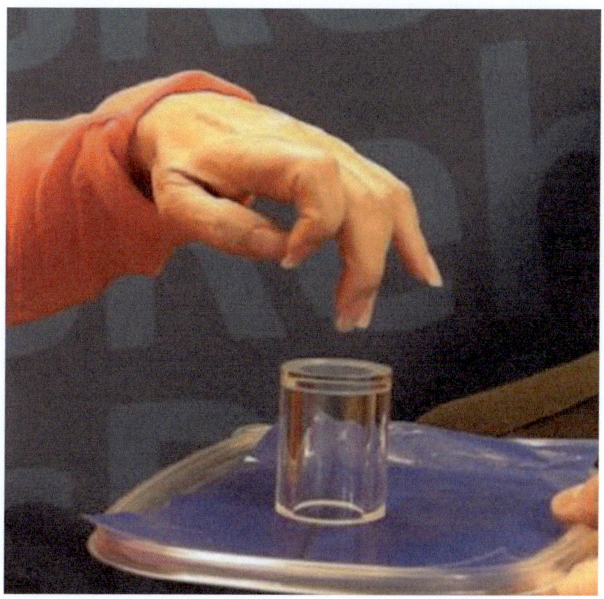

Fig. 7.31 This patient had a flexed thumb of the "FPL type". The thumb with a flexed interphalangeal joint has a narrow web space inlet, affecting "hand as a holder" function. *FPL* flexor pollicis longus

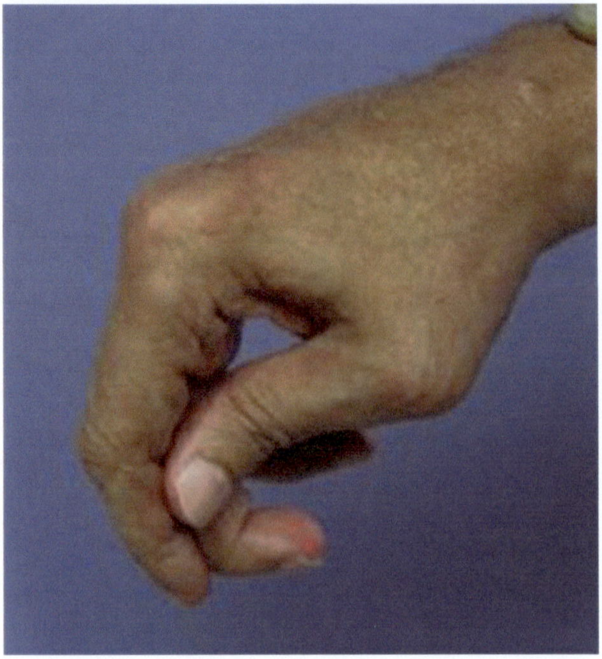

Fig. 7.32 Image of an "FPB type" thumb. An overactive flexor pollicis brevis (FPB) results in flexed metacarpophalangeal and carpometacarpal joints, the interphalangeal joint typically remains extended. The thumb ends up well into the palm, reducing access, and consequently compromising holding function

Neurotoxin injections of thumb flexors may be able to mitigate muscle overactivity but weakness of thumb extensors does not allow the thumb to be a post against which the fingers can compress an object for holding. If this happens, the use of a thumb spica or other type of orthosis for posting the thumb can go a long way toward restoring the function of hand grasp.

Reach Dysfunction

Reaching, as a motor behavior, involves the whole limb. Individuals may have some degree of two-way volitional movement of a given joint when tested in isolation but individuals with spastic paresis may or may not have such movements available for whole limb reaching. However, not all reaching movements are the same because depending on the intent and direction of the reach, the specific muscle ensembles involved are different. Hence, "reaching for a cup" is different from "reaching for a pen," which is different from "reaching for a ball on the right side of the body" [21]. In addition to single joint movements, traditional manual muscle strength testing is also not likely to be predictive of whole limb behavior. Instead, direct testing of tasks that require whole limb actions is recommended, such as reaching to touch a target with the fist or reaching to pick up an object with the hand. The target and the object may be placed sequentially on the left, center, and right side of the individual to allow the observer to make inferences about scapula, shoulder, elbow, forearm, wrist, finger, and thumb movements during whole limb behavior. For the clinical purpose of evaluating whole limb motor behavior in spastic paresis, it is helpful to ask the following questions: (1) Is weakness of one or more components of whole limb movement impeding a specific task? (2) Is co-contraction of muscles across a joint restraining the movement or movement components of a given task? Or (3) are the movement responses the same (or very similar) and stereotypical regardless of the task? See Chaps. 2 and 3 for a full description and functional assessments in spastic movement disorder.

Deficits in reaching behavior may occur due to a primary problem at the scapula, shoulder, elbow, and/or forearm, and secondarily at the wrist, fingers and thumb. Impairment of the latter segments mainly affects grasp and release. Since the purpose of a reaching movement is to place the hand at a given location in space, limitation of movement at one or more joints can affect it.

Inadequate Scapular Rotation

Forward reaching of the arm requires protraction of the scapula, shoulder flexion, and elbow extension. Hand placement across the midline to the contralateral side requires the most protraction of the scapula, and shoulder adduction. Clinical testing of scapular motion can best be observed by asking the patient to place the hand contralaterally on a tabletop or on the opposite knee.

An important agonist of scapular motion is the serratus anterior, the prime protractor of the scapula which enables scapulothoracic motion and forward movement of the arm. Weakness or stiffness in the serratus anterior impairs reaching. The pectoralis minor and major also contribute to protraction of the scapula. The retractors of the scapula are primarily the rhomboids and middle trapezius. During forward reach with the unaffected left arm, note appropriate protraction of the scapula on the left image of Fig. 7.33. The image on the right reveals a retracted scapula on the affected right side. Treatment considerations may include aggressive stretching of muscles retracting the scapula as well as injection treatment to assist with lengthening these muscles. When the scapula does not move during reaching, i.e., when there is no retraction or protraction, a clinician must decide whether this is due to weakness or stiffness in the agonists and/or antagonists, and the net balance of the agonist and antagonist muscles.

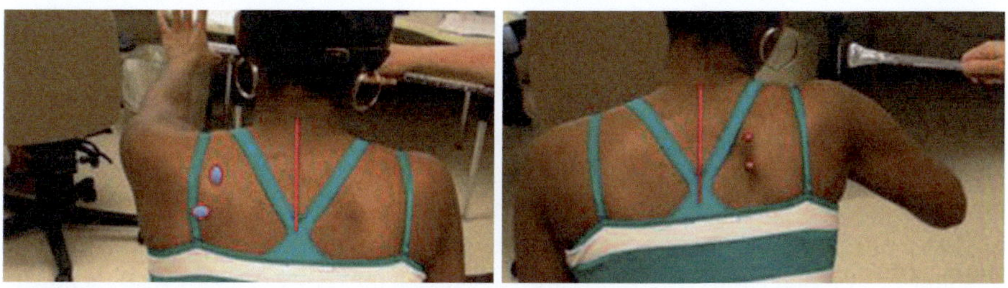

Fig. 7.33 During forward reach of the arm by a patient with right hemiparesis, the left image shows protraction of the scapula on the unaffected side while the right image reveals a retracted scapula on the affected right side which impedes forward reaching

Inadequate Shoulder Movement

Reaching in front of the body requires shoulder flexion and elbow extension against gravity. Therefore, the muscles involved must necessarily activate anti-gravity muscles to support the weight of the arm against gravity and also control the direction of limb placement in forward locations. Shoulder flexion generates upward and forward motion of the arm and may be accompanied by shoulder internal rotation and adduction for hand placement on the contralateral side of the body, or by external rotation and abduction for hand placement away from the body. Clinical testing of shoulder motion can be performed by hand placement at various locations on a tabletop (see placement of objects recommended for the Frenchay Arm Test in Chap. 3). Support of the forearm on a table eliminates gravity to facilitate examination of the directional control of movement. Shoulder external rotation is tested by asking the patient to bring the hand behind the neck or by demonstrating the pre-throwing motion of a football quarterback. Shoulder internal rotation, important for toileting, can be tested by bringing the hand behind the low back. When patients with spastic paresis have a fair degree of recovery, voluntary alternating movements of the shoulder, namely, flexion/extension, abduction/adduction, external/internal rotation movements may reveal potential temporal asymmetries such as slower flexion phase compared to the extension phase, slower abduction compared with adduction, and slower external rotation compared with internal rotation (or vice versa). Temporal asymmetry can point to restraint by co-contracting antagonists or to stiffness that may be palpable by the clinician. It might also reflect weakness of specific agonist muscles rather than antagonist restraint (see Step 5 of the Five-Step Assessment in Chap. 3).

Because the shoulder joint is a shallow ball-and-socket joint with three degrees of freedom, it enables hand placement in the workspace around the body. In spastic paresis, weak descending signals to synergistically acting shoulder muscles result in impairment of hand placement. This can be tested clinically by placing targets to the left, right, and center of the body on a tabletop. When a patient lifts the arm to reach toward a target, two operational problems are present: (1) support of the arm against gravity and (2) placement of the hand in a specific location in the workspace. When descending signals are weak, lifting the arm against gravity becomes strenuous and one can observe all kinds of effortful attempts by the patient to lift and hold the arm against gravity. Effortful behavior tends to activate many compensatory muscles farther away from the more localized muscle ensemble that is activated normally. Such activation may interfere with hand placement because the same muscles may have dual anti-gravity and placement roles. The first goal is to enable arm support against gravity by strengthening muscles that support the weight of the arm. The second goal is restoration of directional control by performing exercises that enable reaching targets in the workspace.

Shortening or co-contraction of shoulder adductors and extensors often leads to restraint of voluntary movement. Figure 7.34 reveals a young woman who has difficulty placing her hand behind her neck. The movement ordinarily requires shoulder abduction by the deltoids and external rotation by the rotator cuff muscles. Shortened or overactive internal rotators of the shoulder including the PM, LD, TM, and

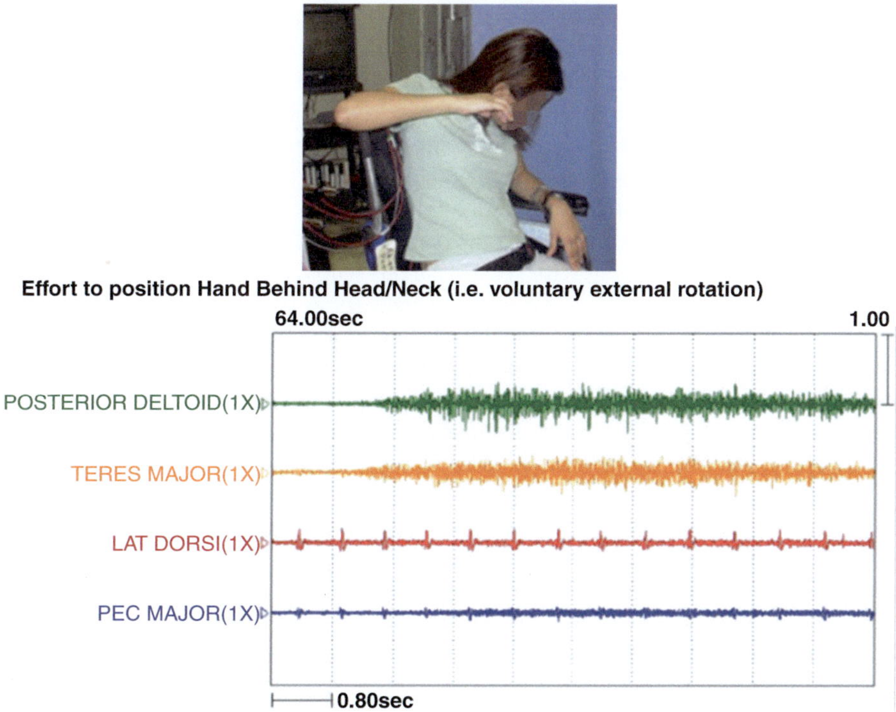

Fig. 7.34 Co-contraction of shoulder adductors often leads to restraint of voluntary movement. This figure reveals a young woman who has difficulty placing her hand behind her neck. The poly-EMG record reveals co-contraction of teres major, an adductor and internal rotator of the shoulder. Latissimus dorsi was not active and pectoralis major was only minimally active. *LAT DORSI* latissimus dorsi, *PEC MAJOR* pectoralis major

subscapularis can stymie this task. In this case, the figure reveals co-contraction of the TM and posterior deltoid (PD) muscles. There was no activation of LD or PM and we do not know whether there was co-contraction of the subscapularis (not recorded) muscle. Weak signals to the external rotators may also be contributory although activation of the PD, an abductor and external rotator of the shoulder, was good. The limitation of dynamic EMG is that it does not reflect the degree of force being generated which must be inferred by the examiner. On the other hand, if one were to treat shortening or overactivity, a good first approach would be to inject the TM based on noted activation of this internal rotator with no activation of other internal rotators (LD and PM). Admittedly, dynamic EMG is not a commonly available tool. Hence, clinical examination including observation and palpation of muscles and tendons must necessarily be relied upon to make inferences regarding the appropriate muscles to select for treatment [22]. It is important to keep in mind that spastic paresis results in variable agonist and antagonist muscle weakness and restraint.

Temporary diagnostic nerve blocks may also be helpful in identifying involuntarily overactive shoulder muscles that restrain movement or cause dysfunctional posturing. Figure 7.35 reveals a patient with stroke who complained of persistent posterior posturing of her shoulder when she walked. Clinical examination revealed a stiff LD by palpation of the muscle and its taut tendon in the axilla. A diagnostic lidocaine block of the thoracodorsal nerve quickly eliminated the posturing, and it was inferred that no other extensors were involved. Phenol application to the thoracodorsal nerve (an entirely motor nerve without sensory component) was performed for long-term treatment of the problem.

More than one shoulder extensor may be co-contracting. Figure 7.36 reveals the polyEMG record of a patient with spastic paresis who had great difficulty performing shoulder flexion. Although he could initiate some flexion at the shoulder, the movement flattened out. The agonist muscle, anterior deltoid, showed a good EMG recruitment pattern. However, co-contraction of the TM and long head of triceps, a two joint muscle that extends the shoulder when the elbow is fixed by flexors, negated the effect of activation of the anterior deltoid in flexing the shoulder. Some activation of the LD, another shoulder extensor, can be seen as well. Treatment of multiple muscles should be considered.

Weakness in the shoulder external rotators and abductors favors the development of stiffness and contracture in the opposing shoulder internal rotators and adductors. Precursors of rheologic change in these muscles include immobility due to severity of the spastic paresis as well as neural phenomena including spastic dystonia, spastic co-contraction, flexor reflex afferent activity, and associated reactions, which bias the shoulder joint toward internal rotation and adduction. The weak descending signals to the external rotators/abductors are insufficient to redress the bias. Two of the internal rotators/adductors are also shoulder extensors (specifically, the LD and TM) so that forward motion of the arm, necessary for reaching, may be significantly affected by extensor shortening and stiffness. Unlike elbow, forearm, wrist, and finger

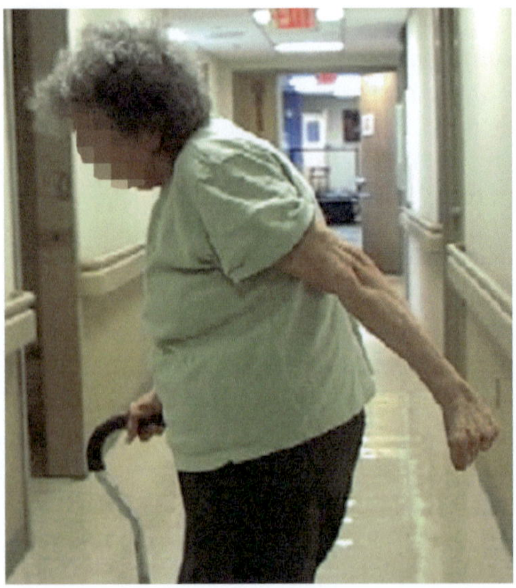

Fig. 7.35 This figure reveals a patient with stroke who complained of persistent posterior posturing of her shoulder when she walked. Clinical examination suggested an overactive latissimus dorsi by palpation, and a diagnostic lidocaine block of the thoracodorsal nerve quickly eliminated the posturing. Temporary nerve blocks may be useful in predicting the outcome of longer-term treatments

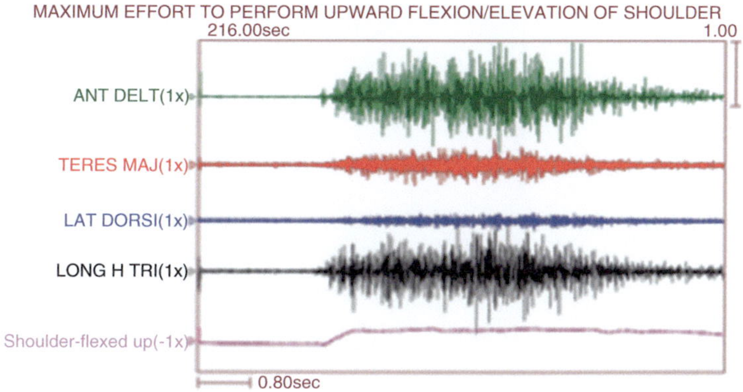

Fig. 7.36 More than one shoulder extensor may be co-contracting. This figure reveals the poly-EMG record of a patient with spastic paresis who had great difficulty performing shoulder flexion. The record reveals co-contraction of multiple shoulder extensors including the teres major and long head of triceps with some activation of the latissimus dorsi as well. *ANT DELT* anterior deltoid, *TERES MAJ* teres major, *LAT DORSI* latissimus dorsi, *LONG H TRI* long head of triceps

contractures, shoulder contracture is not amenable to serial casting. Prevention of such contractures requires positioning the shoulder in external rotation starting early on, and facilitation of shoulder external rotation movements [23, 24]. Surgical intervention is a consideration, especially when skin problems in the axilla are persistent.

Inadequate Elbow Movement

Elbow extension lengthens the upper limb during reaching and elbow flexion shortens it when bringing the hand to the body. A combination of scapular protraction, shoulder flexion, and elbow extension are key movements that place the hand in various spatial locations away from the body.

Paresis of the elbow extensors (triceps and anconeus) results in an impairment of elbow extension during reaching. The patient in Figs. 7.37 and 7.38 illustrates impaired length of reaching in the left paretic upper limb compared with the right. The elbow flexors were not co-contracting or stiff on clinical palpation. Shoulder flexion, tested separately, was good. Incomplete elbow extension was attributed to weak activation of the triceps.

In patients with spastic paresis, it is common for shortening and/or spastic co-contraction of elbow flexors to restrain elbow extension [25]. The result is a strained, slow, and effortful movement which may result in incomplete extension (see Fig. 7.39). The underlying dynamic EMG is seen in Fig. 7.40. Triceps and anconeus are active during the extension phase while biceps has the most activity in the flexion phase. However, antagonist activity in biceps, brachialis, brachioradialis, and pronator teres during the extension phase restrains active elbow extension. Restraint can be seen in the prolonged extension phase compared with the smooth, rapid flexion phase of the movement. Release of the restraining muscles, particularly of the brachioradialis and pronator teres, should be considered.

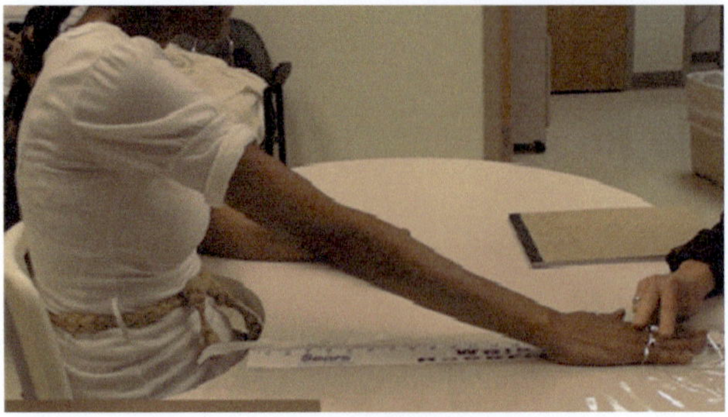

Fig. 7.37 Normal elbow extension during full arm reach

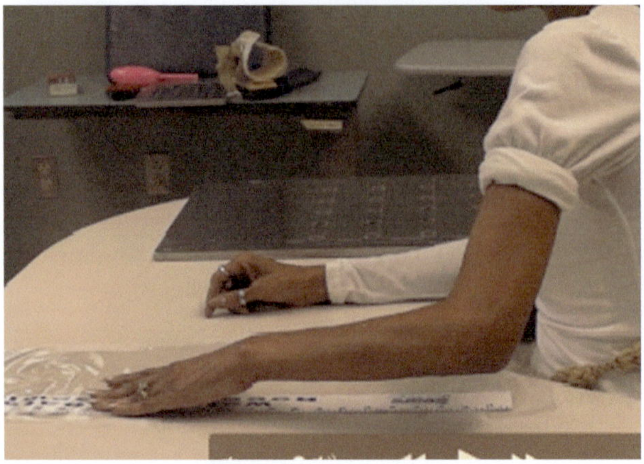

Fig. 7.38 In this figure, paresis of elbow extensors (triceps and anconeus) results in an impairment of elbow extension during reaching. The elbow flexors were not co-contracting and the shoulder flexors, tested separately, were not weak either

A flexion contracture blocks full reaching of the upper limb. Figure 7.41 reveals the impact of a flexion contracture of the elbow in a patient with good neurological recovery from right hemiparesis but with a residual elbow flexion contracture. The patient had to shorten his step length because elbow flexion limited his ability to extend the walker forward during limb advancement. Ambulation speed was necessarily slow and his chief complaint was "I walk slowly."

Elbow extensor overactivity and/or contracture restrain active elbow flexion with a major effect on feeding if the patient is otherwise able to do so. Release of the muscle and serial casting are considerations as treatment. Extensor contracture is sometimes seen after surgical release of a severe elbow flexion contracture. The extensor contracture occurs when it is not recognized that extensor overactivity is

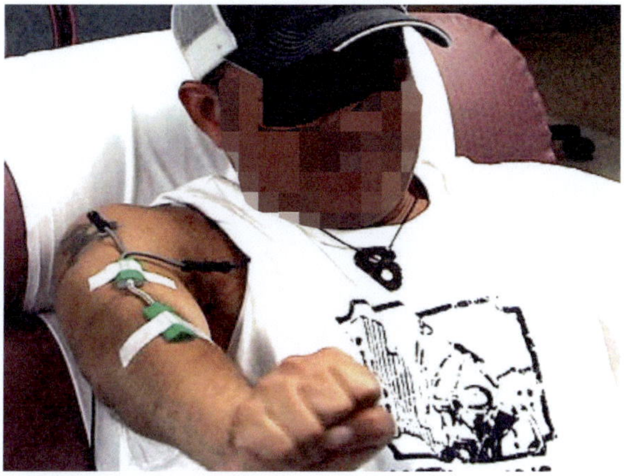

Fig. 7.39 It is common for spastic co-contraction of elbow flexors to restrain elbow extension, resulting in a strained, slow effort to achieve full elbow extension, or more commonly, to achieve only partial elbow extension

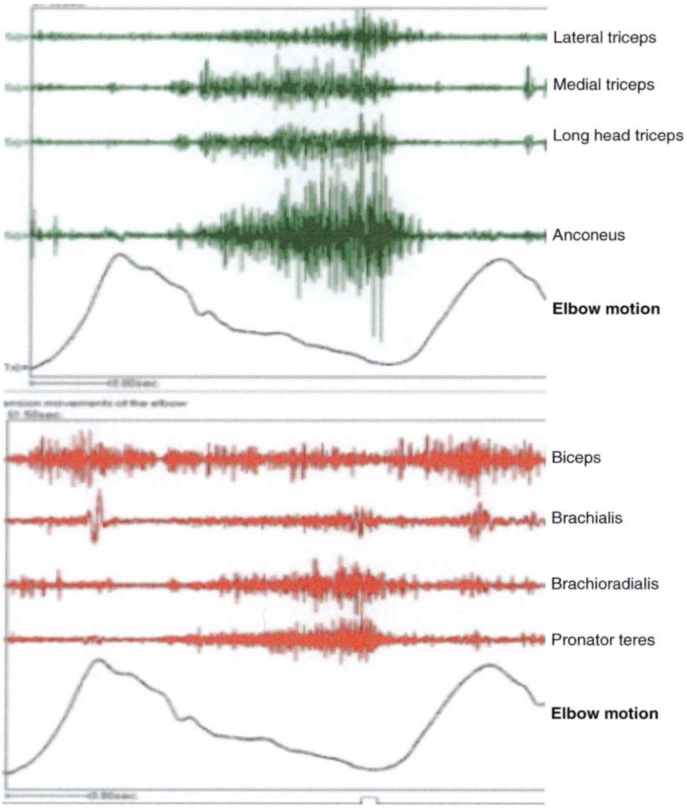

Fig. 7.40 The underlying enlarged dynamic EMG image of the patient in Fig. 7.39 during elbow extension includes agonist activity in the triceps and anconeus muscles (top 4 green traces) during the extension phase along with antagonist activity in the biceps, brachialis, brachioradialis, and pronator teres muscles (bottom 4 red traces), acting to restrain elbow extension. Spastic co-contraction acts like a brake while simultaneously accelerating

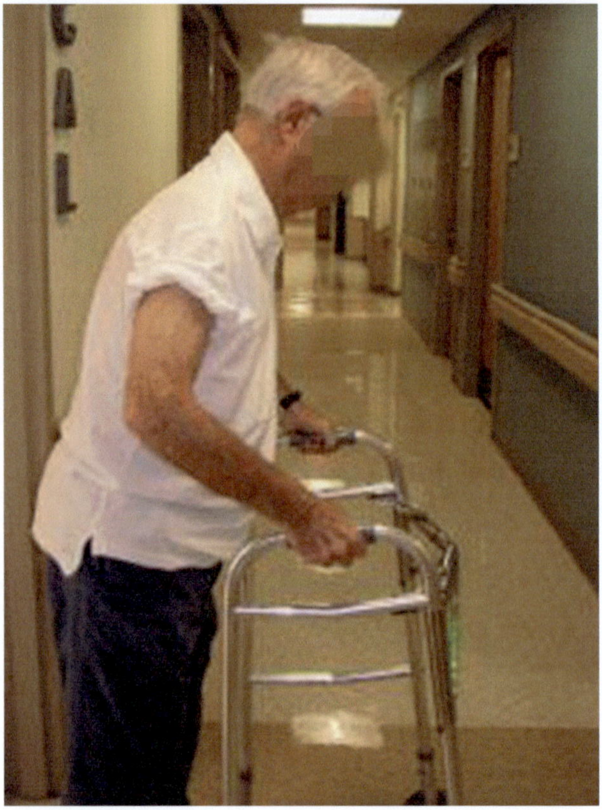

Fig. 7.41 A flexion contracture blocks full reaching of the upper limb. This figure shows a patient with spastic paresis who had to shorten his step length because his elbow flexion contracture limited his ability to extend the walker during limb advancement

present at the time of elbow flexion posturing. Surgical release of flexors changes the postoperative balance of forces that will, in some cases, favor elbow extension. In spastic paresis, it is the net balance of forces across a joint that determines clinical posturing. Clinicians should not assume that severe posturing of a joint in one direction means that there is no muscle activation in the other direction.

Inadequate Forearm Orientation of the Hand

The palm-down (overhand) orientation of the hand occurs due to forearm pronation while the palm-up (underhand) orientation requires forearm supination.

Reaching overhand to pick up an object such as a ball involves active pronation (unless the forearm is already pronated). In spastic paresis, a pronated forearm configuration is seen more often than a supinated one (see Fig. 7.42). Shortening and/or involuntary overactivity of the pronator teres is a major contributor to restraint of supination during reaching but the pronator quadratus needs to be considered as well (see Fig. 7.43). Pronator muscle stiffness and contracture frequently develop when volitional supination is weak. Serial casting can be performed for contracture.

Weakness of pronators is associated with involuntary overactivity and/or stiffness of muscles that supinate (biceps, supinator) and can result in a forearm with a

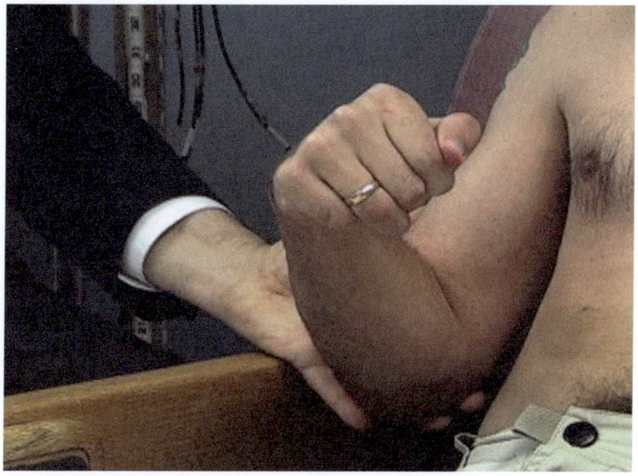

Fig. 7.42 In spastic paresis, a pronated forearm configuration is seen more often than a supinated one. This figure reveals a patient who is attempting voluntary forearm supination

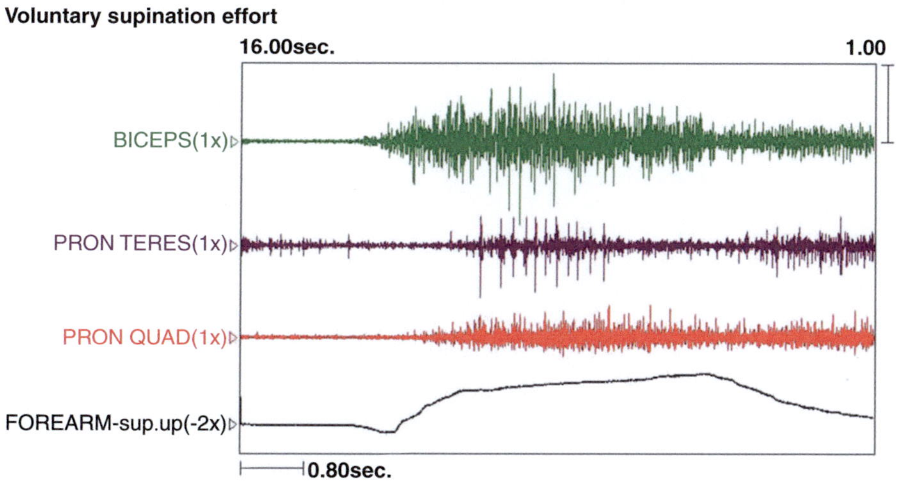

Fig. 7.43 Although the biceps muscle (supinator when the elbow is flexed) is active during supination, so are the pronator teres and pronator quadratus muscles in this polyEMG record corresponding to the patient in the figure above. *PRON TERES* pronator teres, *PRON QUAD* pronator quadratus, *sup* supination

resting supinated configuration. The biceps, in particular, supinates the forearm when the elbow is flexed. A fully extended elbow is supinated by the supinator, not the biceps. If some degree of active pronation is noted clinically, release of the supinating muscles may increase voluntary pronation.

Inadequate Vernier Adjustments of the Wrist

In addition to forearm rotation, the wrist contributes to the orientation of the fingers and thumb to acquire an object. For example, reaching for a small object such as a ball on a table requires wrist, finger, and thumb extension as part of reaching.

Extension of these limb segments typically occurs during the reach phase prior to contact with the object and informs how the hand makes contact and articulates with an object.

The wrist provides vernier (fine adjustment) movements for the reaching arm. This is illustrated in Fig. 7.44 which reveals the flexion adjustment of the wrist required to insert the hand into a receptacle with an upper boundary wall, such as the large box in the figure. A patient who cannot flex the wrist will not be able to make this adjustment as seen in Fig. 7.45.

A more common type of wrist restraint during whole limb movements is co-contraction of wrist flexors that restrain wrist extension. The left image of Fig. 7.46 reveals normal extension of the wrist prior to throwing a ball. The right image reveals a wrist that extends to neutral but is restrained from further extension by spastic co-contraction of the wrist flexors. Co-contraction is a normal phenomenon which refers to simultaneous contraction of the agonist and antagonist muscles by supraspinal drive to stabilize a joint. The co-contracting antagonist muscles are not activated by a stretch reflex but are triggered by their sensitivity to stretch, particularly if the muscle is shortened (see Fig. 7.47). However, it is not easy to

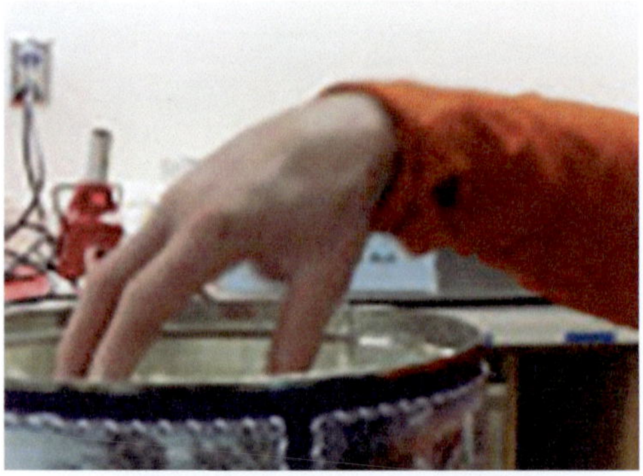

Fig. 7.44 The wrist provides fine adjustment (vernier) for the reaching arm. This figure illustrates flexion adjustment at the wrist required to retrieve a cookie from a large metal box

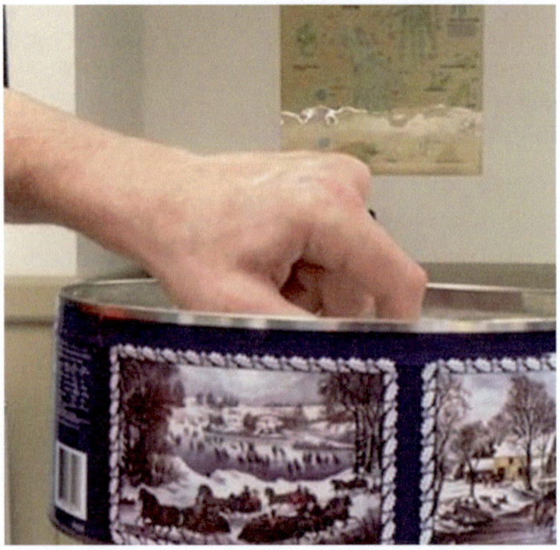

Fig. 7.45 The patient in this figure could not flex his wrist when he put his hand into the metal box to retrieve a cookie

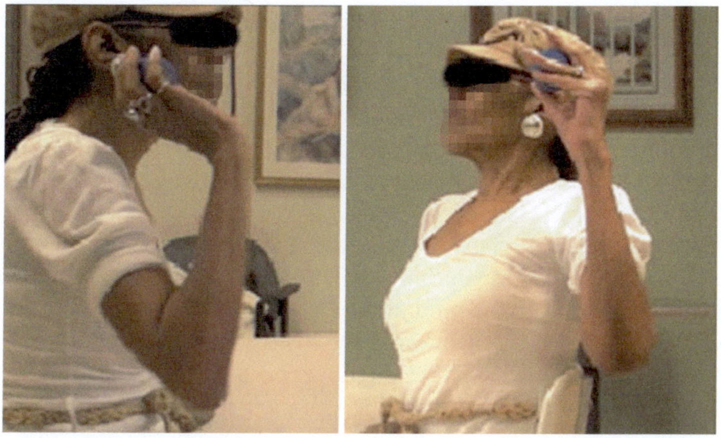

Fig. 7.46 Wrist restraint during whole limb movements may result from co-contraction of wrist flexors that restrain wrist extension. The left image of this figure reveals wrist extension in the unaffected upper limb prior to throwing a ball. The image on the right side reveals a wrist that extends to neutral but is restrained from further extension by spastic co-contraction of the wrist flexors as illustrated in the next figure

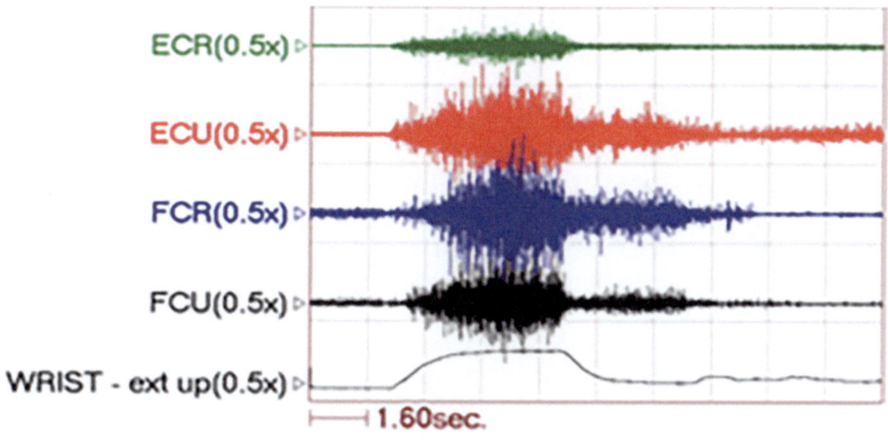

Fig. 7.47 Voluntary wrist extension in a patient with co-contraction of antagonist muscles FCR and FCU accompanying agonist muscles ECR and ECU. Co-contracting antagonist muscles are not initially activated by a stretch reflex but are triggered by their sensitivity to stretch (particularly if the muscle is shortened) and reduce the effect of agonist activation on the movement, hence the term *spastic* co-contraction. *ECR* extensor carpi radialis, *ECU* extensor carpi ulnaris, *FCR* flexor carpi radialis, *FCU* flexor carpi ulnaris, *ext* extension

differentiate whether weakness of the agonist, muscle shortening of the antagonist, or overactivity in the antagonist is the problem. PolyEMG can identify antagonist muscle activity that starts simultaneously with agonist activity, establishing the presence of antagonist co-contraction. Once the movement is underway, superimposed spastic activity due to stretch may or may not contribute.

Functional Consequences in the Lower Limb

The three main functional goals of ambulation are: (1) to move from one place to another, (2) to move safely, and (3) to move efficiently. Gait is characterized by periods of limb loading and unloading in a cyclic and complex pattern. In order to analyze gait, an understanding of basic terminology is needed to identify the components and events of the gait cycle. Considering one limb at a time, the gait cycle has two basic components: a stance phase during which the limb is in contact with the ground, and a swing phase during which the limb is off the ground. During the stance phase, the foot is on the ground for about 60% of a whole symmetrical gait cycle, and the swing phase is approximately 40% of the gait cycle.

The objectives of the stance phase are proper positioning of the limb for stability at initial contact, maintaining a normal loading response, single limb support and forward progression of the body over the stance phase limb, and preparing the lower extremity for the subsequent swing phase. During the swing phase, the objectives are to enable limb clearance and advancement.

Pathological gait can be classified as stance and swing phase abnormalities. For example, observation of hemiparetic gait reveals an overall loss of symmetry with decreased stance time and increased swing time on the affected side, and increased stance time on the unaffected side. A shorter step length on the affected side and increased double support time preserves stability, because more time in double support and more weight-bearing time on the sound limb results in less time spent weight-bearing by the affected limb [26]. Reciprocal arm motion is typically absent or diminished on the affected side, the arm is typically positioned in shoulder adduction and elbow flexion, though it may be flaccid in the early stages of neurological recovery. The affected lower limb appears stiff-legged, showing an extensor synergy pattern with hip extension, adduction, and internal rotation, reduced knee flexion, and plantarflexion/inversion of the foot/ankle (equinovarus). Because extensor posturing lengthens the limb, patients may have difficulty achieving adequate clearance during the swing phase, leading to compensatory maneuvers such as hip hiking (elevation of the hip), circumduction, lateral trunk bending away from the side of the affected swing limb, and less commonly, contralateral vaulting. Initiation of swing phase is delayed, prolonged, or effortful, and is usually associated with a stiff knee and ankle equinus [27].

During stance phase on the affected side, ankle dorsiflexion is decreased at initial contact, and also during the stance and swing phases. Knee hyperextension in the stance phase is seen in most patients, although in some cases, excessive knee flexion is observed. During the swing phase on the affected side, knee flexion is reduced, initiation of hip flexion is delayed, and compensation occurs by means of hip hiking or limb circumduction.

Skin and Footwear Problems

Striatal Toe

Observation of barefoot walking reveals extension of the great toe during the stance and swing phases of gait (Fig. 7.48). When wearing shoes, the patient may report pain at the first metatarsal head, commonly on the tip of the great toe (Fig. 7.49). Shortening or overactivity of the extensor hallucis longus is the mechanism for this problem. However, weakness of the flexor hallucis longus may also contribute. Frequently, patients will complain of pressure on the tip of the big toe resulting from

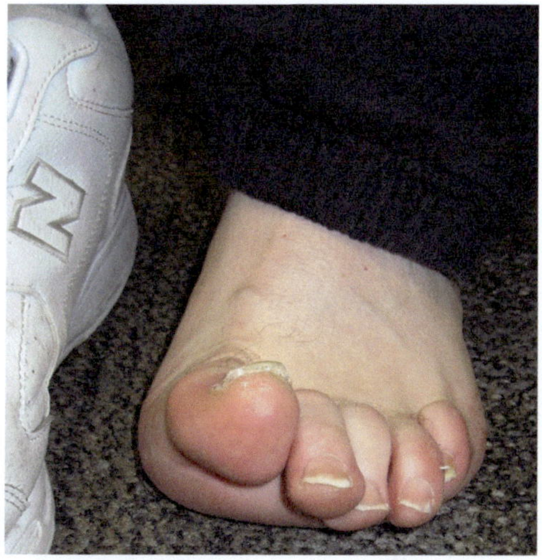

Fig. 7.48 Image of a striatal toe. Observation of barefoot walking reveals that the great toe is held extended during the stance and swing phases of gait

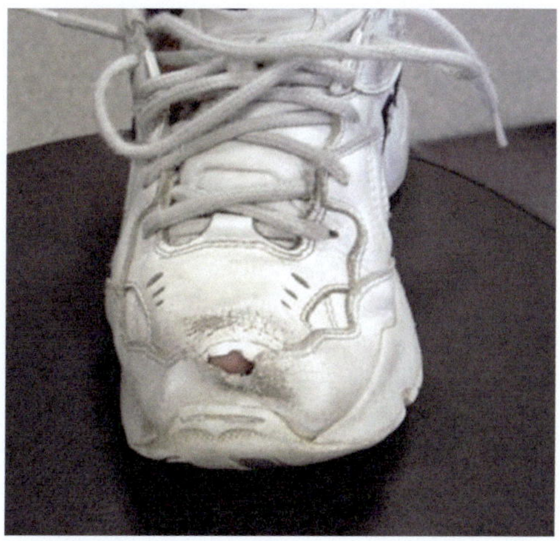

Fig. 7.49 When wearing shoes, the patient with a striatal toe may report pain at the first metatarsal head, commonly on the tip of the great toe

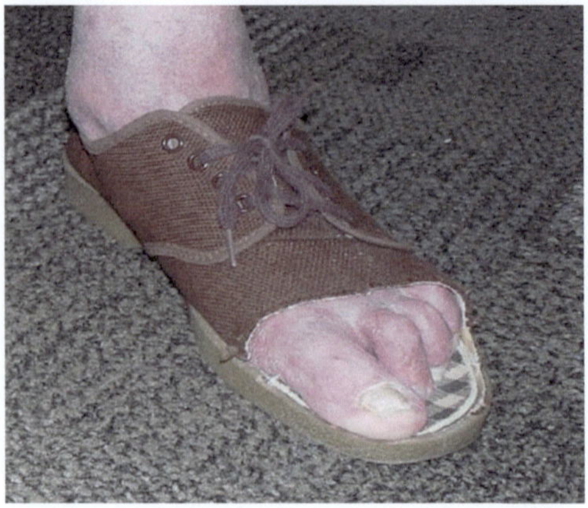

Fig. 7.50 This patient with spastic paresis had painful toe flexion. Observation of barefoot walking revealed the toes to be flexed during the stance phase of gait, producing pain as a symptom that interfered with weightbearing

contact with the top of the shoe's toe box. Ankle equinovarus posture may accompany this deformity, and if present, evaluation of the tibialis anterior, tibialis posterior, gastrocnemius, soleus, and long toe flexors should be performed. Relieving pressure on the tip of the toe inside the shoe can increase comfort.

Painful Toe Flexion

Observation of barefoot walking reveals the toes to be flexed during the stance phase producing pain that interferes with weightbearing (Fig. 7.50). When wearing shoes, the patient may report pain on the dorsal aspect of the toes due to pressure from the shoe's toe box. Pain during standing may impair weightbearing, and interfere with transfers and walking. Shortening or overactivity of the flexor digitorum longus is the cause of this problem. Patients may complain of pressure on the tip of the toes. Evaluation of the long toe flexors should be performed. Pressure relieving toe pads inside the shoe can increase comfort [28].

Problems of Limb Clearance

Stiff Knee with and without Equinovarus

In patients with a stiff knee, the knee is maintained in extension throughout the swing phase. Even when the foot and ankle are adequately positioned, limb clearance can be inadequate due to an inability to bend the swing phase limb. The foot can drag, even if the ankle has adequate dorsiflexion. Compensatory mechanisms involving the trunk, ipsilateral hip (e.g., circumduction), and contralateral limb (e.g., vaulting or early heel rise) may be used by the patient to increase the likelihood of safe ambulation.

Out-of-phase activation of the rectus femoris (RF) during swing phase can be a major contributor to the stiff knee gait, because the RF crosses both the hip and knee joints and can restrict knee flexion. Out-of-phase activation of the vasti (medialis, lateralis, and intermedius) muscles during the swing phase can also contribute to a stiff knee gait. At the hip, a weak iliopsoas muscle can reduce hip flexion in the swing phase, further impairing knee flexion. Shortening or overactivity of the gluteus maximus and hamstring muscles during the swing phase may restrain hip flexion, potentially causing a stiff knee gait.

If a stiff knee is present in the absence of an ankle deformity, a diagnostic lidocaine block of the motor branch of the femoral nerve to the rectus femoris can be performed to help differentiate the contribution of the knee extensors versus the hip extensor muscles and guide the treatment decisions.

Inadequate Hip Flexion

Limited hip flexion is a common finding in individuals with spastic paresis that has functional implications for limb clearance. Inadequate hip flexion may occur due to hip muscle weakness from prolonged sitting, leading to muscle shortening of the hip flexors or overactivity of hip extensor muscles (e.g., gluteus maximus). During walking, a common penalty is reduced step length due to limited hip flexion and an inability to put the affected limb in front of the unaffected limb during the swing phase of gait. Hip adduction may result from shortening and/or overactivity of the adductor longus, adductor brevis, sartorius, and in some cases, from weakness of the gluteus medius.

Problems of Foot Loading

Loading on the Lateral Border of the Foot

Equinovarus foot deformity is the most frequently seen abnormality in the lower limb in individuals with spastic paresis. The foot and ankle are inverted, pointed downward (plantarflexed), and the toes may be curled as well.

The patient frequently complains of pain on the lateral border of the foot during weightbearing (Fig. 7.51). During loading, contact with the ground occurs first with the forefoot, weight is borne primarily on the anterior and lateral border of the foot and may frequently be concentrated in the area under the fifth metatarsal. Limited dorsiflexion during midstance prevents forward progression of the tibia over the stationary foot leading to increased pressure over the metatarsals, promoting lateral ankle instability and potentially causing knee hyperextension. Compensatory hip flexion may occur to maintain ambulation. The presence of an inadequate base of support may result in instability of the whole body and correction of the problem is essential, even for persons with limited ambulation capacity.

Muscles that potentially contribute to the equinovarus deformity include the gastrocnemius, soleus, tibialis posterior, tibialis anterior, long toe flexors, extensor hallucis longus, and peroneus longus.

Forefoot First Loading

Foot equinus deformity is frequently seen during walking in individuals with spastic paresis. The foot and ankle are plantarflexed prior to initial contact. During loading, the patient first touches the ground with the forefoot and contact with the ground may be primarily or exclusively on the forefoot (Fig. 7.52).

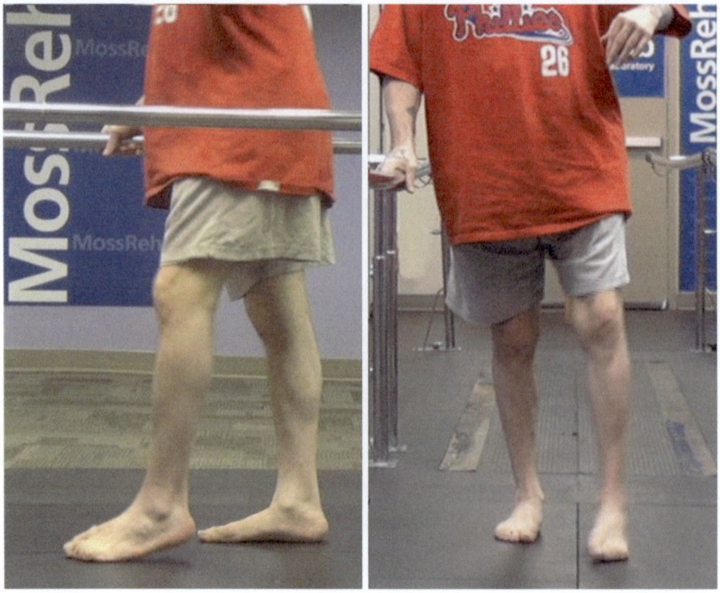

Fig. 7.51 Equinovarus foot is the abnormal posture most frequently seen in the lower limb in individuals with spastic paresis. The foot and ankle are inverted, plantar flexed and the toes may be curled as well. The patient frequently complains of pain on the lateral border of the foot during weightbearing

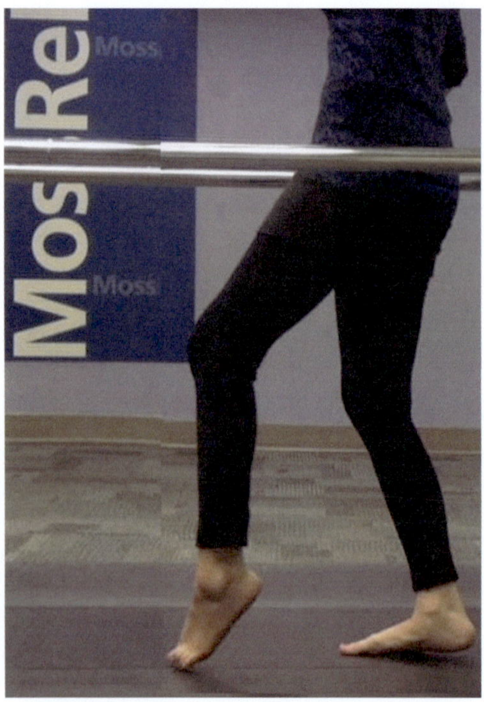

Fig. 7.52 Image of "forefoot first loading." The foot and ankle are plantarflexed prior to initial contact. The patient touches the ground first with the forefoot during loading, and in some patients, contact with the ground may be exclusively or primarily on the forefoot during the subsequent stance phase

Limited dorsiflexion during midstance prevents forward progression of the tibia over the stationary foot leading to increased pressure over the metatarsals. Compensatory hip flexion, and depending on the degree of equinus, knee flexion or extension may occur to accommodate the deformity to maintain ambulation. The presence of equinus may interfere with limb clearance during the swing phase and require contralateral early heel rise (vaulting) or increased hip and knee flexion (steppage). Muscles that potentially contribute to this deformity include the gastrocnemius, soleus, and tibialis anterior.

Problems of Limb Advancement

Insufficient Hip Flexion

Lack of hip flexion not only affects walking by interfering with limb advancement but may also impact floor clearance by the foot. Weakness of hip flexor muscles (e.g., iliacus, psoas, pectineus, and rectus femoris), and in some cases, overactive hip extensors (gluteus maximus and hamstrings) may be the source of lack of hip flexion. Reduced swing phase hip flexion may also promote a more extended knee (akin to a stiff knee gait) because restraint of hip flexion during swing phase reduces limb acceleration needed to generate the pendular motion of the knee.

Impaired hip flexion can also become a significant positioning issue during sitting (Fig. 7.53). In addition to hip extensor tone/spasticity, one should also consider heterotopic ossification, hip dislocation, undiagnosed fractures and other sources of painful stimuli, because pain can increase overactivity of the hip extensors and knee flexors (see Chap. 9).

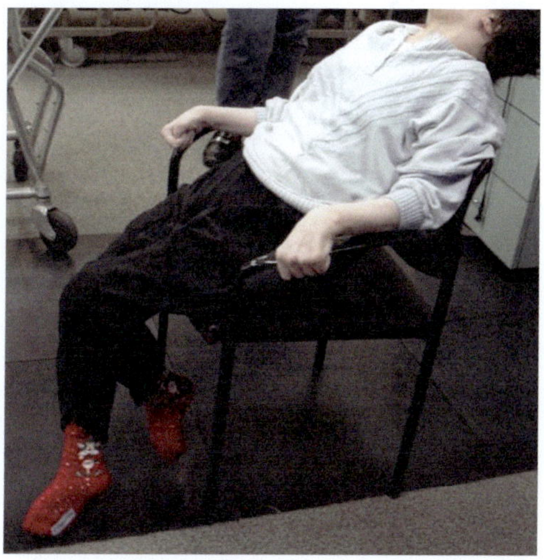

Fig. 7.53 As seen in this image, insufficient hip flexion can cause a significant positioning issue during sitting. In addition to shortening of hip extensors and hip extensor overactivity, one should also consider heterotopic ossification, hip dislocation, undiagnosed fractures and other sources of painful stimuli, because pain can increase overactivity of the hip extensors and knee flexors

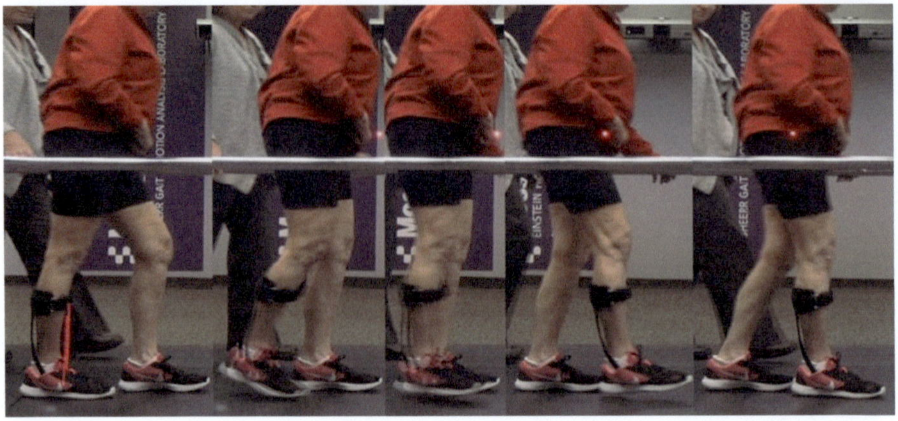

Fig. 7.54 Image of a patient with a stiff knee gait. The knee is maintained in a largely or completely extended position throughout the swing phase and the moment of inertia of the lower limb is increased, further impairing hip flexion

Stiff Knee (Inadequate Knee Flexion in Swing Phase)

In this gait deviation, the knee is maintained in a largely or completely extended position throughout the swing phase and the moment of inertia of the lower limb is increased, further impairing hip flexion (Fig. 7.54). In the context of spastic paresis, a stiff knee gait results from a dynamic deformity created by muscle shortening or contraction and external moments rather than a structural deformity of the knee joint. The resulting lack of adequate limb clearance due to reduced hip and knee flexion can result in a foot drag, even if the ankle has adequate dorsiflexion. Compensatory mechanisms in the trunk, ipsilateral hip (e.g., circumduction), and contralateral limb (e.g., vaulting or early heel rise) may be present, leading to increased effort during walking.

Out-of-phase activation of the RF during the swing phase can be a major contributor to the stiff knee pattern because the RF crosses both the hip and knee joint and can restrict knee flexion. Out-of-phase activation of the vasti muscles in the swing phase can also contribute to this gait deviation. At the hip, overactivity of the gluteus maximus and hamstrings during the swing phase may restrain hip flexion, resulting in a stiff knee gait. A weak iliopsoas can also reduce hip flexion in the swing phase, further impairing knee flexion. Ankle equinus can contribute to knee hyperextension in the stance phase by preventing forward progression of the tibia and delaying knee flexion. In general, when a concomitant ankle deformity is observed, the ankle should be addressed first, as this may ameliorate the stiff knee gait pattern.

Toe Drag

During the swing phase, five different mechanisms facilitate limb clearance so that the limb can be advanced. These include: (1) swing limb hip flexion, (2) swing limb knee flexion, (3) swing limb ankle dorsiflexion, (4) stance limb

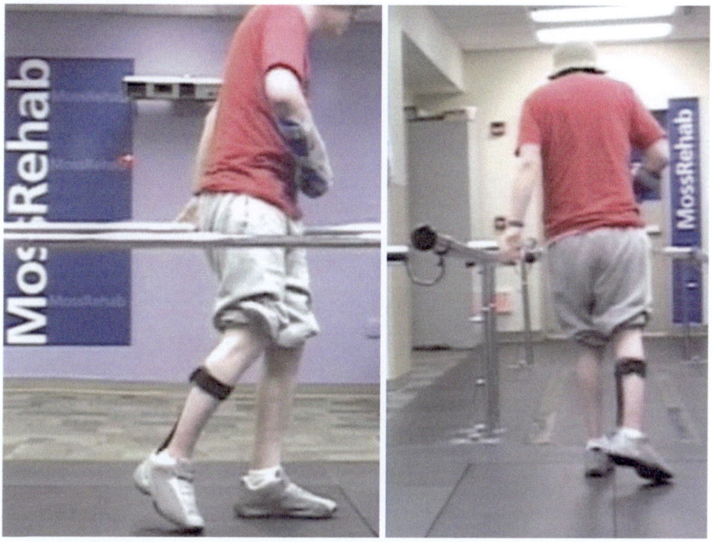

Fig. 7.55 Image of a patient with toe drag. In its most frequent presentation, toe drag is present during the early swing phase. It can also be seen at the end of the swing phase or throughout swing. When it is present throughout swing, toe drag impairs limb clearance and restrains limb advancement. When it occurs in the early swing phase, the penalty is limited limb advancement

extension control (controlled forward progression of the tibia), and (5) stance limb control of pelvic tilt. If toe drag occurs, it is because of the loss of three or more of the five identified mechanisms, possibilities for compensation having been lost. In its most frequent presentation, toe drag manifests during the early swing phase (Fig. 7.55). It can also be evident at the end of the swing phase or throughout swing. When it is present throughout swing, toe drag impairs limb clearance and restrains limb advancement. When it occurs in early swing phase, the penalty is limited limb advancement [29].

Inadequate Knee Extension in Terminal Swing

Limited knee extension is a common physical finding that has functional implications for walking (Fig. 7.56). It may occur due to contracture from prolonged sitting or overactivity of knee flexor muscles (e.g., hamstrings and gastrocnemius). When severe, heterotopic ossification, knee dislocation, and undiagnosed fractures should be ruled out. During walking, a common penalty is reduced step length due to limited knee extension. Hip flexion deformities may also contribute to knee flexion posturing when the patient lies supine. Hip flexion deformities can restrain hip acceleration during the swing phase, reducing the inertial forward displacement of the tibia. Hamstring and gastrocnemius stretching should increase knee extension in this phase of walking [30].

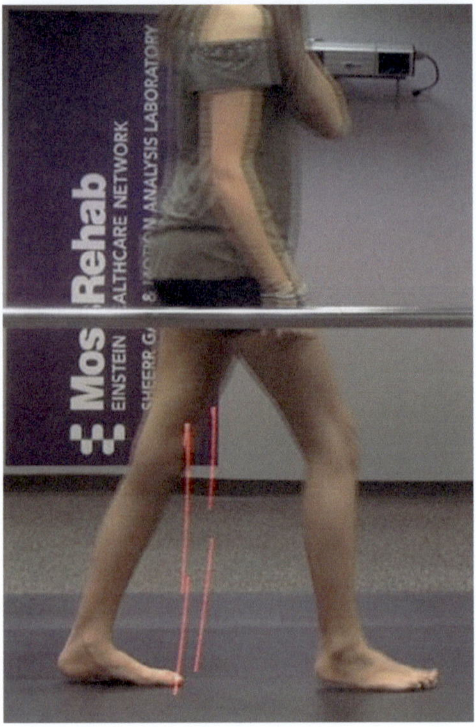

Fig. 7.56 Limited knee extension of the right lower limb at the very end of terminal swing (virtually at initial contact), with resulting limited limb advancement and a short step length

Problems of Single Limb Support

Knee Flexion in Stance

The flexed knee deformity may refer to the flexed posture of the knee in both the stance and swing phases. Not only does a flexed knee deformity impair limb stability and contralateral limb clearance, but the lack of knee extension in terminal swing also limits limb advancement. This gait pattern is often associated with hamstring muscle shortening, overactivity, or contracture. Other factors that contribute to this dysfunction include shortening or overactivity of the gastrocnemius in the stance phase and of the iliopsoas in the swing phase.

Weak Knee Extensors

Profound weakness of the knee extensors, hip extensors, or ankle plantar flexors may also lead to knee flexion in the stance phase with marked limb instability that forces the patient to rely on upper limb support (Fig. 7.57). The patient's sense of instability shortens the contralateral step length and substantially reduces walking velocity and tolerance [31]. Bracing may be the only alternative because the lack of motor control may prevent strengthening. Bracing the knee to prevent flexion appears to be the most sensible intervention, but this unfortunately also limits knee flexion during the swing phase and interferes with limb clearance. Newer

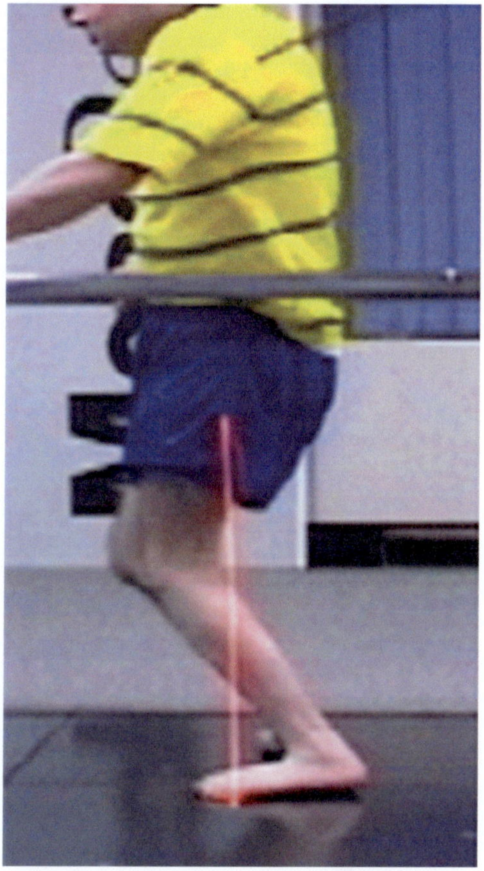

Fig. 7.57 Image of weak knee extensors. Profound weakness of knee extensors, hip extensors, or ankle plantar flexors may also lead to knee flexion in the stance phase with marked limb instability that forces the patient to rely on upper limb support. The sense of instability shortens the contralateral step length and substantially reduces walking velocity and tolerance

devices that provide support only during the stance phase would work best, but these devices tend to be heavier and more expensive. The use of a limited motion ankle foot orthosis with a dorsiflexion stop and rear entry design may be a suitable solution for this problem (Fig. 7.58).

Painful Toe Flexors During Loading and Weightbearing

When the toe flexors are painful, observation of barefoot walking may reveal that the lesser toes and/ or hallux are held in flexion during the phases of terminal stance and terminal swing (Fig. 7.59). The patient will complain of pain at the tip of the toes, demonstrate prolonged limb loading, and reduced stance phase duration. When wearing shoes, the patient may report pain at the tip of the toes and pressure from the shoe upper. Shortening or overactivity of the flexor digitorum longus and flexor hallucis longus muscles is the principal mechanism for this problem. However, weakness of the extensor muscles may also contribute. Toe flexion has a deleterious effect on late stance propulsion and can reduce limb clearance and advancement

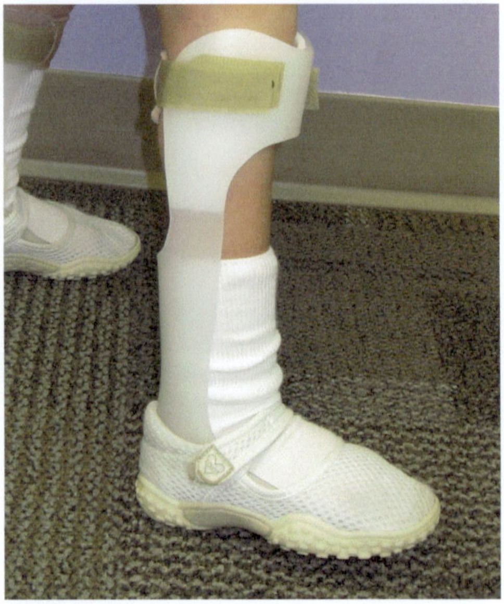

Fig. 7.58 Bracing may be the only alternative for weak knee extensors because lack of motor control may prevent extensor strengthening. Bracing the knee to prevent flexion appears to be the most sensible intervention, but it also limits knee flexion during the swing phase and interferes with limb clearance. As depicted in this figure, the use of a limited motion ankle foot orthosis with a dorsiflexion stop and rear entry design may be a suitable solution for weak knee extensors

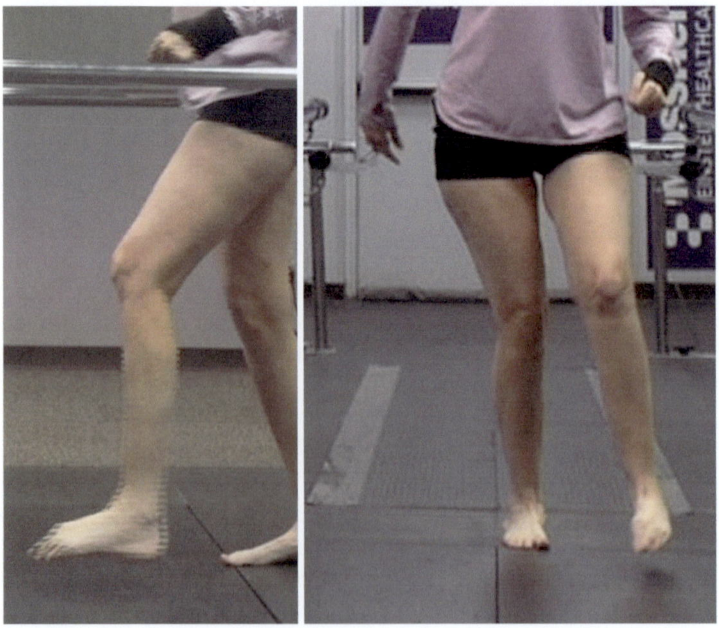

Fig. 7.59 Painful toe flexors during loading and weightbearing. Observation of barefoot walking reveals that the lesser toes and/ or hallux are held in flexion during the phases of terminal stance and terminal swing. The patient will complain of pain at the tip of the toes, demonstrate prolongation of the loading response during the period of double support, and reduced stance duration because of shortened single limb support

during swing. Ankle equinus posture may accompany this deformity, and if present, evaluation of the gastrocnemius and soleus muscles should be performed [32].

Conclusions

This chapter outlines the abnormal limb postures that affect the upper and lower limbs as a result of long-standing spastic paresis, and attempts to describe the various muscles that contribute to these postures. We have also reviewed the functional consequences of these abnormal postures to set reasonable goals for treatment.

References

1. Mayer NH, Esquenazi A. Upper limb skin and musculoskeletal consequences of the upper motor neuron syndrome. In: Jankovic J, Albanese A, Atassi M, Dolly O, Hallett M, Mayer NH, editors. Botulinum toxin: therapeutic clinical practice & science. Philadelphia: Saunders; 2009. p. 131–47.
2. Mayer NH, Herman R. Phenomenology of muscle overactivity in the upper motor neuron syndrome. Eura Medicophys. 2004;40(2):85–110.
3. Sheean G. The pathophysiology of spasticity. Eur J Neurol. 2002;9(Suppl 1):3–9.
4. Lannin NA, Novak I, Cusick A. A systematic review of upper extremity casting for children and adults with central nervous system motor disorders. Clin Rehabil. 2007;21(11):963–76.
5. Pappas N, Baldwin K, Keenan MA. Treatment of the non-functional contracted hand. UPOJ. 2011;21:90–2.
6. Steinberg FU, Ferguson KL. Effect of dantrolene sodium on spasticity associated with hemiplegia. J Am Geriatr Soc. 1975;23(2):1532–5415.
7. Herman R, Mayer N, Mecomber SA. Clinical pharmaco-physiology of dantrolene sodium. Am J Phys Med. 1972;51(6):296–311.
8. Zucchi R, Ronca-Testoni S. The sarcoplasmic reticulum Ca2+ channel/ryanodine receptor: modulation by endogenous effectors, drugs and disease states. Pharmacol Rev. 1997;49(1):1–51.
9. Herman R, Freedman W, Mayer N. Neurophysiologic mechanisms of hemiplegic and paraplegic spasticity: implications for therapy. Arch Phys Med Rehabil. 1974;55(8):338–43.
10. Chang E, Ghosh N, Yanni D, Lee S, Alexandru D, Mozaffar T. A review of spasticity treatments: pharmacological and interventional approaches. Crit Rev Phys Rehabil Med. 2013;25(1–2):11–22.
11. Walshe FMR. On certain tonic or postural reflexes in hemiplegia with special reference to the so called associated movements. Brain. 1923;46:1–37.
12. Bakheit AM, Sawyer J. The effects of botulinum toxin treatment on associated reactions of the upper limb on hemiplegic gait–a pilot study. Disabil Rehabil. 2002;24(10):519–22.
13. Mayer N, Esquenazi A. Muscle overactivity and movement dysfunction in the upper motoneuron syndrome. Phys Med Rehabil Clin N Am. 2003;14:855–83.
14. Thorley M, Donaghey S, Edwards P, Copeland L, Kentish M, McLennan K, Lindsley J, Gascoigne-Pees L, Sakzewski L, Boyd RN. Evaluation of the effects of botulinum toxin A injections when used to improve ease of care and comfort in children with cerebral palsy whom are non-ambulant: a double blind randomized controlled trial. BMC Pediatr. 2012;12:120–32. https://doi.org/10.1186/1471-2431-12-120.
15. Francisco GE, Li S. Spasticity. In: Cifu DX, editor. Physical medicine and rehabilitation. Philadelphia: Elsevier; 2016. p. 487–9.

16. Jeannerod M. The formation of finger grip during prehension. A cortically mediated visuomotor pattern. Behav Brain Res. 1986;19:99–116.
17. Miczak K, Padova J. Muscle overactivity in the upper motor neuron syndrome: assessment and problem solving for complex cases: the role of physical and occupational therapy. Phys Med Rehab Clinics NA. 2018;29(3):529–36.
18. Frank C, Akeson WH, Woo S, Arniel D, Coutts RD. Physiology and therapeutic value of passive joint motion. Clin Orthop Relat Res. 1984;185:113–25.
19. Keenan MAE. Management of the spastic upper extremity in the neurologically impaired adult. Clin Orthop Relat Res. 1988;233:116–25.
20. Rhagavan P, Lu Y, Mirchandani M, Stecco A. Human recombinant hyaluronidase injections for upper limb muscle stiffness in individuals with cerebral injury: a case series. EBioMedicine. 2016;9:306–13. https://doi.org/10.1016/j.ebiom.2016.05.014.
21. Nazarpour K, Barnard A, Jackson A. Flexible cortical control of task-specific muscle synergies. J Neurosci. 2012;32(36):12349–60.
22. Pathak MS, Nguyen HT, Graham HK, Moore AP. Management of spasticity in adults: practical application of botulinum toxin. Eur J Neurol. 2006;13(1s):42–50.
23. Ada L, Goddard E, McCully J, Stavrinos T, Bampton J. Thirty minutes of positioning reduces the development of shoulder external rotation contracture after stroke: a randomized controlled trial. Arch Phys Med Rehabil. 2005;86(2):230–4.
24. Raghavan P, Aluru V, Milani S, Thai P, Geller D, Bilaloglu S, Lu Y, Weisz DJ. Coupled bimanual training using a non-powered device for individuals with severe hemiparesis: a pilot study. Int J Phys Med Rehabil. 2017;5(3):404.
25. Mayer NH. Spasticity and other signs of the upper motor neuron syndrome. In: Brashear A, Elovic E, editors. Spasticity diagnosis & management. 2nd ed. New York: Demos Medical Publishing; 2016. p. 17–32.
26. Brandstater ME, Debruin H, Gowland C. Hemiplegic gait: analysis of temporal variables. Arch Phys Med Rehabil. 1983;64:583–7.
27. Ochi F, Esquenazi A, Hirai B. Temporal-spatial features of gait after traumatic brain injury. J Head Trauma Rehabil. 1999;14:105–15.
28. Mayer NH, Esquenazi A, Keenan MAE. Analysis and management of spasticity, contracture and impaired motor control. In: Horn LJ, Zasler ND, editors. Medical rehabilitation of traumatic brain injury. Philadelphia: Hanley & Belfus; 1996. p. 411–58.
29. Vachranukunkiet T, Esquenazi A. Pathophysiology of gait disturbance in neurologic disorders and clinical presentations. Phys Med Rehabil Clin N Am. 2013;24(2):233–46.
30. Esquenazi A. Assessment of spasticity and other consequences of the upper motor neuron syndrome affecting the lower limb. In: Brashear A, Elovic E, editors. Spasticity diagnosis & management. 2nd ed. New York: Demos Medical Publishing; 2016. p. 91–100.
31. Esquenazi A, Mayer NH. Clinical experience and recent advances in the management of gait disorders with botulinum neurotoxin. In: Jankovic J, Albanese A, Atassi M, Dolly O, Hallett M, Mayer NH, editors. Botulinum toxin: therapeutic clinical practice & science. Philadelphia: Saunders; 2009. p. 192–203.
32. Esquenazi A, Mayer NH. Instrumented assessment of muscle overactivity and spasticity with dynamic polyelectromyographic and motion analysis for treatment planning. Am J Phys Med Rehabil. 2004;83(suppl10):S19–29.

Part II

Treatment

Framework for the Treatment of Spasticity and Muscle Stiffness

8

Preeti Raghavan

New frameworks are like climbing a mountain - the larger view encompasses rather than rejects the more restricted view.
– Albert Einstein, 1879–1955.

- This chapter provides a brief overview of a framework for the treatment of spasticity and muscle stiffness in the context of the overall rehabilitation plan for patients with spastic paresis. A key aspect of any treatment of spasticity and muscle stiffness is to restore mobility and function as early as possible, and to the greatest extent possible, to mitigate the negative effects of weakness, immobility, and inactivity.
- Central to the framework is a comprehensive evaluation including a patient-centered history and physical examination, as well as a five-step assessment which incorporates upper and lower limb functional ability, passive range of motion, and active range of motion with repetition of movement.
- The purpose of the assessment is to set collaborative patient-centered goals for treatment and to evaluate the treatment response in a consistent and repeatable manner. The history and physical should enable the assessment of medical conditions exacerbating spasticity that must be treated first and include body diagrams to determine the degree to which the symptoms are generalized or focal for appropriate selection of treatment(s).

P. Raghavan (✉)
Departments of Physical Medicine and Rehabilitation and Neurology, The Johns Hopkins University School of Medicine, Baltimore, MD, USA
e-mail: praghavan@jhmi.edu

P. Raghavan (ed.), *Spasticity and Muscle Stiffness*,
https://doi.org/10.1007/978-3-030-96900-4_8

- The assessment can aid in distinguishing between generalized hyperexcitability amenable to intervention with oral spasmolytics and intrathecal baclofen in severe cases, predominantly neural muscle overactivity that can be treated with focal neurolysis and/or chemodenervation using botulinum toxins, and predominantly non-neural muscle shortening that can be treated with focal pharmacologic release using hyaluronidase injections.

Introduction

Damage to the central nervous system (CNS) leads to negative symptoms such as weakness and loss of selective control of muscles, limb segments, and finger dexterity [1]. In addition, positive symptoms of hyperreflexia and spasticity are hallmarks of the movement dysfunction [2]. The co-existence of weakness and spasticity make the syndrome of spastic paresis particularly challenging to treat as the treatment of the positive symptoms can exacerbate the negative symptoms [3, 4].

Weakness, immobility, and inactivity affect several organ systems adversely, including the skin, vascular, and musculoskeletal systems [5], and individuals with spasticity are not protected from these adverse effects [6–8]. Immobility and inactivity produce secondary musculoskeletal changes including muscle atrophy, fatty infiltration, weakness, osteoporosis, muscle stiffness, and contractures through complex biophysical and endocrine interactions [9]. Furthermore, the degree to which patients are mobile influences decision-making about how to treat spasticity and the ensuing spastic movement disorder as discussed in Chap. 2. In turn, spasticity and muscle stiffness contribute to persistent motor dysfunction and impaired motor control [10]. Early mobilization after neurological stability has been found to be beneficial in promoting motor recovery, for example, after stroke [11, 12]. Even individuals who are severely impaired and in the chronic stage poststroke benefit from frequent therapy provided over long durations [13, 14]. Therefore, to reduce the complications related to weakness, immobility, and inactivity, rehabilitation therapy is the cornerstone of treatment after CNS injury due to stroke, traumatic brain injury, spinal cord injury, cerebral palsy, and multiple sclerosis [7, 8, 15–17].

Rehabilitation Based on Principles of Motor Learning

The goal of rehabilitation is to restore function which requires recovery of movement and performance to the extent possible. The management of spasticity and/or muscle stiffness should thus aim to facilitate the process of rehabilitation, i.e., facilitate therapy and caregiving and restore function [18]. Functional training with task-specific practice also requires sensory feedback for task-appropriate intra- and interlimb coordination [19, 20], which is frequently impaired in individuals with spastic movement disorder as discussed in Chap. 2. Individuals with severe motor impairment generally demonstrate greater spasticity and/or muscle stiffness [21]. However, even in these individuals skill acquisition can be accomplished based on the principles of motor learning using a stepwise logical approach. The focus should first be on recovery of the movement components composing functional tasks, such as: muscle activation in synergy, then single joint movements in synergy, followed by single joint movements out of synergy to restore full isolated movement, first in one direction and then using alternating joint movements in both directions, progressing to task component practice, and then eventually to full functional task practice [14, 22, 23]. Attempting to engage severely impaired patients in complex functional task practice early on invariably leads to the use of compensatory strategies [24], which if reinforced can be detrimental to long-term recovery [25]. Therefore, it may not be productive to practice complex functional tasks at the beginning of treatment. However, individual movement components, including finger extension and somatosensory function, have been shown to continue to recover over the long term [26, 27]. As isolated movements of the scapula, shoulder, elbow, forearm, wrist, fingers, and thumb improve, they can be incorporated into functional task components and subsequently into whole task practice. The idea is to practice movements that are as close to normal as possible [28], and to gradually increase the ability to repeat the movements without compromising movement quality [29–31]. It is also important to allow room for variability in practice to enable self-correction based on explicit knowledge about the task and sensory feedback [32–37].

Operationalizing motor learning strategies for recovery of movement and skill in the context of spasticity and/or muscle stiffness requires setting small accomplishable goals, and education of and partnership with patients and their caregivers to achieve these goals. Technology can be used to aid this process using the A3E framework which stands for Accessibility, Adaptability, Accountability, and Engagement [38] (Fig. 8.1). Accessibility encompasses awareness of the benefits of rehabilitation, access to the appropriate frequency of visits, intensity of prescribed activities, duration of therapy, availability of technological resources needed, and affordability of rehabilitation services. Adaptability refers to the ability of

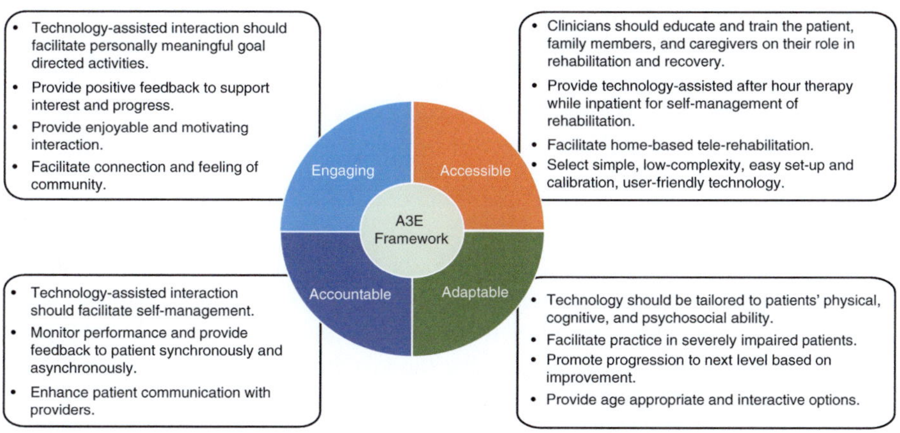

Fig. 8.1 The A3E framework for technology-aided rehabilitation can extend rehabilitation services beyond conventional care settings. (From Jayasree-Krishnan (2020), with permission)

technological solutions to serve patients with varying impairment levels in the physical, cognitive, and psychosocial domains. Accountability refers to patients' willingness to accept responsibility to continue rehabilitation even when they are not in direct contact with the provider, and engagement represents all the efforts that patients make during rehabilitation to derive benefit. Regardless of the specific technology used, a staged stepwise approach should target preservation of muscle length and range of motion, muscle strengthening, and functional performance, with frequent evaluation of progress to address any barriers that arise [39]. One example of a patient-provider partnership is the use of guided self-rehabilitation contracts (GSCs), a diary-based rehabilitation strategy where specific muscles are identified for self-stretching. A combination treatment using GSC for stretching and botulinum toxin injections for muscle overactivity demonstrated high compliance with GSC and improvement in composite active range of motion in adults with chronic spastic paresis [40]. In this study, the GSCs did not use any specific technology to aid stretching. Also, no direct comparisons were made between treatment with injections alone, GSCs alone, and the combined approach. However, the results favor the argument that the purpose of pharmacologic and technologic approaches in the treatment of spasticity and muscle stiffness should be to facilitate the process of rehabilitation beyond the clinic, and that patient education and engagement are key aspects in doing so. This study also points to the usefulness of the five-step assessment for selection of the appropriate treatment and for post-treatment evaluations as discussed below and detailed in Chap. 3 [41].

Medical and Pharmacologic Treatment Algorithm

As described above, the first line of treatment for individuals with spasticity and muscle stiffness is rehabilitation to restore and maintain movement capability. Medical and pharmacologic interventions are an adjunct to facilitate mobility and function. Figure 8.2 outlines a medical and pharmacologic treatment algorithm. Central to the algorithm is evaluation of the patient by a careful history and physical examination and the setting of collaborative patient-centered SMART (specific, measurable, achievable, relevant, and timely) goals based on the patient's experience of their symptoms and limitations [42].

The Patient's Experience

It is important to understand the patient's experience of spasticity and muscle stiffness as it has been shown to differ from the clinician's assessment [43–46]. For example, the vocabulary used to describe the symptoms of 'muscle tightness' by patients includes words such as 'tight', 'stiff', 'sore', and 'tender'. Patients may use metaphorical descriptors such as 'rock feeling', 'Charlie horse', and 'locked feeling' that contain pain and sensory experiences. On the other hand, clinicians may

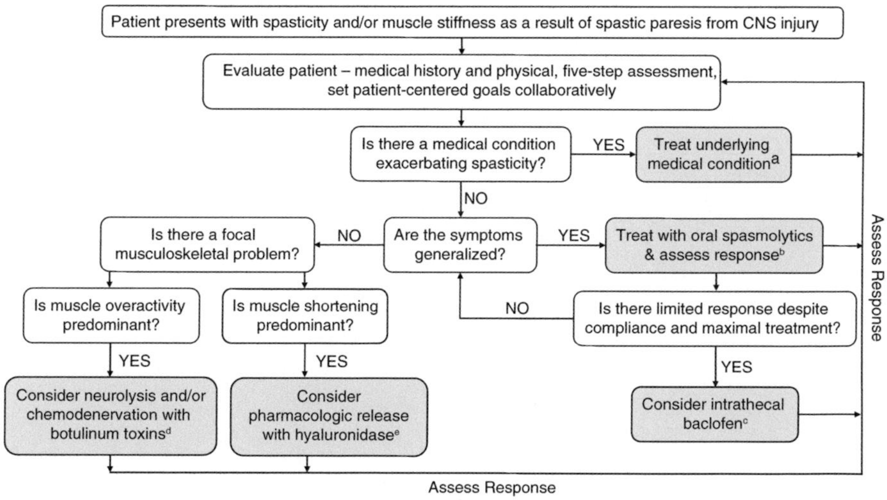

Fig. 8.2 Medical and pharmacologic algorithm for clinical decision-making regarding treatment. *CNS* central nervous system; [a]see Chap. 9; [b]see Chap. 10; [c]see Chap. 11; [d]see Chap. 12; [e]see Chap. 13

describe muscle tightness from a functional perspective using words such as 'restricted range of motion', 'contracted muscles', 'soreness', and 'fibrous band' which contain few descriptors of pain and sensory input. Overlapping vocabulary across patients and clinicians includes words such as 'stiffness', 'inflexible', 'spasm', 'tingling', 'knots', 'hard', and 'movement restrictions' [47]. Understanding the symptoms from the patient's perspective can enable appropriate goal setting, shared decision-making, and a successful response to treatment. A body diagram (Fig. 8.3) may assist in determining whether the symptoms are generalized or localized.

The medical history and physical should also include a thorough review of systems to determine whether a medical condition, such as a pressure sore, urinary tract infection, or constipation could be exacerbating spasticity and need to be treated first. Chapter 9 provides details on the medical exacerbation of spasticity and its treatment.

Many patients with spasticity, for example those with multiple sclerosis, may have multiple co-morbidities and interrelated symptoms such as fatigue, pain, and difficulty sleeping that may have to be assessed carefully to develop an individualized treatment strategy [48, 49]. It is also critical to reconcile medications as a sudden change in dose or frequency of spasmolytics can lead to symptoms of withdrawal and exacerbation of spasticity, as detailed in Chap. 10. Patients may also use non-medicinal cannabinoids via various routes such as smoking, vaping, topicals, tinctures and oils, and/or edibles, including foods, chocolate, and candy that may influence their symptoms and their treatment [50].

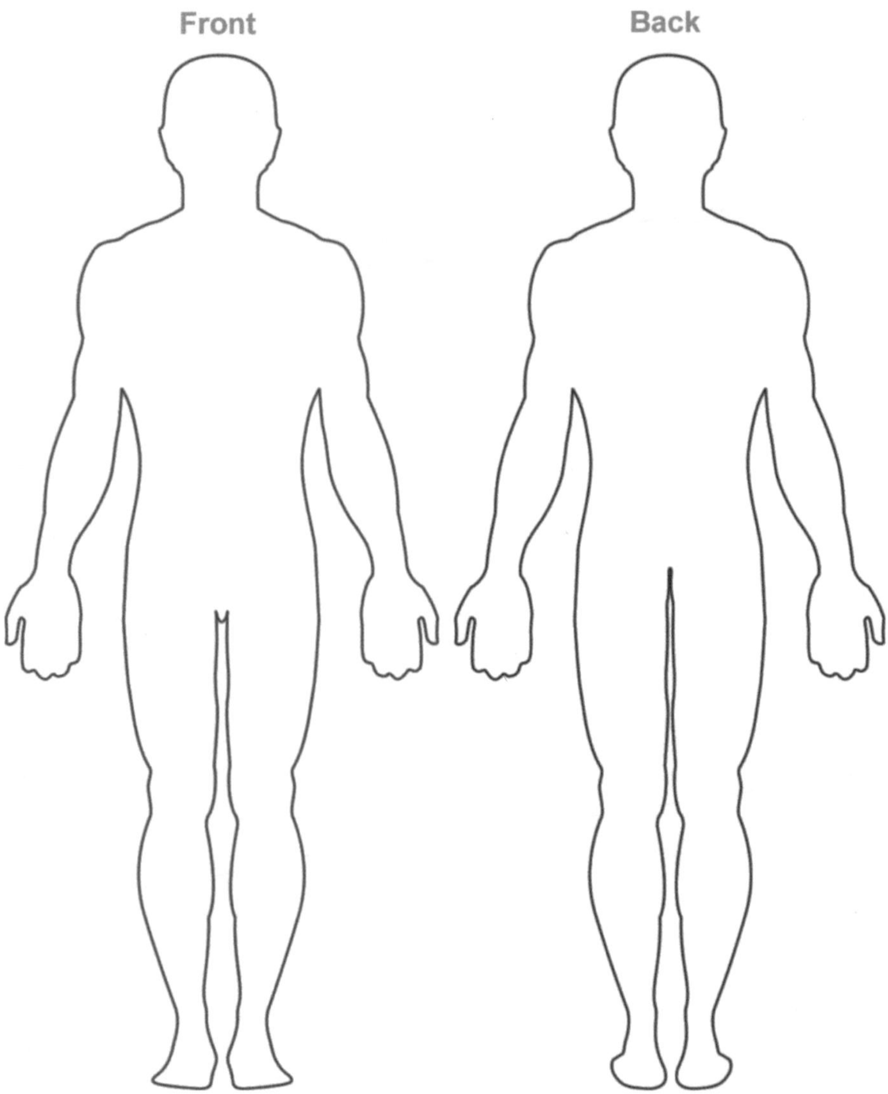

Fig. 8.3 A body diagram can be used to indicate areas of pain, discomfort, tightness or restriction to determine the degree to which the symptoms are generalized or localized for appropriate goal setting, shared decision-making, and assessment of treatment response. A blank body diagram is provided here as an example for the patient to fill out

Spasticity Versus Muscle Stiffness

Since the syndrome of spastic paresis consists of both neural and non-neural components as detailed in Chaps. 1, 2, 3, 4, 5, 6 and 7 in Part I of this book, accurate identification of the dominant component can assist with effective treatment. Spasticity is a neural phenomenon which can have both generalized manifestations such as hyperexcitability to sensory stimuli, exaggerated stretch reflexes, muscle spasms, and clonus, as well as focal manifestations such as overactivity of the antagonist muscle and/or hypoactivity of the agonist muscle across a joint, which together limit active movement. In contrast, muscle stiffness is a non-neural consequence of spasticity characterized by loss of extensibility of the muscle tissue due to increased muscle viscosity, which if untreated can eventually lead to contracture as detailed in Chap. 6. The affected muscles become physically shortened and demonstrate increased resistance to both active and passive movement [51], often producing deforming after-effects that are described in Chap. 7. Distinguishing between symptoms related predominantly to spasticity versus those related predominantly to muscle stiffness can be helpful to optimize focal treatment.

The Five-Step Assessment

Traditionally, the Modified Ashworth Scale (MAS) has been used to assess spasticity at the bedside and in the clinic. Although widely used, the MAS is limited in both inter- and intra-rater reliability, and cannot differentiate between the neural and non-neural components underlying the movement limitation, as demonstrated in Chap. 4. The five-step clinical assessment proposed by Gracies et al. is a comprehensive assessment that incorporates functional assessments as well as the Tardieu test and attempts to distinguish between predominantly neural and non-neural focal components contributing to the functional limitation [41]. *Step 1* assesses function using a standard test such as the 10 m walk test for the lower limb or the Modified Frenchay Scale for the upper limb. *Steps 2 and 3* assess passive range of motion at slow and fast speeds to differentiate between muscle shortening/stiffness (non-neural resistance at slow speed, X_{V1}) and spasticity (neural resistance at fast speed, X_{V3}) relative to the expected total range of motion at a given joint (X_N). *Steps 4 and 5* assess maximal active range of motion, X_A (due to neural weakness), and the decrement in range of motion with repetition X_R (due to fatigability and/or mild non-neural resistance). Coefficients of impairment can be derived based on these measurements to provide clinical guidance regarding treatment as detailed in Chap. 3 and summarized in Table 8.1.

Although these coefficients are theoretically derived, they provide a means to test the effect of specific treatments on the various coefficients of impairment. For example, the baseline coefficient of shortening was used to create a guided self-stretching program that resulted in increased passive range of motion in the stretched versus non-stretched muscles and increased ambulation speed [52]. However, there are a few caveats to bear in mind with the five-step assessment in the context of the quantitative data presented in Chap. 4. For example, the speed of elbow joint rotation did not clearly

Table 8.1 Coefficients of impairment derived from the five-step assessment, their interpretation, and implications for treatment

Coefficient of impairment	Interpretation	Treatment implication
Coefficient of shortening	Represents greater limitation in passive range of motion at slow speed suggesting non-neural passive resistance	Consider stretching, pharmacologic release of shortened/ stiff muscles, or surgical release in case of contracture
Coefficient of spasticity	Represents greater limitation in passive range of motion at fast speed likely due to neural muscle overactivity	Consider nerve (phenol or alcohol) or muscle (botulinum toxin) blocks to overactive muscles
Coefficient of weakness	Represents reduced active range of motion due to weakness	Consider strengthening using rehabilitation therapy and/or electrical stimulation
Coefficient of fatigability	Represents movement fatigability due to a combination of weakness and mild non-neural resistance	Consider combination treatment to strengthen appropriate muscle groups and reduce resistance/ stiffness by pharmacologic release

distinguish between passive resistance arising from neurally driven EMG overactivity versus non-neural stiffness associated with a minimal EMG response (see Chap. 4). This may make it difficult to differentiate between the coefficients of shortening and spasticity. In fact, patients who showed an EMG response showed a decreased catch angle as a function of joint rotation speed (i.e., the catch angle became smaller indicating greater extension with increasing speed of joint rotation), which is contrary to what is expected with spasticity. The acquisition of EMG signals along with joint motion data may provide a better understanding of the origins of the perceived resistance as demonstrated in Chap. 7, although it is highly likely that both neurally driven muscle overactivity and non-neural muscle stiffness coexist in most patients as they reinforce each other as explained in Chap. 6. Hence, consistent and periodic assessments of the response to treatment using objective measurements of function and active and passive range of motion may be the most practical manner of delineating neural and non-neural contributions to the movement restriction, and planning the next course of treatment in a staged manner. Diagnostic short-acting local anesthetic nerve blocks can also be a valuable screening tool in deciding whether to treat with longer-acting nerve blocks or botulinum toxin injections [53, 54]. New guidelines for the use of these agents in the treatment of spasticity have recently been released [55].

Generalized and Focal Treatments

Should the patient's symptoms be generalized, treatment may be initiated with oral spasmolytics individually or in combination. Chapter 10 details the various classes of medication, their mechanisms of action, clinical use, dosing and pharmacology, side-effect profile, and case studies to highlight salient aspects of treatment. Should symptoms remain generalized and severe despite compliance with maximal oral treatment, intrathecal baclofen may be considered. Chapter 11 details the components of intrathecal baclofen therapy, patient selection, the advantages, and disadvantages of the treatment, as well as the intrathecal baclofen trial, pump implantation, maintenance, troubleshooting, and pump explantation. Generalized treatments alone may be insufficient if there are focal musculoskeletal symptoms that contribute to discomfort and/or dysfunction, such as those described in Chap. 7.

If symptoms are localized to specific limb(s) or muscle group(s), it is helpful to ask if the symptoms can be attributed predominantly to muscle overactivity or to muscle shortening using the five-step assessment or its equivalent, measurement of EMG and resistance using instrumented tools, and/or screening using short-acting local anesthetics. Although these may be difficult to do precisely for several reasons discussed above, a consistent set of assessments will be most helpful to test the treatment hypothesis. If muscle overactivity is found to be a key driver of the focal symptoms, the treating clinician must decide if treatment-induced focal muscle weakness could potentially exacerbate the dysfunction as outlined in Chap. 2. Here, collaborative patient-centered decision-making may be helpful [42]. Partial nerve blocks using phenol or alcohol and/or chemodenervation using botulinum toxin injections to partially weaken overactive muscles may be appropriate. Details on the use of neurolysis using phenol and alcohol and newer techniques are outside the scope of this book, although the reader is referred to several pertinent sources [56–62]. Chapter 12 provides details on the use and guidelines for botulinum toxin injections.

Muscle shortening can be caused by immobility and inactivity, but also by muscle overactivity as discussed in detail in Chap. 6. Pharmacologic release of shortened stiff muscles using hyaluronidase injections is a new tool that shows promise in increasing passive and active range of motion in the upper limb [63, 64]. Chapter 13 provides details on the selection of patients and the available evidence using this new tool. Here, the treating clinician must decide if the muscle shortening is reversible. Should the patient already have irreversible contracture, referral for surgical treatment with or without serial casting in combination with other focal treatments may be warranted [65, 66].

Emerging Non-Pharmacologic Treatments

As our understanding of the neural basis and pathophysiology of spasticity and its consequences such as muscle stiffness and contracture continue to evolve, new treatments are likely to emerge. Chapter 14 discusses the many potentially promising emerging non-pharmacologic treatments available. These include peripheral electrical stimulation at the level of the skin (transcutaneous electrical nerve stimulation, TENS) and muscle (neuromuscular electrical stimulation, NMES; functional electrical stimulation, FES; breathing-controlled electrical stimulation, BreEStim), spinal cord stimulation (SCS), transcranial direct current stimulation (tDCS), transcranial magnetic stimulation (TMS), acupuncture, whole body vibration, and extracorporeal shockwave therapy, which have been studied in various populations such as stroke, spinal cord injury, multiple sclerosis, and cerebral palsy.

Conclusion

A key aspect of the framework for the treatment of spasticity and/or muscle stiffness from CNS injury is the stepwise restoration of movement and function to mitigate the negative effects of weakness, immobility, and inactivity. This requires a comprehensive evaluation including a patient-centered history and physical examination, as well as a five-step assessment which incorporates upper and lower limb functional ability, passive range of motion, and active range of motion with repetition of movement to determine the degree to which the symptoms are generalized or focal for appropriate selection of treatment(s). The evaluation may help distinguish between neural muscle overactivity versus non-neural muscle shortening for clinical decision-making about focal treatment with chemodenervation using neurolytic agents and botulinum toxins versus pharmacologic release with hyaluronidase injections, and assess the treatment response in a consistent and repeatable manner.

References

1. Kuypers HGJM. Anatomy of the descending pathways. In: Brooks VB, editor. Handbook of physiology. Bethesda: American Physiological Society; 1981.
2. Lance JW. Symposium synopsis. In: Feldman RG, Young RR, Koella WP, editors. Spasticity: disordered motor control. Chicago: Year Book Medical Publishers; 1980.
3. Pandyan AD, Gregoric M, Barnes MP, Wood D, Van Wijck F, Burridge J, et al. Spasticity: clinical perceptions, neurological realities and meaningful measurement. Disabil Rehabil. 2005;27(1–2):2–6.
4. Li S, Francisco GE, Rymer WZ. A new definition of poststroke spasticity and the interference of spasticity with motor recovery from acute to chronic stages. Neurorehabil Neural Repair. 2021;35:601. https://doi.org/10.1177/15459683211011214.
5. Kortebein P. Rehabilitation for hospital-associated deconditioning. Am J Phys Med Rehabil. 2009;88(1):66–77.
6. Jaul E, Factor H, Karni S, Schiffmiller T, Meiron O. Spasticity and dementia increase the risk of pressure ulcers. Int Wound J. 2019;16(3):847–51.
7. de Bruin M, Smeulders MJ, Kreulen M. Why is joint range of motion limited in patients with cerebral palsy? J Hand Surg Eur. 2013;38(1):8–13.
8. Qin W, Bauman WA, Cardozo C. Bone and muscle loss after spinal cord injury: organ interactions. Ann N Y Acad Sci. 2010;1211:66–84.
9. Herrmann M, Engelke K, Ebert R, Muller-Deubert S, Rudert M, Ziouti F, et al. Interactions between muscle and bone-where physics meets biology. Biomol Ther. 2020;10(3):432.
10. Pundik S, McCabe J, Skelly M, Tatsuoka C, Daly JJ. Association of spasticity and motor dysfunction in chronic stroke. Ann Phys Rehabil Med. 2019;62(6):397–402.
11. Oyanagi K, Kitai T, Yoshimura Y, Yokoi Y, Ohara N, Kohara N, et al. Effect of early intensive rehabilitation on the clinical outcomes of patients with acute stroke. Geriatr Gerontol Int. 2021;21(8):623–8.
12. Yen HC, Jeng JS, Chen WS, Pan GS, Chuang Pt Bs WY, Lee YY, et al. Early mobilization of mild-moderate intracerebral hemorrhage patients in a stroke center: a randomized controlled trial. Neurorehabil Neural Repair. 2020;34(1):72–81.
13. Boissoneault C, Grimes T, Rose DK, Waters MF, Khanna A, Datta S, et al. Innovative Long-dose neurorehabilitation for balance and mobility in chronic stroke: a preliminary case series. Brain Sci. 2020;10(8):555.

14. Daly JJ, McCabe JP, Holcomb J, Monkiewicz M, Gansen J, Pundik S. Long-dose intensive therapy is necessary for strong, clinically significant, upper limb functional gains and retained gains in severe/moderate chronic stroke. Neurorehabil Neural Repair. 2019;33(7):523–37.
15. Gaber TA. Significant reduction of the risk of venous thromboembolism in all long-term immobile patients a few months after the onset of immobility. Med Hypotheses. 2005;64(6):1173–6.
16. Hagen EM. Acute complications of spinal cord injuries. World J Orthop. 2015;6(1):17–23.
17. LaBan MM, Martin T, Pechur J, Sarnacki S. Physical and occupational therapy in the treatment of patients with multiple sclerosis. Phys Med Rehabil Clin N Am. 1998;9(3):603–14, vii.
18. Galea MP. Physical modalities in the treatment of neurological dysfunction. Clin Neurol Neurosurg. 2012;114(5):483–8.
19. Logan LR. Rehabilitation techniques to maximize spasticity management. Top Stroke Rehabil. 2011;18(3):203–11.
20. Dietz V. Proprioception and locomotor disorders. Nat Rev Neurosci. 2002;3(10):781–90.
21. Andringa A, Meskers C, van de Port I, van Wegen E, Kwakkel G. Time course of wrist hyper-resistance in relation to upper limb motor recovery early post stroke. Neurorehabil Neural Repair. 2020;34(8):690–701.
22. Daly JJ, McCabe JP, Gansen J, Rogers J, Butler K, Brenner I, et al. Gait coordination protocol for recovery of coordinated gait, function, and quality of life following stroke. J Rehabil Res Dev. 2012;49(8):xix–xxviii.
23. McCabe J, Monkiewicz M, Holcomb J, Pundik S, Daly JJ. Comparison of robotics, functional electrical stimulation, and motor learning methods for treatment of persistent upper extremity dysfunction after stroke: a randomized controlled trial. Arch Phys Med Rehabil. 2015;96(6):981–90.
24. van Kordelaar J, van Wegen EE, Nijland RH, Daffertshofer A, Kwakkel G. Understanding adaptive motor control of the paretic upper limb early poststroke: the EXPLICIT-stroke program. Neurorehabil Neural Repair. 2013;27(9):854–63.
25. Raghavan P. Upper limb motor impairment after stroke. Phys Med Rehabil Clin N Am. 2015;26(4):599–610.
26. Winters C, Kwakkel G, Nijland R, van Wegen E. Consortium EX-s. When does return of voluntary finger extension occur post-stroke? A prospective Cohort Study. PLoS One. 2016;11(8):e0160528.
27. Zandvliet SB, Kwakkel G, Nijland RHM, van Wegen EEH, Meskers CGM. Is recovery of somatosensory impairment conditional for upper-limb motor recovery early after stroke? Neurorehabil Neural Repair. 2020;34(5):403–16.
28. Levin MF, Kleim JA, Wolf SL. What do motor "recovery" and "compensation" mean in patients following stroke? Neurorehabil Neural Repair. 2009;23(4):313–9.
29. Butefisch C, Hummelsheim H, Denzler P, Mauritz KH. Repetitive training of isolated movements improves the outcome of motor rehabilitation of the centrally paretic hand. J Neurol Sci. 1995;130(1):59–68.
30. Kitago T, Krakauer JW. Motor learning principles for neurorehabilitation. Handb Clin Neurol. 2013;110:93–103.
31. Plautz EJ, Milliken GW, Nudo RJ. Effects of repetitive motor training on movement representations in adult squirrel monkeys: role of use versus learning. Neurobiol Learn Mem. 2000;74(1):27–55.
32. Halsband U, Lange RK. Motor learning in man: a review of functional and clinical studies. J Physiol Paris. 2006;99(4–6):414–24.
33. Vidoni ED, Boyd LA. Achieving enlightenment: what do we know about the implicit learning system and its interaction with explicit knowledge? J Neurol Phys Ther. 2007;31(3):145–54.
34. Stanley J, Krakauer JW. Motor skill depends on knowledge of facts. Front Hum Neurosci. 2013;7:503.
35. Subramanian SK, Massie CL, Malcolm MP, Levin MF. Does provision of extrinsic feedback result in improved motor learning in the upper limb poststroke? A systematic review of the evidence. Neurorehabil Neural Repair. 2010;24(2):113–24.

36. Ranganathan R, Lee MH, Newell KM. Repetition without repetition: challenges in understanding behavioral flexibility in motor skill. Front Psychol. 2020;11:2018.
37. Lee TD, Swanson LR, Hall AL. What is repeated in a repetition? Effects of practice conditions on motor skill acquisition. Phys Ther. 1991;71(2):150–6.
38. Jayasree-Krishnan V, Ghosh S, Palumbo A, Kapila V, Raghavan P. Developing a framework for designing and deploying technology-assisted rehabilitation after stroke: a qualitative study. Am J Phys Med Rehabil. 2021;100(8):774–9.
39. Richardson D. Physical therapy in spasticity. Eur J Neurol. 2002;9(Suppl 1):17–22. discussion 53-61
40. Gracies JM, Francisco GE, Jech R, Khatkova S, Rios CD, Maisonobe P, et al. Guided self-rehabilitation contracts combined with AbobotulinumtoxinA in adults with spastic paresis. J Neurol Phys Ther. 2021;45(3):203–13.
41. Gracies JM. Coefficients of impairment in deforming spastic paresis. Ann Phys Rehabil Med. 2015;58(3):173–8.
42. Turner-Stokes L, Ashford S, Esquenazi A, Wissel J, Ward AB, Francisco G, et al. A comprehensive person-centered approach to adult spastic paresis: a consensus-based framework. Eur J Phys Rehabil Med. 2018;54(4):605–17.
43. Bhimani RH, Peden-McAlpine C, Gaugler J, Anderson LC. Spasticity over time during acute rehabilitation: a study of patient and clinician scores. Appl Nurs Res. 2016;30:16–23.
44. Bhimani RH, McAlpine CP, Henly SJ. Understanding spasticity from patients' perspectives over time. J Adv Nurs. 2012;68(11):2504–14.
45. Mahoney JS, Engebretson JC, Cook KF, Hart KA, Robinson-Whelen S, Sherwood AM. Spasticity experience domains in persons with spinal cord injury. Arch Phys Med Rehabil. 2007;88(3):287–94.
46. Morley A, Tod A, Cramp M, Mawson S. The meaning of spasticity to people with multiple sclerosis: what can health professionals learn? Disabil Rehabil. 2013;35(15):1284–92.
47. Bhimani RH, Gaugler JE, Skay C. Understanding symptom experiences of muscle tightness from patients' and clinicians' perspectives. J Clin Nurs. 2017;26(13–14):1927–38.
48. Barin L, Salmen A, Disanto G, Babacic H, Calabrese P, Chan A, et al. The disease burden of Multiple Sclerosis from the individual and population perspective: which symptoms matter most? Mult Scler Relat Disord. 2018;25:112–21.
49. Gustavsen S, Olsson A, Sondergaard HB, Andresen SR, Sorensen PS, Sellebjerg F, et al. The association of selected multiple sclerosis symptoms with disability and quality of life: a large Danish self-report survey. BMC Neurol. 2021;21(1):317.
50. Rice J, Hildebrand A, Spain R, Senders A, Silbermann E, Wooliscroft L, et al. A cross-sectional survey of cannabis use by people with MS in Oregon and Southwest Washington. Mult Scler Relat Disord. 2021;55:103172.
51. Baude M, Nielsen JB, Gracies JM. The neurophysiology of deforming spastic paresis: a revised taxonomy. Ann Phys Rehabil Med. 2019;62(6):426–30.
52. Pradines M, Baude M, Marciniak C, Francisco G, Gracies JM, Hutin E, et al. Effect on passive range of motion and functional correlates after a Long-term lower limb self-stretch program in patients with chronic spastic paresis. PM R. 2018;10(10):1020–31.
53. Picelli A, Battistuzzi E, Filippetti M, Modenese A, Gandolfi M, Munari D, et al. Diagnostic nerve block in prediction of outcome of botulinum toxin treatment for spastic equinovarus foot after stroke: a retrospective observational study. J Rehabil Med. 2020;52(6):jrm00069.
54. Gracies JM, Elovic E, McGuire J, Simpson DM. Traditional pharmacological treatments for spasticity. Part I: local treatments. Muscle Nerve Suppl. 1997;6:S61–91.
55. Yelnik AP, Hentzen C, Cuvillon P, Allart E, Bonan IV, Boyer FC, et al. French clinical guidelines for peripheral motor nerve blocks in a PRM setting. Ann Phys Rehabil Med. 2019;62(4):252–64.
56. Karri J, Zhang B, Li S. Phenol neurolysis for management of focal spasticity in the distal upper extremity. PM R. 2020;12(3):246–50.

57. Kaymak B, Kara M, Gurcay E, Aydin G, Ozcakar L. Selective peripheral neurolysis using high frequency ultrasound imaging: a novel approach in the treatment of spasticity. Eur J Phys Rehabil Med. 2019;55(4):522–5.
58. Gonnade N, Lokhande V, Ajij M, Gaur A, Shukla K. Phenol versus Botulinum toxin a injection in ambulatory cerebral palsy spastic Diplegia: a comparative study. J Pediatr Neurosci. 2017;12(4):338–43.
59. Ploypetch T, Kwon JY, Armstrong HF, Kim H. A retrospective review of unintended effects after single-event multi-level Chemoneurolysis with botulinum toxin-A and phenol in children with cerebral palsy. PM R. 2015;7(10):1073–80.
60. Kocabas H, Salli A, Demir AH, Ozerbil OM. Comparison of phenol and alcohol neurolysis of tibial nerve motor branches to the gastrocnemius muscle for treatment of spastic foot after stroke: a randomized controlled pilot study. Eur J Phys Rehabil Med. 2010;46(1):5–10.
61. Elovic EP, Esquenazi A, Alter KE, Lin JL, Alfaro A, Kaelin DL. Chemodenervation and nerve blocks in the diagnosis and management of spasticity and muscle overactivity. PM R. 2009;1(9):842–51.
62. Zafonte RD, Munin MC. Phenol and alcohol blocks for the treatment of spasticity. Phys Med Rehabil Clin N Am. 2001;12(4):817–32, vii.
63. Raghavan P, Lu Y, Mirchandani M, Stecco A. Human recombinant hyaluronidase injections for upper limb muscle stiffness in individuals with cerebral injury: a case series. EBioMedicine. 2016;9:306–13.
64. Harlaar J. Diagnosis and treatment of spasticity and stiff muscles. EBioMedicine. 2016;9:23–4.
65. Long JT, Cobb L, Garcia MC, McCarthy JJ. Improved clinical and functional outcomes in Crouch gait following minimally invasive hamstring lengthening and serial casting in children with cerebral palsy. J Pediatr Orthop. 2020;40(6):e510–e5.
66. Leung J, King C, Fereday S. Effectiveness of a programme comprising serial casting, botulinum toxin, splinting and motor training for contracture management: a randomized controlled trial. Clin Rehabil. 2019;33(6):1035–44.

Medical Exacerbation of Spasticity

9

Steven R. Flanagan, Cynthia Hung, Robert Petrucelli, and Mark Ragucci

The coordinated physiological processes which maintain most of the steady states in the organism are so complex and so peculiar to living beings—involving, as they may, the brain and nerves, the heart, lungs, kidneys and spleen, all working cooperatively...
– Walter Bradford Cannon, The Wisdom of the Body, 1932.

- Spasticity is a common problem resulting from injury to or disease of the central nervous system (CNS). It can be exacerbated by common comorbidities associated with CNS dysfunction that disrupt autonomic nervous system homeostasis, creating an imbalance between parasympathetic and sympathetic outflow to the visceral organs.
- The pathophysiology may be similar to that underlying brain injury-related dysautonomia, also known as paroxysmal sympathetic hyperactivity (PSH).
- Medical exacerbation of spasticity commonly involves the genitourinary, gastrointestinal, musculoskeletal, vascular, and neurological systems.
- Successful management of medical exacerbation of spasticity requires an understanding of the underlying pathophysiology, early identification of the triggering factors, and timely implementation of treatment.

S. R. Flanagan (✉) · C. Hung · R. Petrucelli · M. Ragucci
Department of Rehabilitation Medicine, NYU Grossman School of Medicine, New York, NY, USA
e-mail: Steven.Flanagan@nyumc.org; cyhung@montefiore.org; Robert.Petrucelli@nyumc.org; Mark.Ragucci@nyumc.org

P. Raghavan (ed.), *Spasticity and Muscle Stiffness*,
https://doi.org/10.1007/978-3-030-96900-4_9

Introduction

Spasticity, broadly characterized by sensorimotor hyperexcitability, is a common feature of central nervous system (CNS) injury observed in individuals with multiple sclerosis, traumatic and non-traumatic brain injury, spinal cord injury, cerebral and spinal neoplasms, and cerebral palsy (see Chap. 1). It is estimated to affect between 40% and 80% of patients with spinal cord injury (SCI) and multiple sclerosis, up to 80% of patients with traumatic brain injury (TBI), and as many as 40% of patients poststroke [1]. It frequently has adverse consequences on functional ability and maintenance of hygiene and skin integrity, although in certain circumstances it may facilitate mobility and transfers.

Management of spasticity is challenging, and requires a thoughtful approach to assess its impact on function followed by a decision on whether and how to implement treatment, with the goal of optimizing function, hygiene, and pain control. Assessment begins with a thorough history and physical examination. Patients may complain of increased tone in the extremities, worsening pain, or a decline in mobility and/or ability to effectively perform activities of daily living. Caregivers may notice increased difficulty positioning the limbs that interferes with the ease of providing care. The physical exam and appropriate diagnostic tests provide additional information to guide treatment decisions as detailed in Chap. 8. A change in previously controlled spasticity should warrant an investigation of possible noxious, physiologic, and psychological triggers (see Table 9.1).

Many conditions that aggravate spasticity are common to all CNS injuries, whereas some such as posttraumatic syringomyelia, are specific to SCI. Practitioners

Table 9.1 Factors aggravating spasticity

Autonomic dysfunction
Bladder dysfunction
Body posture/position
Bowel dysfunction
Change in weather
Infectious process
Medication withdrawal
Menstrual cycle, pregnancy, labor and delivery
Orthopedic conditions
Pain
Poor fitting orthotics
Posttraumatic syringomyelia
Psychological conditions
Skin conditions
Thromboembolic disease
Time of day

need to consider the potential contribution of these exacerbating factors in planning treatment. Once identified, the aggravating factors need to be addressed, followed by an assessment as to whether additional intervention for persistent spasticity is warranted. Patient and caregiver education on identification of the potential causes of worsening spasticity is another important component in the overall care of the patient.

Although avoiding and treating the potential exacerbating conditions is part of a comprehensive rehabilitation plan, most conditions that increase spasticity have been reported in the literature as anecdotal observations. Scientific studies on the effects of medical conditions on spasticity are limited and have focused primarily on persons with SCI and autonomic dysfunction [2, 3]. Hence, this chapter will discuss the pathophysiology of autonomic dysfunction in individuals with spasticity and the medical conditions that lead to its exacerbation. Strategies for spasticity management associated with these exacerbating conditions are also presented.

Pathophysiology of Autonomic Dysfunction in Individuals with Spasticity

The autonomic nervous system maintains homeostasis through a balance between the parasympathetic and sympathetic outflow to the visceral organs. Although the precise reasons certain medical conditions exacerbate spasticity is unclear, the pathophysiology may be similar to that underlying brain injury-related dysautonomia, also known as paroxysmal sympathetic hyperactivity (PSH). PSH leads to hypertonia along with varying degrees of hyperthermia, hypertension, tachycardia, agitation, and diaphoresis [4]. The condition itself is a diagnosis of exclusion, requiring other medical causes to be ruled out [5]. Episodes of PSH can be caused by noxious stimuli such as endotracheal suctioning, passive movement, constipation, and urinary retention [6]. The same procedures and medical problems often exacerbate spasticity in individuals with other CNS disorders as well.

One theory underlying the pathophysiology of PSH suggests that it occurs as a result of dysfunction of autonomic centers of the brain, such as the thalamus, hypothalamus, and upper brainstem, including their connections to areas that mediate autonomic function [7]. It has been experimentally demonstrated in cats that stimulating the lateral hypothalamus elicits increased blood pressure, raised body hair and tail, pupillary constriction, and arching of the back [8]. The cerebral structures underlying autonomic control can be disinhibited due to injury to cortical and subcortical regions [9–11], resulting in what is often referred to as a disconnection syndrome. In a case series of nine patients with PSH reported by Rossitch and Bullard, a variety of etiologies induced PSH, including hydrocephalus, intracranial hemorrhage, and trauma [11]. The authors hypothesized that disinhibition of the diencephalon by increased intracranial pressure caused by these conditions leads to PSH. Boeve et al. further suggested that disinhibition of any of the sympathetic centers, including the paraventricular hypothalamic nucleus, lateral periaqueductal gray substance, lateral parabrachial nucleus, or rostral ventrolateral medulla may contribute to PSH [10].

Another theory is the excitatory-inhibitory ratio (EIR) model proposed by Baguley. It provides a pathophysiological explanation for several conditions in addition to PSH, including autonomic dysreflexia, neuroleptic malignant syndrome, malignant hyperthermia, serotonin syndrome, and stiff man syndrome [12]. The EIR model proposes that in the healthy state, there is a balance between the excitatory and inhibitory signals at the level of the brain stem and spinal cord. An imbalance of signals favoring excitation leads to motor and sympathetic hyperactivity. This may be derived from an "allodynic tendency." Allodynia results from sensitization of the spinal cord which makes non-painful stimuli become painful [13]. In this model, insufficient inhibitory signals from the brainstem and diencephalon result in allodynia [7]. The allodynic tendency model is supported by several case reports demonstrating the effectiveness of intrathecal baclofen (ITB) in ameliorating PSH [14, 15]. ITB acts predominantly at the level of the spinal cord to potentiate inhibition and may hence suppress allodynia which also occurs at the level of the spinal cord.

The sympathetic output from the CNS flows through sympathetic preganglionic neurons (SPNs) that lie mainly in the lateral regions of the thoracolumbar cord. These neurons innervate postganglionic sympathetic neurons to visceral organs or directly innervate certain organs, such as the adrenal glands. A series of elegant experiments in animals using viral tracers, which cross the synapses between sympathetic preganglionic neurons and interneurons, found spinal autonomic interneurons, which likely integrate information and help coordinate the precise and complex control of autonomic outflow to many end organs [16, 17]. The level of activity of these autonomic interneurons is influenced by a number of descending, local, and afferent inputs that together shape the final sympathetic output from the spinal cord [18]. These interneurons are located in laminae V, VII, and X and within the intermediolateral cell column (see Chap. 1) and have both inhibitory and excitatory roles [19, 20]. In addition, there are interneurons in lamina X, which are GABAergic and provide monosynaptic inhibitory inputs to SPNs [21]. These interneurons form part of the descending inhibitory control of SPNs that arises from the medial prefrontal cortex [22]. Stimulation of descending axons results in both monosynaptic excitatory and inhibitory responses in spinal autonomic interneurons [23, 24]. GABAergic pathways originating in the rostral ventrolateral medulla and caudal ventrolateral medulla may also provide direct input to the SPNs [25, 26]. Furthermore, axons from the rostral ventrolateral medulla and corticospinal tract closely appose both SPNs and interneurons [27] and can amplify or modulate spinal responses.

The GABAergic inputs onto SPNs, whether from local sources or from descending pathways, provide both tonic and phasic inhibition of sympathetic outflow. Tonic GABAergic inhibition is mediated via extrasynaptic GABA-A receptors that are sensitive to low GABA concentrations [28]. This can be of functional relevance especially in situations where there is increased sympathetic activity that may be detrimental to health. Diazepam acts on these receptors and enhances tonic inhibition, causing hypotension and reduced muscle sympathetic activity [29]. GABA-B receptors also play a role in controlling SPN activity and are present on the postsynaptic membrane as well as on the presynaptic terminals arising from both descending and local GABAergic inputs to SPNs [30]. Activation of somatic and visceral afferent inputs has a major influence on sympathetic activity, and these inputs always utilize interneurons. Stimulation of visceral afferents elicits mainly polysynaptic excitatory potentials in single sympathetic preganglionic neurons. In contrast, stimulation of somatic afferents inhibits the activity of sympathetic preganglionic neurons, an effect that persists in cats even after spinal cord transection [31]. However, the interneurons show exaggerated responses to somatic and visceral afferent stimulation especially in the chronic stage after spinal cord injury reflecting elevated levels of spinal excitability [32].

The interneurons in the sacral spinal cord play major roles in a number of reflexes, including micturition, defecation, and sexual function [20]. Micturition and defecation involve distinct spatially segregated populations of sympathetic preganglionic neurons, parasympathetic preganglionic neurons, and afferent terminations. During micturition, relaxation of the external urethral sphincter (EUS) is controlled by an excitatory pathway from the pontine micturition center to inhibitory interneurons in the sacral dorsal gray commissure mediated via glycine- and GABA-ergic interneurons [33, 34]. Many of the neurons lying between the parasympathetic preganglionic neurons and sympathetic preganglionic neurons are interneurons that may be critical links in coordinating the antagonistic excitation/inhibition of parasympathetic preganglionic neurons involved in the micturition and defecation reflexes. Some spinal interneurons may also be vital in orchestrating autonomic components of responses to, for example, pain [35] and so may have roles in addition to those mediating conventional autonomic reflexes.

The contribution of interneurons to spinal sympathetic activity can change considerably after injury to the CNS. For example, immediately after spinal cord injury, there is a decrease in sympathetic activity because of spinal shock [3]. An exaggerated hypotensive response without reflex tachycardia indicates loss of supraspinal pathways that would normally enable a reflex compensatory response. Two to four months post-injury, autonomic dysreflexia occurs in patients in whom the injury is above the sixth thoracic level [3]. It is thought that plasticity in local interneuronal networks provides the drive to these sympathetic circuits in the absence of supraspinal pathways [36]. There is evidence of local axonal sprouting from afferent inputs and local interneurons after spinal cord lesions [37], and interneurons themselves may show exaggerated responses to somatic and visceral stimulation due to elevated levels of spinal excitability [32, 38]. Given the pathophysiology described above, it is not surprising that intrathecally delivered baclofen, a GABA agonist, has been shown to be helpful in severe autonomic dysfunction associated with SCI [39–41] (see also Chaps. 10 and 11).

Medical Conditions that Exacerbate Spasticity

The Genitourinary Tract

An inadequately managed neurogenic bladder can have an adverse impact on spasticity and quality of life. People with neurological conditions constitute a large proportion of those requiring institutionalized care. Individuals confined to institutions also have a high rate of urinary incontinence that ranges from 30% to 70% [42]. This has societal, epidemiologic, and financial implications. For example, many stroke survivors cannot return home due to incontinence, and chronic spinal cord injury survivors report worsening of incontinence years after injury [43, 44].

The urinary bladder is the focus of most of the genitourinary (GU) tract dysfunction related to spasticity. The primary function of the urinary bladder is the storage of urine and coordinated bladder emptying. The innervation of the human urinary bladder is dense and complex. The process of elimination of urine or micturition begins when the proper time, place, and bladder volume signals the pontine micturition center (PMC), which initiates the contraction of the detrusor muscle and relaxation of the urinary sphincter [45]. The contraction of the detrusor muscle is initiated by the phosphorylation of light myosin chains and terminates with their dephosphorylation. Contraction also involves the release of calcium from intracellular stores within the detrusor muscle, which is controlled by calcium-specific channels in addition to an influx of potassium into the detrusor muscle cells [45]. In healthy individuals, the detrusor muscle consists of 50% smooth muscle. In contrast, the pelvic floor and bladder neck consist mostly of skeletal muscle for the conscious control of micturition [45].

It is well documented in the literature that individuals with neurological conditions, such as stroke and spinal cord injury, experience exacerbation of spasticity related to bladder infections and dysfunction. Approximately 76.9% of patients with spinal cord injury show increased spasticity in association with active infection, which commonly occurs in the urinary tract, and 50% of the same sample reported worsened spasticity in the presence of a full bladder [46]. In another study on individuals with spinal cord injury, 30% of urinary tract infections led to spasticity [47]. Incomplete bladder emptying in individuals with stroke was also commonly associated with worsened spasticity [48].

Urinary tract infection-induced spasticity can be relieved with appropriate antibiotic therapy. First-line antibiotics for uncomplicated urinary tract infections typically include nitrofurantoin, trimethoprim/sulfamethoxazole, and fosfomycin tromethamine [49]. Once culture and sensitivity results are available, antibiotics can be adjusted as needed to address the sensitivity profile of the bacteria. Traditionally, bacteriuria greater than 100,000 CFU/ml in urine culture is considered significant [49]. However, asymptomatic bacteriuria does not require treatment. Therefore, treatment based on symptoms, rather than solely on urinalysis or culture and sensitivity results, is generally recommended. The treatment duration for uncomplicated urinary tract infection typically ranges from 3 to 7 days depending on the antibiotic used, although longer treatment durations may be required for complicated infections [49].

Neurogenic bladder should be managed aggressively to prevent spasticity and GU system pathology. The bladder functions in a fairly predictable manner based on the anatomical location of the CNS lesion. Suprapontine lesions above the pontine micturition center, such as from a stroke usually lead to detrusor overactivity, causing patients to complain of urgency. Suprasacral lesions from injury to the spinal cord often lead to detrusor-external sphincter dyssynergia, characterized by poorly coordinated detrusor and sphincter activity that leads to incomplete bladder emptying and high intra-bladder pressures. Damage to the sacral spinal cord leads to an acontractile or flaccid bladder. Formal determination of the type of neurogenic bladder is achieved through urodynamic testing. Other tests to consider when assessing the status of the urinary system include renal and bladder ultrasound, cystography, cystoscopy, and serum creatinine levels [50]. The goal of treatment is to prevent urinary tract infections and upper urinary tract damage while maintaining a balanced bladder, i.e., avoiding over distention of the bladder by controlled regular emptying [51].

For those with urinary urgency, for example from incomplete spinal cord injury, who have the capacity to empty their bladder voluntarily, timed voiding can be tried. With timed voiding, patients are cued to empty their bladder at regular intervals to prevent uncontrolled bladder evacuation that would otherwise occur as the bladder becomes distended. In certain circumstances and for limited periods of time, a Credé maneuver can be performed which involves applying manual pressure on the bladder to facilitate voiding. Similarly, a Valsalva maneuver, where the patient breathes out strongly while holding the nose and mouth tightly closed, can also facilitate voiding. However, these techniques should not be used long term as they can lead to back flow of urine into the kidneys and result in pyuria, urinary lithiasis, ureteral distention, hydronephrosis, and renal damage [51]. For individuals with trouble emptying their bladder, intermittent catheterization may be performed, and it is the preferred method of bladder emptying in persons with spinal cord injury who do not have voluntary control of micturition. Intermittent catheterization is generally performed every 4–6 hours with the goal of keeping the bladder volume below 500 mL [50]. If bladder volumes exceed 500 mL, fluid restriction or increasing the frequency of catheterizations may be required. The main complication of intermittent catheterization is urinary tract infection, but the risk is acceptably low when using proper technique. Patients with poor cognition are not good candidates for intermittent catheterization unless they have a caretaker that can perform the procedure.

An indwelling urinary catheter can also be used for bladder emptying; however, complications such as renal/bladder stones, urethral fistulas, strictures, urethral erosions, renal failure, and bladder cancer are increased. An indwelling urinary catheter may be a preferred option for women with upper-level spinal cord injury and poor hand function [50].

Surgical options include the insertion of a suprapubic tube; this option avoids urethral trauma as there is no need to repeatedly pass a catheter through the urethra several times a day. This is a reasonable option for individuals with tetraplegia who do not have a caretaker to perform intermittent catherization [50]. The complications rates of urinary tract infections, bladder/renal calculi, and cancer are similar to that with indwelling urinary catheters [52]. When conservative measures have failed, other surgical options can be considered. External urethral sphincterotomy involves making an incision into the 12 o'clock area of the bulbar urethra. This is a potential option for individuals with detrusor sphincter dyssynergia or for those who fail intermittent catheterization [50].

Augmentation cystoplasty involves increasing the size of the bladder to lower bladder pressures that would otherwise result in renal injury over time [50]. Urinary diversion can be achieved with an ileal conduit where the ureters are connected to a detached portion of the ileum. The ileum is brought out through a stoma in the abdomen that connects to a urine collecting bag [53]. Urinary diversion may be considered for individuals with tetraplegia who cannot perform intermittent catheterization and for those with recurrent urinary tract infections due to an indwelling catheter [50]. Sacral nerve stimulation is another option for which an electrode is placed at the 3rd sacral root. A neurostimulator located subcutaneously can be activated to trigger bladder emptying [54]. An artificial urinary sphincter can also be placed; the sphincter occludes the urethra from the inside, and is controlled by a pump in the labia or scrotum [54].

Pharmacologic interventions can also be used to manage a neurogenic bladder and may decrease the risk of worsening spasticity. Anticholinergic medications, such as tolterodine and oxybutynin, are considered the mainstay of treatment for detrusor overactivity [55]. They work by inhibiting detrusor contraction and increasing bladder compliance. Their anticholinergic actions are the source of side effects, which include dry mouth and constipation. Alpha-adrenoreceptor antagonists, or alpha blockers such as tamsulosin or terazosin, relax the smooth muscle of the prostate and bladder neck allowing for better urine flow. Studies have shown that they can improve bladder compliance leading to lower intravesical pressures, decrease detrusor overactivity, and promote more complete bladder emptying. These medications work best in individuals who retain some ability to void. A beta-3 agonist, mirabegron, relaxes the detrusor muscle, and has a similar impact on bladder function as anticholinergics. Its major side effects are small increases in blood pressure and heart rate. There is a paucity of studies of mirabegron in the neurogenic bladder population, but it is used occasionally. Cholinergics like bethanechol are used for areflexic bladders but can cause bronchospasm and miosis as side effects [55].

Botulinum toxin injections have also been used to treat detrusor overactivity [54]. The toxin binds to the muscle nerve terminal and prevents the presynaptic release of acetylcholine, thus inhibiting bladder contraction. The effects of botulinum toxin wear off in 3–6 months, hence repeat injections are often needed. Other less commonly used medications include imipramine and desmopressin [55]. Imipramine relaxes the detrusor muscle and decreases bladder overactivity. However, it must be used with caution in the elderly due to the risk of adverse cardiac events. Desmopressin is used for nocturnal polyuria.

The Gastrointestinal System

Persons with SCI often have problems with fecal elimination [56]. Gastrointestinal (GI) dysfunction associated with spasticity is predominantly characterized by constipation and fecal impaction. Upper GI problems such as bloating, nausea, and early satiety occur less commonly. Significant advancements have recently been made in understanding the physiology of GI tract motility, including the interactions between the brain, spinal cord, and the autonomic and enteric nervous systems. Normal functioning of the stomach and intestines requires coordinated muscle contraction, digestion, absorption of nutrients, and regulation of blood flow. This coordination is much more complex than previously realized. The enteric nervous system (ENS) is a distinct nervous system consisting of its own set of neurons that coordinates sensory and motor functions of the GI tract. ENS ganglia are interconnected, creating highly organized circuitry that processes sensory input from the gut and generates reflex responses to various stimuli [57].

The vagus nerve relays sensory information from the ENS to the medullary nuclei in the brainstem. Multiple neurotransmitters are involved in the connections of the vagus nerve complex including acetylcholine, biogenic amines, amino acids, nitric oxide, and various peptides. Spinal afferent and efferent neurons are responsible for sending signals via the pudendal nerve to coordinate the process of defecation. The musculature of the pelvic floor, including the internal anal sphincter, puborectalis, external anal sphincter, and levator ani, in addition to those involved in squatting that open the distal anal canal, are involved in normal defecation [56].

There is sparse information in the medical literature regarding spasticity-related GI complications [58]. In one study on manifestations of GI fullness in spinal cord injury, about 30% of patients reported increased spasticity with the sensation of defecation [59]. Neurogenic bowel caused by SCI is initially managed with conservative measures to promote regular emptying without accidents, which include dietary modifications, adequate fluid intake, and bowel movement habits. Increasing dietary fiber and fluid intake helps to prevent constipation, and timing bowel movements after eating takes advantage of the gastrocolic reflex that promotes bowel evacuation [60]. Although increasing dietary fiber is a mainstay for preventing constipation in the general population, a small case series of subjects with a spinal cord injury indicated that it may actually slow GI motility [61]. Digital rectal stimulation, which increases motility in the left colon by activating the anorectal colonic reflex, can serve as an adjunct to laxatives and enemas to promote bowel emptying [60]. Abdominal massage has also been shown to increase the frequency of bowel movements in a pre-post study in 24 individuals with spinal cord injury [62].

Oral laxatives are often used in the management of neurogenic bowel and are categorized into bulking agents, osmotic laxatives, stimulant laxatives, and stool softeners [63]. Bulking agents include bran, wheat husk, and psyllium fiber, which promote increased fluid retention in the colon and contribute to stool softness, although as previously noted, they may slow GI motility. Osmotic laxatives include mannitol, sorbitol, lactulose, polyethylene glycol, and magnesium citrate, which retain water in the feces to facilitate colonic transport. Stimulant laxatives such as bisacodyl, senna, and glycerol act on the intestinal mucosa to increase GI motility. Docusate, a commonly prescribed stool softener, reduces stool firmness. A newer drug called prucalopride is a selective serotonin receptor agonist that has been shown in a small randomized controlled trial of 12 subjects to increase bowel movement frequency and improve stool consistency [64]. However, moderate-to-severe abdominal pain was noted as a side effect in four subjects.

Suppositories are often used to prevent constipation due to neurogenic bowel. Bisacodyl, which is most often prescribed in this category, acts directly on the mucosa to stimulate the sensory fibers, leading to a parasympathetic response, which results in increased peristalsis in the large intestine and also stimulates fluid and electrolyte accumulation in the colon for softening effects [63].

Other techniques that have been investigated include transanal irrigation and external electrical stimulation of the abdomen. Transanal irrigation was shown to improve incontinence and constipation in a randomized controlled trial (RCT) with 87 subjects with spinal cord injury [65]. External electrical stimulation of the abdomen, with an abdominal belt, increased colonic transit time in an RCT in 10 subjects with SCI [66].

For refractory constipation, surgical options may be considered. These include sacral anterior root stimulation, colostomy, and the malone antegrade continence enema (MACE) where an entry point into the colon is created for irrigation [60]. These options are typically not considered until at least after one year post spinal cord injury, as bowel habits will likely have stabilized by that time.

Skin Conditions

Skin is the largest organ system in the body. It is composed of two broad layers—the epidermis and dermis. Both acute and chronic spasticity can be exacerbated by noxious stimuli, such as ingrown toenails, infections, decubitus ulcers, and ill-fitting clothing. Proper identification and treatment of skin-related problems can reduce the intensity of spasticity in susceptible patients [46, 67].

Preventing the development of pressure sores is key to averting the exacerbation of spasticity in those with neurological disability. Regular repositioning throughout the day is critical to preventing decubitus ulcers. However, once skin breakdown has occurred, the avoidance of pressure on the affected area becomes of paramount importance [68]. A high protein diet (25% protein diet) is helpful in ensuring skin health as well as in healing existing pressure sores [69]. Proper skin cleansing that includes debridement of necrotic tissue on established sores, avoidance of excessive friction, and maintenance of adequate hydration are mandatory components of a comprehensive prevention and treatment plan to promote healthy skin [68]. Vacuum-assisted wound closure can also assist with healing of decubitus ulcers [68].

Cleaning decubitus ulcers is important for wound healing. It helps prevent infection and promotes a healthy environment for healing. Cleaning is typically achieved with tap water or normal saline, although dilute 0.5% acetic acid can be used as an anti-microbial cleansing medium for short periods of time [68]. Other topical antimicrobials that can be used for superficially-infected wounds include dilute povidone iodine, cadexomer iodine, metronidazole gel, silver-containing products, and manuka honey. However, these products should be stopped once the wound is clean to discourage the development of bacterial resistance [68]. The presence of sepsis or osteomyelitis requires systemic antibiotics [69].

Managing decubitus ulcers requires debridement of nonviable tissue, which can be achieved by mechanical, surgical, enzymatic, autolytic, or biological methods [68]. Surgical debridement with a scalpel or scissors may require anesthesia. Surgical debridement should be avoided in ischemic limbs or heel ulcers due to the already poor blood supply which may further impede healing. Mechanical debridement may involve packing with saline moistened gauze or the "wet-to-dry" technique, whirlpool, pulsed lavage, ultrasound, and debridement pads with monofilaments. This can be painful, requiring proper selection of patients as well as possible pretreatment with analgesics. Autolytic debridement uses endogenous enzymes to break down nonviable wound tissue, which can be achieved by keeping the wound moist in its own fluid. Enzymatic debridement uses enzymes such as collagenase to break down devitalized tissue. Biologic debridement uses insect larvae, such as maggots, to remove nonviable tissue; it is reserved for very difficult fibrinous wounds and may be painful.

Appropriate moisture balance is important in wound healing as moisture promotes keratinocyte migration [68]. Various types of moisture retentive dressings are readily available and include films, foams, hydrocolloids, alginates, and hydrogels. Films are thin layers of elastic polyurethane that provide good coverage of donor sites of split thickness skin grafts. Foams are useful for mild-to-moderate exudative wounds and are especially helpful over bony prominences. Hydrocolloids are useful in the presence of mild amounts of exudate and are waterproof. Alginates are derived from algae or kelp, and are used for wounds with heavy exudates. Hydrogels can be squeezed onto a wound or made into sheets that are placed on the surface for dry necrotic wounds.

Heterotopic Ossification

Heterotopic ossification (HO) is the formation of mature, lamellar bone in extraskeletal soft tissue. It occurs around joints such as the hip, knee, shoulder, and elbow following CNS injury, and commonly co-occurs with spasticity [70, 71]. It can also be associated with non-neurological conditions such as burns, fractures, and after total joint arthroplasty. It is often painful, providing a noxious stimulus that can further exacerbate spasticity.

The reported incidence of HO varies widely from 11% to 75% following severe TBI and SCI [72, 73]. The difference in reported rates is likely due to differences in the methodology used in the epidemiological studies. The joints most commonly involved in patients with TBI are the hips, elbows, shoulders, and knees. After a stroke, the joints commonly involved are the elbows and shoulders. In patients with SCI, HO usually occurs below the neurological level of injury, commonly at the hip, knee, shoulder, and elbow.

The exact etiology and pathophysiologic mechanisms of HO are not well delineated. Proposed mechanisms include an alteration of neuronal control over the differentiation of mesenchymal cells into osteoblasts which form bone. Both CNS and local factors likely play a role, leading to inflammation and increased blood flow to the affected tissues [74, 75].

HO can occur as early as two weeks post-injury, but it is more commonly observed 1–4 months post-injury [75]. The signs and symptoms include local soft tissue swelling, erythema, heat/warmth around the joint, pain, and decreased range of motion which may be associated with low-grade fever. The differential diagnosis of a painful, swollen limb, or joint includes infection, trauma, and venous thrombosis, all of which need to be systematically ruled out. The three-phase bone scan remains the gold standard for detecting early HO, with positive findings observed at the time clinical signs and symptoms develop. X-ray findings typically take weeks to show abnormal bone formation after clinical signs appear. Abnormal laboratory tests include elevated serum alkaline phosphatase, which is nonspecific, and thus supports rather than confirms the diagnosis. Alkaline phosphatase levels rise as early as two weeks after the process begins and reach a peak at approximately 10 weeks, returning to normal as the heterotopic bone matures [76].

Non-surgical and surgical treatments can be used to manage HO, and include early joint mobilization which may be achieved with range of motion exercises. The goal of joint mobilization is to prevent contractures and maintain functional range of motion [77]. Medications are often used for prophylaxis and treatment. Nonsteroidal anti-inflammatory drugs (NSAIDs) are commonly used to reduce bone formation by the inhibition of prostaglandin synthase and they also reduce inflammation [78]. Indomethacin is the most widely used NSAID for this indication. Etidronate disodium, a bisphosphonate, has been shown to reduce progression of the ossification process [78]. However, it does not eliminate bone that has already formed.

The only definitive treatment for mature HO is surgical excision. Common indications for surgical resection of HO include immobile joints that significantly impair activities of daily living, mobility, maintenance of adequate hygiene, or lead to skin breakdown, pain, and/or the development of peripheral neuropathies [71]. The optimal timing of surgical resection is not well-defined; note that the resection of immature HO may result in its reoccurrence. Some have proposed waiting for a period of 12–18 months prior to resection [79, 80]. However, others have suggested that earlier resection can be performed with similar rates of reoccurrence, thus avoiding the physical limitations and pain associated with HO as well as the potential complications of long-term joint immobility [81, 82].

Venous Thromboembolism

In patient populations at risk for developing spasticity, venous thromboembolism (VTE), which encompasses deep venous thrombosis (DVT) and pulmonary embolism, are major causes of mortality and morbidity. Virchow's triad, i.e., venous stasis, endothelial injury, and hypercoagulability, is thought to be the basis for VTE development, although the existence of all three components of the triad is not necessary for thrombosis. The risk of VTE varies based on the underlying medical and surgical comorbidities and specific characteristics of each individual patient [83]. In the population at risk for spasticity, where early immobility post-onset is common (e.g., stroke, CNS trauma, and non-traumatic neurological conditions), the risk of VTE is high. The risk further increases in these conditions following neurological surgery, in the presence of concurrent orthopedic injures, or with marked paralysis of the lower limbs [83].

Prophylaxis against VTE is of primary importance and is considered standard of care in hospitalized settings. The most appropriate choice of prophylaxis is guided by a thorough risk-benefit analysis for each patient. Chemical prophylaxis should be initiated as soon as it is deemed acceptable. Options for chemical prophylaxis include low molecular weight or unfractionated heparin, fondaparinux, new oral anticoagulants, or warfarin. Options for mechanical prophylaxis include intermittent pneumatic compression devices and/or graduated compression stockings. The duration of prophylaxis varies by the underlying diagnosis and the length of immobility.

Common symptoms of DVT include pain, fever, warmth, and edema of the affected limb, although there may not be any signs or symptoms. Therefore, practitioners must be mindful of the potential presence of DVT and regularly assess for the signs and symptoms of DVT during bedside examination. Calf tenderness, edema, warmth, or a positive Homans sign suggest the presence of a DVT which requires pursuing definitive tests, and appropriate management if the diagnosis is confirmed. Pulmonary embolism is a complication of DVT, and a leading cause of early mortality that requires vigilance in prevention and early diagnosis. The signs and symptoms of pulmonary embolism typically include shortness of breath, tachycardia, and hypoxia.

The diagnosis of DVT is made by venous ultrasonography, which is easy to obtain and has high sensitivity and specificity for detecting proximal vein thrombosis. Contrast venography is considered the gold standard, although it is rarely used as an initial screening test. D-Dimer assay is a serum laboratory test that can be employed for the detection of DVT. It has high sensitivity but low specificity, and thus is a useful tool for ruling out DVT. However, the assay can be elevated in many other conditions including trauma, post-surgery, hemorrhage, sepsis, and malignancy making a positive test non-diagnostic for DVT.

Once a DVT has been diagnosed, the goals of treatment are to prevent pulmonary embolism and late vascular complications, including post-thrombotic syndrome. The American College of Chest Physicians has published anticoagulation guidelines for treatment that ranges between three months to indefinite use based on the inciting event and the risk factors [84]. Inferior vena cava filters are reserved for patients who have a contraindication to anticoagulation as there is a risk of thrombosis around the filter, and an increased risk of DVT in individuals with filters.

Fractures

Bone fractures are common comorbidities in patients with neurological trauma and stroke, which can exacerbate spasticity. Fractures often occur at the time of the injury, although physical and cognitive impairments that occur as a result of the neurological injury also place patients at risk for fall-related fractures. Falls are a leading cause of fractures; hence, patients with neurological disability should be carefully assessed to establish their fall risk, followed by specific interventions to mitigate the risk. Interventions to mitigate fall risk include, but are not limited to, physical therapy to improve balance, mobility skills, and strength in addition to home and other environmental modifications that may decrease the rate of falls and fractures [85].

Immobility-related osteopenia due to neurological impairment and the ensuing inactivity also increases the risk of fractures. Thus, resumption of weight-bearing activities and mobility should be initiated as soon as is medically appropriate post-injury to reduce bone loss [86]. Supplementation with ergocalciferol and oral bisphosphonates has been shown to be helpful in preventing hip fractures following stroke [87, 88]. In certain neurological conditions, including TBI, excessive callus formation at the site of the fracture can result in additional noxious stimulation to surrounding soft tissues, potentially resulting in exacerbation of spasticity.

Patients with stroke are at increased risk for fractures, especially at the hip [89]. Hip fractures are associated with high morbidity and mortality in the elderly. A large study found that the risk of fractures increased sevenfold during the first year after stroke, largely due to falls that significantly increased during this time [90]. Elderly patients with stroke are also likely to have age-associated osteopenia in addition to paresis which results in reduced weight bearing and accelerates bone loss [91].

Prolonged immobilization after SCI also results in osteopenia and increases the risk for fractures [92]. Decreased bone density is initially observed during the first few weeks after injury, and occurs below the neurological level of injury [93]. Bone loss is most pronounced during the first two years after injury but can be prolonged for up to seven years [94]. Fractures observed after SCI commonly occur from low energy injuries and in bones distal to the level of injury, most often in the femur, tibia, and fibula [95, 96].

Patients suspected of a fracture require prompt physical assessment and appropriate imaging including X-rays and/or computerized tomography. Orthopedic consultation should be obtained and followed by fracture management that is guided by the nature of the fracture as well as other clinical considerations. In patients with chronic SCI who do not use the fractured extremity for functional mobility, the goal of management is to minimize complications [97]. This may include non-operative management with splinting, such as with a knee immobilizer for a femoral shaft fracture. Surgery and casting may not be indicated due to potential complications such as skin breakdown in limbs that are insensate. Appropriate management of a patient's hip fracture may also include operative fixation.

Management of Paroxysmal Sympathetic Hyperactivity

Paroxysmal sympathetic hyperactivity (PSH) is a condition that occurs after brain injury, characterized by episodes of hypertension, tachypnea, tachycardia, diaphoresis, hyperthermia, and motor posturing or dystonia, often in response to external stimuli [4, 98]. Several terms have been used to describe this condition, including dysautonomia, autonomic storms, sympathetic storms, diencephalic seizures, and paroxysmal autonomic instability with dystonia (PAID) [98, 99]. It is associated with elevated serum levels of cortisol, adrenocorticotropic hormone, norepinephrine, epinephrine, and dopamine, suggesting that the term PSH most appropriately describes the condition. Eighty percent of the cases of PSH are associated with acquired cerebral pathology [99].

The pathophysiology of PSH is poorly understood. Initial studies suggested a relationship to epileptic activity; however, electroencephalographic data revealed no causative seizure activity and anti-epileptics fail to ameliorate PSH [9, 100]. PSH is a diagnosis of exclusion, requiring practitioners to assess for other possible conditions that share similar clinical signs. Infection, intracranial hypertension, hydrocephalus, agitation, pain, opioid or sedative withdrawal, malignant hyperthermia, seizures, and systemic inflammatory response syndrome should be considered in the differential diagnosis. Other conditions that can worsen spasticity should also be ruled out including heterotopic ossification and fractures [100, 101].

An international panel of brain injury experts was recently formed to develop a consensus-based term for the condition and to provide diagnostic guidelines for research and clinical purposes [101]. The experts agreed on the term PSH and defined it as "a syndrome, recognized in a sub-group of survivors of severe acquired brain injury, of simultaneous, paroxysmal transient increases in sympathetic (elevated heart rate, blood pressure, respiratory rate, temperature, sweating) and motor (posturing) activity." The panel recognized that PSH would need to remain a diagnosis of exclusion but agreed to develop a two-part tool called the Paroxysmal Sympathetic Hyperactivity—Assessment Measure consisting of the Clinical Feature Scale based on symptom severity, and the Diagnosis Likelihood Tool to establish the likelihood of the diagnosis based on the presence of specific criteria (Table 9.2).

For the Clinical Feature Scale, heart rate, respiratory rate, systolic blood pressure, temperature, sweating, and posturing are assessed. Scores for each clinical sign range from 0 to 3 based on the degree of aberration in vitals and presentation of the clinical signs. Table 9.2 outlines the thresholds for each category. Sweating is categorized as 0 if there is no sweating, as 1 if there is mild sweating seen as moist or glistening skin, as 2 if there is moderate sweating seen as beads of sweat, and as 3 if there is profuse sweating. Posturing is categorized as 0 if there is no increased tone, as 1 if there is mildly increased tone that is easily breakable, as 2 if there is moderate tone that is hard to overcome, and as 3 if there is rigidity. On the Diagnosis Likelihood Tool, one point is provided for each criterion that is present. Some of the criteria are redundant and intended to give more points when more criteria are met. For example, a duration of two weeks will automatically give two points since it meets two criteria. The two subsection scores are added to provide a score that ranges from 0 to 29. Scores less than 8 indicate that PSH is unlikely, whereas scores between 8 and 16 indicate a possible diagnosis. Scores greater than 17 indicate a probable diagnosis of PSH. The tool is also useful for assessing the severity of PSH, as well as the response to treatment, and can help smooth transitions in care.

Table 9.2 Paroxysmal sympathetic hyperactivity—assessment measure

Clinical Feature Scale (CFS)					
	0	1	2	3	Score
Heart rate	<100	100–119	120–139	≥140	
Respiratory rate	<18	18–23	24–29	≥30	
Systolic blood pressure	<140	140–159	160–179	≥180	
Temperature (°C)	<37	37–37.9	38–38.9	≥39.0	
Sweating	Nil	Mild	Moderate	Severe	
Posturing	Nil	Mild	Moderate	Severe	
				CFS subtotal	
			Nil	0	
Severity of clinical features			Mild	1–6	
			Moderate	7–12	
			Severe	≥13	
Diagnosis Likelihood Tool (DLT)					
Clinical features occur simultaneously					
Episodes are paroxysmal in nature					
Sympathetic over-reactivity to normally non-painful stimuli					
Features persist ≥3 consecutive days					
Features persist ≥2 weeks post-brain injury					
Features persist despite treatment of alternative differential diagnoses					
Medication administered to decrease sympathetic features					
≥2 episodes daily					
Absence of parasympathetic features during episodes					
Absence of other presumed cause of features					
Antecedent acquired brain injury					
(Score 1 point for each feature present)				DLT subtotal	
Combined total (CFS + DLT)					
			Unlikely	<8	
PSH diagnostic likelihood			Possible	8–16	
			Probable	>17	

Republished with permission of Mary Ann Liebert, Inc. Publishers, from Baguley et al. [101]
PSH paroxysmal sympathetic hyperactivity

Treatments for PSH are supported only by low-quality evidence consisting predominantly of case reports and case series. There have been no published randomized controlled trials. Furthermore, it is unclear whether early aggressive intervention impacts the long-term outcome of patients. PSH is often elicited in susceptible patients by noxious or painful stimuli. Thus, prophylactic treatment, particularly prior to a stimulus known to exacerbate PSH, may prevent or ameliorate the intensity of the response. Gabapentin, which binds to presynaptic calcium channels, prevents the excitatory neurotransmission of pain signals and has been used predominantly for prevention of PSH [98]. Gabapentin is typically started at 300 mg daily and the dose is gradually increased to three times daily. Thereafter, the dose can be increased by 100–300 mg per dose per day, up to a maximum dose of 3600 mg per day [100].

Opioids are considered a first-line option for treatment of PSH [98]. Oxycodone can be started at 5 mg and titrated up in 5 mg increments every 4 h as needed. Morphine can be given at a dose of 1–2 mg intravenously every 1 or 2 hours, and titrated to control clinical signs [100]. However, one must watch for respiratory depression, sedation, hypotension, ileus, and nausea and vomiting [102].

Benzodiazepines, which are $GABA_A$ receptor agonists, can also be used in the prevention and treatment PSH [102]. They are used as muscle relaxants and anxiolytic agents [100]. Diazepam, lorazepam, or midazolam can treat acute episodes of PSH whereas longer-acting clonazepam can be used for prevention [98]. Side effects include respiratory depression, sedation, and hypotension; hence, caution is advised when using with opioids or other sedating drugs [102].

β-blockers and α2-agonists suppress sympathetic overactivity and are predominantly used for the prevention of PSH. α2-agonists used for PSH include clonidine and dexmedetomidine. β-blockers include propranolol and labetalol. Of these, propranolol is used most frequently, in part because its lipophilic properties permit it to easily penetrate the blood-brain barrier. The starting dose is usually 40 mg daily given every 12 hours. The dose can be increased by 20–40 mg per dose per day up to a maximum dose of 640 mg/day. However, once a dose of 80 mg every 8 hours is reached, an alternative medication such as clonidine should be considered [100]. For acute episodes, labetalol can be started at 10–20 mg intravenously given over 3–5 min. It can be given up to every 10 min if needed to a maximum dose of 300 mg/day. β-blocker use needs to be monitored for bradycardia, hypotension, bronchospasm, sleep disturbance, and hypoglycemia [102]. Clonidine can be used for patients with asthma as β-blockers are contraindicated. It can be started at 0.1 mg daily with titration every 12 hours [100]. Thereafter, the dose is increased by 0.1–0.3 mg per day to a maximum dose of 2.4 mg daily. Clonidine can cause hypotension, sedation, bradycardia, constipation, and depression. It must be systematically tapered once deemed no longer necessary in order to prevent rebound hypertension [102]. Dexmedetomidine is given by infusion and is particularly useful in the intensive care unit due to its rapid onset and titratability with close monitoring for respiratory depression.

Dopamine agonists such as bromocriptine can also be used to inhibit profuse sweating and increased temperature. However, bromocriptine may lower seizure threshold and is contraindicated in patients with uncontrolled hypertension. It can also lead to confusion, agitation, nausea, dyskinesia, and orthostatic hypotension. Treatment is typically initiated at 2.5 mg daily and titrated up every 8 hours. The dose may be increased by 2.5–7.5 mg per day every 2–3 days, up to a maximum daily dose of 100 mg [100].

Baclofen, a $GABA_B$ receptor agonist, can also be used to treat PSH. Baclofen can be started at 5 mg every 8 hours, and titrated up to a maximum of 80 mg daily. Intrathecal baclofen (ITB) can also be used, and effective dosages are reported to range between 100 and 500 μg a day [98]. Side effects of baclofen include muscle weakness, sedation, liver enzyme elevation, bronchial hyperactivity, and abnormal movements. Abrupt withdrawal from ITB is dangerous and must be avoided by carefully screening patients and/or their caretakers to ensure that they will be compliant with scheduled pump refills. They also need to be informed of the signs and symptoms of withdrawal, including fever, rigidity, dystonia/increased spasticity, seizures, pruritus, and mood changes [102]. See Chap. 11 for details on ITB treatment.

Dantrolene, which is used to treat malignant hyperthermia and spasticity, can also help treat episodes of PSH by reducing posturing. However, one must monitor liver function and breathing as it can cause hepatotoxicity and respiratory depression [98, 102]. Liver function should be checked prior to initiating treatment and periodically thereafter for as long as the patient receives the drug. It works by preventing calcium release from the muscle sarcoplasmic reticulum, thereby inhibiting muscle contraction.

For pediatric patients, pharmacologic agents are used less frequently. Nursing interventions such as repositioning and soothing are typical first-line interventions [102]. When medications are used, acetaminophen is prescribed most commonly, followed by niaprazine. Benzodiazepines such as clonazepam and delorazepam can also be used. Hydroxyzine is used less frequently.

Miscellaneous Causes

Pain and spasticity are highly interrelated; spasticity is an acknowledged source of pain and pain is well-known to exacerbate spasticity. As described above, the most well-known scenario of pain triggering spasticity is seen in PSH. Other causes of worsening spasticity include time of day, change in weather, body posture/positioning, poor fitting orthotics, and tight clothing. Psychological conditions/emotional state, menstrual cycle, and labor and delivery can also potentially exacerbate spasticity. All of these potential causes should be kept in mind if there is a change in previously controlled spasticity, followed by appropriate timely intervention(s).

Conclusion

A comprehensive understanding of the medical conditions that exacerbate spasticity is vital to managing patients with spasticity. Exacerbating medical conditions involving the genitourinary, gastrointestinal, musculoskeletal, vascular, and neurological systems are very common in individuals with CNS injury, and need to be thoroughly investigated as part of a spasticity management program. Early identification followed by timely removal or treatment of the exacerbating factors and conditions can improve spasticity, pain control, hygiene, and function.

References

1. Watkins CL, et al. Prevalence of spasticity post stroke. Clin Rehabil. 2002;16(5):515–22.
2. McKinley WO, Tewksbury MA, Godbout CJ. Comparison of medical complications following nontraumatic and traumatic spinal cord injury. J Spinal Cord Med. 2002;25(2):88–93.
3. Karlsson AK. Autonomic dysfunction in spinal cord injury: clinical presentation of symptoms and signs. Prog Brain Res. 2006;152:1–8.
4. Blackman JA, et al. Paroxysmal autonomic instability with dystonia after brain injury. Arch Neurol. 2004;61(3):321–8.
5. Baguley IJ. Autonomic complications following central nervous system injury. Semin Neurol. 2008;28(5):716–25.
6. Baguley IJ, et al. Diagnosing dysautonomia after acute traumatic brain injury: evidence for overresponsiveness to afferent stimuli. Arch Phys Med Rehabil. 2009;90(4):580–6.
7. Baguley IJ, et al. A critical review of the pathophysiology of dysautonomia following traumatic brain injury. Neurocrit Care. 2008;8(2):293–300.
8. Kandel ER, Schwartz JH, Jessell TM. Principles of neural science. 4th ed. New York: McGraw-Hill; 2000.
9. Bullard DE. Diencephalic seizures: responsiveness to bromocriptine and morphine. Ann Neurol. 1987;21(6):609–11.
10. Boeve BF, et al. Paroxysmal sympathetic storms ("diencephalic seizures") after severe diffuse axonal head injury. Mayo Clinic proceedings. 1998;73(2):148–52. https://doi.org/10.4065/73.2.14.
11. Rossitch E, Bullard DE. The autonomic dysfunction syndrome: aetiology and treatment. Br J Neurosurg. 1988;2(4):471–8.
12. Baguley IJ. The excitatory: inhibitory ratio model (EIR model): an integrative explanation of acute autonomic overactivity syndromes. Med Hypotheses. 2008;70(1):26–35.
13. Cervero F, Laird JM. Mechanisms of touch-evoked pain (allodynia): a new model. Pain. 1996;68(1):13–23.
14. Cuny E, Richer E, Castel JP. Dysautonomia syndrome in the acute recovery phase after traumatic brain injury: relief with intrathecal baclofen therapy. Brain Inj. 2001;15(10):917–25.
15. Becker R, et al. Intrathecal baclofen alleviates autonomic dysfunction in severe brain injury. J Clin Neurosci. 2000;7(4):316–9.
16. Joshi S, et al. Identification of spinal interneurons antecedent to adrenal sympathetic preganglionic neurons using trans-synaptic transport of herpes simplex virus type 1. Neuroscience. 1995;65(3):893–903.
17. Cabot JB, et al. Spinal cord lamina V and lamina VII interneuronal projections to sympathetic preganglionic neurons. J Comp Neurol. 1994;347(4):515–30.
18. Deuchars SA. How sympathetic are your spinal cord circuits? Exp Physiol. 2015;100(4):365–71.
19. Deuchars SA. Multi-tasking in the spinal cord--do 'sympathetic' interneurones work harder than we give them credit for? J Physiol. 2007;580(Pt.3):723–9.
20. Deuchars SA. Spinal interneurons in the control of autonomic function. In: Llewellyn-Smith IJ, Verberne AJM, editors. Central regulation of autonomic functions. New York: Oxford University Press; 2011. p. 140–60.
21. Deuchars SA, et al. GABAergic neurons in the central region of the spinal cord: a novel substrate for sympathetic inhibition. J Neurosci. 2005;25(5):1063–70.
22. Bacon SJ, Smith AD. A monosynaptic pathway from an identified vasomotor centre in the medial prefrontal cortex to an autonomic area in the thoracic spinal cord. Neuroscience. 1993;54(3):719–28.
23. Deuchars SA, Brooke RE, Deuchars J. Adenosine A1 receptors reduce release from excitatory but not inhibitory synaptic inputs onto lateral horn neurons. J Neurosci. 2001;21(16):6308–20.

24. Brooke RE, Deuchars J, Deuchars SA. Input-specific modulation of neurotransmitter release in the lateral horn of the spinal cord via adenosine receptors. J Neurosci. 2004;24(1):127–37.
25. Miura M, Takayama K, Okada J. Distribution of glutamate- and GABA-immunoreactive neurons projecting to the cardioacceleratory center of the intermediolateral nucleus of the thoracic cord of SHR and WKY rats: a double-labeling study. Brain Res. 1994;638(1–2):139–50.
26. Deuchars SA, Spyer KM, Gilbey MP. Stimulation within the rostral ventrolateral medulla can evoke monosynaptic GABAergic IPSPs in sympathetic preganglionic neurons in vitro. J Neurophysiol. 1997;77(1):229–35.
27. Pan B, Kim EJ, Schramm LP. Increased close appositions between corticospinal tract axons and spinal sympathetic neurons after spinal cord injury in rats. J Neurotrauma. 2005;22(12):1399–410.
28. Lee V, Maguire J. The impact of tonic GABAA receptor-mediated inhibition on neuronal excitability varies across brain region and cell type. Front Neural Circuits. 2014;8:3.
29. Kitajima T, et al. Diazepam reduces both arterial blood pressure and muscle sympathetic nerve activity in human. Neurosci Lett. 2004;355(1–2):77–80.
30. Wang L, et al. GABA(B) mediated regulation of sympathetic preganglionic neurons: pre- and postsynaptic sites of action. Front Neurol. 2010;1:142.
31. Wyszogrodski I, Polosa C. The inhibition of sympathetic preganglionic neurons by somatic afferents. Can J Physiol Pharmacol. 1973;51(1):29–38.
32. Krassioukov AV, Johns DG, Schramm LP. Sensitivity of sympathetically correlated spinal interneurons, renal sympathetic nerve activity, and arterial pressure to somatic and visceral stimuli after chronic spinal injury. J Neurotrauma. 2002;19(12):1521–9.
33. Sie JA, et al. Ultrastructural evidence for direct projections from the pontine micturition center to glycine-immunoreactive neurons in the sacral dorsal gray commissure in the cat. J Comp Neurol. 2001;429(4):631–7.
34. Blok BF, de Weerd H, Holstege G. The pontine micturition center projects to sacral cord GABA immunoreactive neurons in the cat. Neurosci Lett. 1997;233(2–3):109–12.
35. Tracey I, Mantyh PW. The cerebral signature for pain perception and its modulation. Neuron. 2007;55(3):377–91.
36. Schramm LP. Spinal sympathetic interneurons: their identification and roles after spinal cord injury. Prog Brain Res. 2006;152:27–37.
37. Weaver LC, et al. Changes in immunoreactivity for growth associated protein-43 suggest reorganization of synapses on spinal sympathetic neurons after cord transection. Neuroscience. 1997;81(2):535–51.
38. Hou S, et al. Plasticity of lumbosacral propriospinal neurons is associated with the development of autonomic dysreflexia after thoracic spinal cord transection. J Comp Neurol. 2008;509(4):382–99.
39. Kofler M, Poustka K, Saltuari L. Intrathecal baclofen for autonomic instability due to spinal cord injury. Auton Neurosci. 2009;146(1–2):106–10.
40. Del Fabro AS, Mejia M, Nemunaitis G. An investigation of the relationship between autonomic dysreflexia and intrathecal baclofen in patients with spinal cord injury. J Spinal Cord Med. 2018;41(1):102–5.
41. Delhaas EM, Frankema SPG, Huygen F. Intrathecal baclofen as emergency treatment alleviates severe intractable autonomic dysreflexia in cervical spinal cord injury. J Spinal Cord Med. 2021;44(4):617–20.
42. Omli R, et al. Pad per day usage, urinary incontinence and urinary tract infections in nursing home residents. Age Ageing. 2010;39(5):549–54.
43. Harari D, et al. New-onset fecal incontinence after stroke: prevalence, natural history, risk factors, and impact. Stroke. 2003;34(1):144–50.
44. Stiens SA, Bergman SB, Goetz LL. Neurogenic bowel dysfunction after spinal cord injury: clinical evaluation and rehabilitative management. Arch Phys Med Rehabil. 1997;78(3 Suppl):S86–102.
45. Kaynan AM, Agarwal M, Perkash I. Chapter 137 Neurogenic bladder. In: Frontera WR, Silver JK, Rizzo Jr TD, editors. Essentials of physical medicine and rehabilitation. Philadelphia: Saunders, an imprint of Elsevier Inc.; 2015.

46. Fleuren JF, et al. Perception of lower limb spasticity in patients with spinal cord injury. Spinal Cord. 2009;47(5):396–400.
47. Ronco E, et al. Diagnostic criteria of urinary tract infection in male patients with spinal cord injury. Neurorehabil Neural Repair. 2011;25(4):351–8.
48. Meng NH, et al. Incomplete bladder emptying in patients with stroke: is detrusor external sphincter dyssynergia a potential cause? Arch Phys Med Rehabil. 2010;91(7):1105–9.
49. Chu CM, Lowder JL. Diagnosis and treatment of urinary tract infections across age groups. Am J Obstet Gynecol. 2018;219(1):40–51.
50. Goldmark E, Niver B, Ginsberg DA. Neurogenic bladder: from diagnosis to management. Curr Urol Rep. 2014;15(10):448.
51. Taweel WA, Seyam R. Neurogenic bladder in spinal cord injury patients. Res Rep Urol. 2015;7:85–99.
52. Katsumi HK, et al. Urethral versus suprapubic catheter: choosing the best bladder management for male spinal cord injury patients with indwelling catheters. Spinal Cord. 2010;48(4):325–9.
53. Spencer ES, Lyons MD, Pruthi RS. Patient selection and counseling for urinary diversion. Urol Clin North Am. 2018;45(1):1–9.
54. Pellatt GC, Geddis T. Neurogenic continence. Part 2: Neurogenic bladder management. Br J Nurs. 2008;17(14):904, 906, 908–913.
55. Cameron AP. Medical management of neurogenic bladder with oral therapy. Transl Androl Urol. 2016;5(1):51–62.
56. Perkash I, Agarwal M. Chapter 138 Neurogenic bowel. In: Frontera WR, Silver JK, Rizzo Jr TD, editors. Essentials of physical medicine and rehabilitation. Philadelphia: Saunders, an imprint of Elsevier Inc.; 2015. p. 726–32.
57. Wood JD. Neuropathophysiology of functional gastrointestinal disorders. World J Gastroenterol. 2007;13(9):1313–32.
58. Phadke CP, et al. Revisiting physiologic and psychologic triggers that increase spasticity. Am J Phys Med Rehabil. 2013;92(4):357–69.
59. Haas U, Geng V. Sensation of defecation in patients with spinal cord injury. Spinal Cord. 2008;46(2):107–12.
60. Krassioukov A, et al. Neurogenic bowel management after spinal cord injury: a systematic review of the evidence. Spinal Cord. 2010;48(10):718–33.
61. Cameron KJ, et al. Assessment of the effect of increased dietary fibre intake on bowel function in patients with spinal cord injury. Spinal Cord. 1996;34(5):277–83.
62. Ayas S, et al. The effect of abdominal massage on bowel function in patients with spinal cord injury. Am J Phys Med Rehabil. 2006;85(12):951–5.
63. House JG, Stiens SA. Pharmacologically initiated defecation for persons with spinal cord injury: effectiveness of three agents. Arch Phys Med Rehabil. 1997;78(10):1062–5.
64. Krogh K, et al. Efficacy and tolerability of prucalopride in patients with constipation due to spinal cord injury. Scand J Gastroenterol. 2002;37(4):431–6.
65. Christensen P, et al. A randomized, controlled trial of transanal irrigation versus conservative bowel management in spinal cord-injured patients. Gastroenterology. 2006;131(3):738–47.
66. Hascakova-Bartova R, et al. Neuromuscular electrical stimulation of completely paralyzed abdominal muscles in spinal cord-injured patients: a pilot study. Spinal Cord. 2008;46(6):445–50.
67. Hassan NF, Nasser I, Bennett MM. Increased spasticity in a chronic spinal cord injury patient after scabies infestation: a case report. Arch Phys Med Rehabil. 1997;78(12):1384–5.
68. Powers JG, et al. Wound healing and treating wounds: chronic wound care and management. J Am Acad Dermatol. 2016;74(4):607–25; quiz 625–6.
69. Cannon BC, Cannon JP. Management of pressure ulcers. Am J Health Syst Pharm. 2004;61(18):1895–905; quiz 1906–7.
70. Balboni TA, Gobezie R, Mamon HJ. Heterotopic ossification: pathophysiology, clinical features, and the role of radiotherapy for prophylaxis. Int J Radiat Oncol Biol Phys. 2006;65(5):1289–99.
71. Botte MJ, et al. Heterotopic ossification in neuromuscular disorders. Orthopedics. 1997;20(4):335–41; quiz 342–3.

72. Spielman G, Gennarelli TA, Rogers CR. Disodium etidronate: its role in preventing heterotopic ossification in severe head injury. Arch Phys Med Rehabil. 1983;64(11):539–42.
73. Garland DE. Clinical observations on fractures and heterotopic ossification in the spinal cord and traumatic brain injured populations. Clin Orthop Relat Res. 1988;233:86–101.
74. Pape HC, et al. Current concepts in the development of heterotopic ossification. J Bone Joint Surg Br. 2004;86(6):783–7.
75. Vanden Bossche L, Vanderstraeten G. Heterotopic ossification: a review. J Rehabil Med. 2005;37(3):129–36.
76. Buschbacher R. Heterotopic ossification: a review. Crit Rev Phys Rehabil Med. 1992;4(3):4.
77. Venier LH, Ditunno JF Jr. Heterotopic ossification in the paraplegic patient. Arch Phys Med Rehabil. 1971;52(10):475–9.
78. Banovac K, et al. Advanced clinical solutions prevention and treatment of heterotopic ossification after spinal cord injury. J Spinal Cord Med. 2004;27(4):376.
79. Aubut J-AL, et al. A comparison of heterotopic ossification treatment within the traumatic brain and spinal cord injured population: an evidence based systematic review. NeuroRehabilitation. 2011;28(2):151–60.
80. Mavrogenis AF, Soucacos PN, Papagelopoulos PJ. Heterotopic ossification revisited. Orthopedics. 2011;34(3):177.
81. He SK, et al. Appropriate excision time of heterotopic ossification in elbow caused by trauma. Acta Orthop Traumatol Turc. 2018;52(1):27–31.
82. Chalidis B, Stengel D, Giannoudis PV. Early excision and late excision of heterotopic ossification after traumatic brain injury are equivalent: a systematic review of the literature. J Neurotrauma. 2007;24(11):1675–86.
83. Eapen BC. Deep venous thrombosis. In: Frontera WR, Silver JK, Rizzo Jr TD, editors. Essentials of physical medicine and rehabilitation. Philadelphia: Saunders, an imprint of Elsevier Inc.; 2015. p. 653–9.
84. Kearon C, et al. Antithrombotic therapy for VTE disease. Chest. 2016;149(2):315–52.
85. Kumar S, Selim MH, Caplan LR. Medical complications after stroke. Lancet Neurol. 2010;9(1):105–18.
86. Jorgensen L, et al. Walking after stroke: does it matter? Changes in bone mineral density within the first 12 months after stroke. A longitudinal study. Osteoporos Int. 2000;11(5):381–7.
87. Sato Y, et al. Low-dose vitamin D prevents muscular atrophy and reduces falls and hip fractures in women after stroke: a randomized controlled trial. Cerebrovasc Dis. 2005;20(3):187–92.
88. Sato Y, et al. Risedronate therapy for prevention of hip fracture after stroke in elderly women. Neurology. 2005;64(5):811–6.
89. Dennis MS, et al. Fractures after stroke: frequency, types, and associations. Stroke. 2002;33(3):728–34.
90. Kanis J, Oden A, Johnell O. Acute and long-term increase in fracture risk after hospitalization for stroke. Stroke. 2001;32(3):702–6.
91. Ramnemark A, et al. Progressive hemiosteoporosis on the paretic side and increased bone mineral density in the nonparetic arm the first year after severe stroke. Osteoporos Int. 1999;9(3):269–75.
92. Gifre L, et al. Incidence of skeletal fractures after traumatic spinal cord injury: a 10-year follow-up study. Clin Rehabil. 2014;28(4):361–9.
93. Jiang SD, Jiang LS, Dai LY. Mechanisms of osteoporosis in spinal cord injury. Clin Endocrinol. 2006;65(5):555–65.
94. Lazo MG, et al. Osteoporosis and risk of fracture in men with spinal cord injury. Spinal Cord. 2001;39(4):208–14.
95. Keating JF, Kerr M, Delargy M. Minimal trauma causing fractures in patients with spinal cord injury. Disabil Rehabil. 1992;14(2):108–9.
96. Vestergaard P, et al. Fracture rates and risk factors for fractures in patients with spinal cord injury. Spinal Cord. 1998;36(11):790–6.

97. Giangregorio L, McCartney N. Bone loss and muscle atrophy in spinal cord injury: epidemiology, fracture prediction, and rehabilitation strategies. J Spinal Cord Med. 2006;29(5):489–500.
98. Meyfroidt G, Baguley IJ, Menon DK. Paroxysmal sympathetic hyperactivity: the storm after acute brain injury. Lancet Neurol. 2017;16(9):721–9.
99. Perkes I, et al. A review of paroxysmal sympathetic hyperactivity after acquired brain injury. Ann Neurol. 2010;68(2):126–35.
100. Lump D, Moyer M. Paroxysmal sympathetic hyperactivity after severe brain injury. Curr Neurol Neurosci Rep. 2014;14(11):494.
101. Baguley IJ, et al. Paroxysmal sympathetic hyperactivity after acquired brain injury: consensus on conceptual definition, nomenclature, and diagnostic criteria. J Neurotrauma. 2014;31(17):1515–20.
102. Feng Y, Zheng X, Fang Z. Treatment progress of paroxysmal sympathetic hyperactivity after acquired brain injury. Pediatr Neurosurg. 2015;50(6):301–9.

Oral Spasmolytics

10

Elaine Magat, Isaac Hernandez Jimenez, Haresh Sampathkumar, Joanne Delgado, and Gerard E. Francisco

In modern pharmacology it's so clear that even if you have a fixed dose of a drug, the individuals respond very differently to one and the same dose.
– Arvid Carlsson, 1923–2018.

- The more common oral medications currently used for the treatment of spasticity are baclofen and benzodiazepines such as diazepam (GABA agonists), tizanidine (alpha 2 receptor agonist), and dantrolene sodium (peripherally acting, decreases calcium release in the skeletal muscle).
- Other medications control spasticity by blocking voltage-gated ion channels. Sodium channel blockers that have been studied for spasticity management are primarily anti-epileptic drugs (phenytoin, oxcarbazepine, levetiracetam, and lamotrigine). Calcium channel blockers include gabapentin and pregabalin. Tolperisone acts by blocking both the sodium and calcium channels.

E. Magat · I. H. Jimenez · G. E. Francisco (✉)
Department of Physical Medicine and Rehabilitation, McGovern Medical School, The University of Texas Health Science Center at Houston, Houston, TX, USA
e-mail: Elaine.M.Magat@uth.tmc.edu; Isaac.hernandezjimenez@uth.tmc.edu; Gerard.E.Francisco@uth.tmc.edu

H. Sampathkumar
PAM Health Rehabilitation Hospital of Dover, Dover, DE, USA
e-mail: haresh@jhrehabilitation.com

J. Delgado
Department of Physical Medicine and Rehabilitation, Memorial Physician Group at Memorial Healthcare System, Hollywood, FL, USA
e-mail: joannedelgado@gmail.com

P. Raghavan (ed.), *Spasticity and Muscle Stiffness*,
https://doi.org/10.1007/978-3-030-96900-4_10

- Other medications used in the management of spasticity and/or spasms, whose mechanism of action is not well defined, include cannabis, cyclobenzaprine, orphenadrine, and mexiletine.
- Tiagabine (a GABA-mimetic agent), 4-aminopyridine (a potassium channel blocking agent), and cyproheptadine (a serotonin/alpha receptor antagonist) have also been studied for the treatment of spasticity.

Introduction

Oral spasmolytics primarily target neural hyperexcitability that leads to a lowered stretch reflex threshold due to reduced suppression of the synapses between the Ia afferent and the efferent alpha motor neurons in the spinal cord [1–3]. The various classes of anti-spasticity medications act on specific receptors and ion channels in the stretch reflex circuitry to reduce neural excitability. Figure 10.1 shows the receptors sites where the medications discussed in this chapter exert their actions. Table 10.1 lists the more commonly used oral anti-spasticity medications, and Table 10.2 lists the FDA-approved medications for the treatment of spasticity.

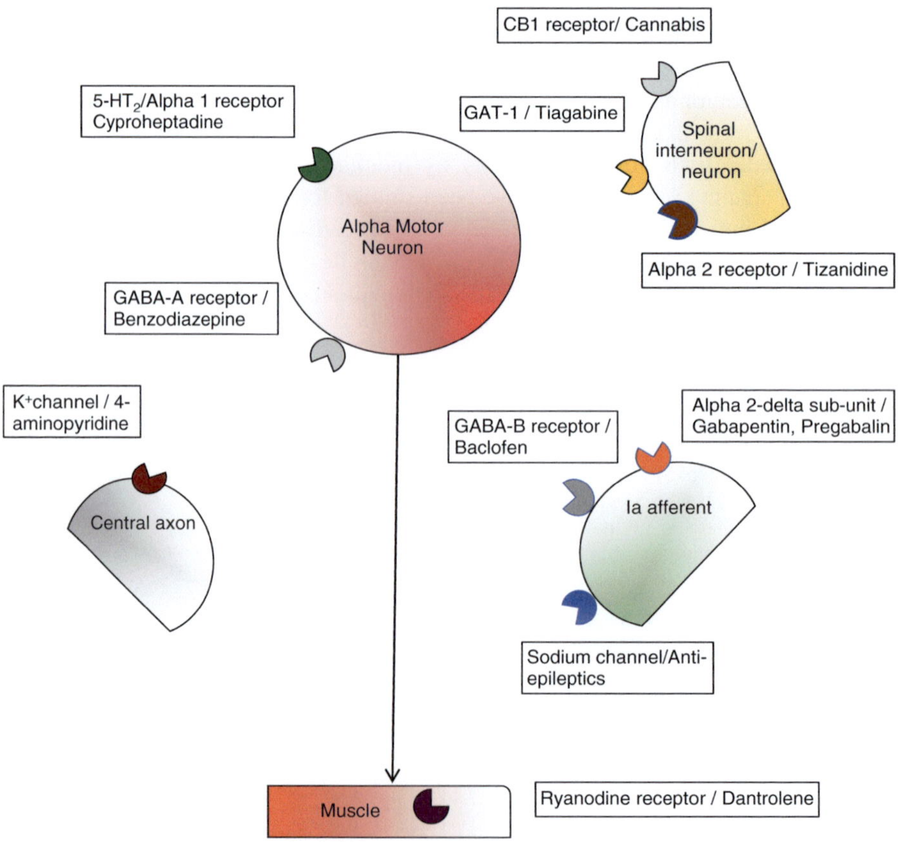

Fig. 10.1 Proposed sites of action of oral anti-spasticity agents

Table 10.1 Commonly used oral anti-spasticity medications: clinical application

Drug	Mechanism of action	Usual starting dose	Maximum dose	Monitoring/comments
Baclofen	GABA agonist – binds GABA-B receptors	5 mg TID or 10 mg TID	80 mg/day	Use a lower starting dose for elderly and brain-injured patients Consider starting at bedtime first then titrate up Abrupt discontinuation can cause withdrawal symptoms
Benzodiazepine Diazepam	GABA agonist – works through GABA-A receptors	2 mg BID or 5 mg at bedtime for nighttime symptoms	30 mg/day; usual dose range is 2–10 mg per day, divided into three or four doses	Abrupt discontinuation after prolonged high dose may cause withdrawal symptoms Commonly used as an adjunct to baclofen for spasticity management Rarely recommended as first- or second-line agent for brain-injured patients
Clonazepam		0.25–1 mg at bedtime		Commonly used for nighttime spasms
Tizanidine	Alpha 2 receptor agonist	1–4 mg at bedtime	36 mg/day, divided every 8 hours	Check liver enzymes for the first 6 months and then periodically thereafter Use with caution in patients with renal and hepatic impairment Start at a lower dose and titrate slowly with close monitoring Avoid use with antihypertensive medications due to possible hypotension Capsule and tablet form are not equivalent. Exercise care when switching formulation
Dantrolene sodium	Decreases calcium release in the skeletal muscle (peripherally-acting)	12.5–25 mg daily	400 mg/day (100 mg every 6 hours)*	Obtain baseline liver function tests, then monitor regularly Titrate dose every 7 days Discontinue if no response after 45 days **Hepatic dysfunction* has a dose-response relationship – 23% incidence of hepatic failure with dose between *200 and 400 mg per day* **Significantly lower incidence* of hepatic dysfunction with *≤100 mg per day* Monitor for respiratory disease – unusual but can include sterile pleural effusion

Table 10.2 Indications, warnings, and precautions for FDA-approved oral medications for spasticity

Drug	Indications	Warnings/precautions
Baclofen [4]	Spasticity from MS Efficacy in stroke, CP, and Parkinson's disease has not been established	Abrupt drug withdrawal Impaired renal function Pregnancy Stroke (poor tolerance)
Diazepam [5]	Spasticity caused by upper motor neuron disorders (like CP, paraplegia) Adjunct for skeletal muscle spasm from local pathology (trauma or inflammation of the muscles or joints)	Risk of respiratory depression, sedation, coma, and death, if used with opioids Advice patients against ingestion of alcohol and other CNS depressant medications Increased risk of teratogenic effects has been suggested Non-teratogenic risks may also be associated (neonatal flaccidity, respiratory and feeding difficulties, hypothermia, neonatal withdrawal symptoms) Breast-feeding is not recommended
Tizanidine [6]	Spasticity	Hypotension Risk of liver injury Sedation Hallucinations Renal impairment (creatinine clearance <25 ml/min): use with caution, monitor for potential overdose (dry mouth, somnolence, asthenia, and dizziness)
Dantrolene sodium [7]	Chronic spasticity from upper motor neuron disorders (SCI, stroke, CP, or MS)	Fatal and non-fatal liver disorders may occur. Use with caution in females and those over 35 years old: greater likelihood of drug induced hepatocellular disease Long-term safety in humans has not been established It is not known if it can cause fetal harm Should not be used in nursing mothers Use with caution if patient has impaired pulmonary and cardiac function. Associated with pleural effusion with eosinophilia

MS multiple sclerosis, *CP* cerebral palsy, *SCI* spinal cord injury

GABA Agonists/GABA Mimetics

Gamma aminobutyric acid (GABA) is the major inhibitory neurotransmitter in the mammalian central nervous system (CNS) [8]. GABA receptors are found pre-synaptically and post-synaptically in both the central and the peripheral nervous system [9]. CNS locations include areas within the brainstem, dorsal horn of the spinal cord, alpha motor neurons, and other sites [9, 10]. In the peripheral nervous system, GABA receptors can be found in Ia sensory afferent neurons, the primary afferent fibers of the muscle spindle [9].

Baclofen

Baclofen is a chlorophenyl derivative of GABA [11]. Its chemical name is 4-amino-3-(4-chlorophenyl) butanoic acid [12]. Baclofen was developed in the 1970s and was the first marketed anti-spastic agent [13]. It remains one of the most commonly used drugs for the treatment of spasticity over the long term [14], and some consider it the most preferred oral anti-spasticity drug [15].

Mechanisms of Action

Baclofen is a GABA-B agonist. It binds to GABA-B receptors [16] and inhibits spinal reflexes [17] by several mechanisms. It binds pre- and post-synaptically to the receptors leading to membrane hyperpolarization [18]. It interferes with the release of excitatory neurotransmitters from afferent fibers by interfering with the movement of calcium and potassium ions [11, 17, 19]. It alters membrane properties in the interneuron pool and may also stimulate the release of glycine by inhibitory neurons, with overall reduction of motor output from the spinal cord [11]. This includes the output of the gamma motor neuron, which regulates the tension in the muscle spindles, and hence may decrease spindle sensitivity [19]. All of these mechanisms may lead to a decrease in neural hyperexcitability (Fig. 10.2).

Clinical Use

Baclofen is used for the treatment of spasticity in persons with spinal cord injury, cerebral palsy, multiple sclerosis, stroke, and traumatic brain injury. Most of the studies show benefit in persons with spinal cord injury and multiple sclerosis for the control of muscle spasms. The NICE (National Institute for Clinical Excellence) guidelines recommend baclofen as a first-line drug for the treatment of spasticity in multiple sclerosis [20].

Dosing

Oral baclofen is available in 5 mg, 10 mg, and 20 mg tablets. The time to reach maximum concentration of the drug in the plasma is 1 hour [21]. The mean half-life is 4 hours [21]. Tissue half-life in the CNS is about 3–5 hours [19]. Mean bioavailability is 74%, as 25% of the drug is either not absorbed or undergoes first-pass metabolism prior to reaching the circulation [21]. The liver metabolizes 6–15%, and the remainder is excreted by the kidney (70–80% unchanged).

It is common practice to start the medication at a low dose and frequency (e.g., once or twice daily). The dose is gradually increased until the desired effect is achieved—usually at doses of 40–80 mg daily, if tolerated by patients. The determination of optimal dosage requires individual titration. It is commonly started at 10 mg three times a day. However, with certain populations like brain-injured patients or the elderly, starting at 5 mg three times a day is common as well. Dose increases have been suggested every 3 days. Some consider starting at a lower frequency, such as a 5–10 mg bedtime dose for three nights, slowly titrating up in frequency or dosing as the patient tolerates.

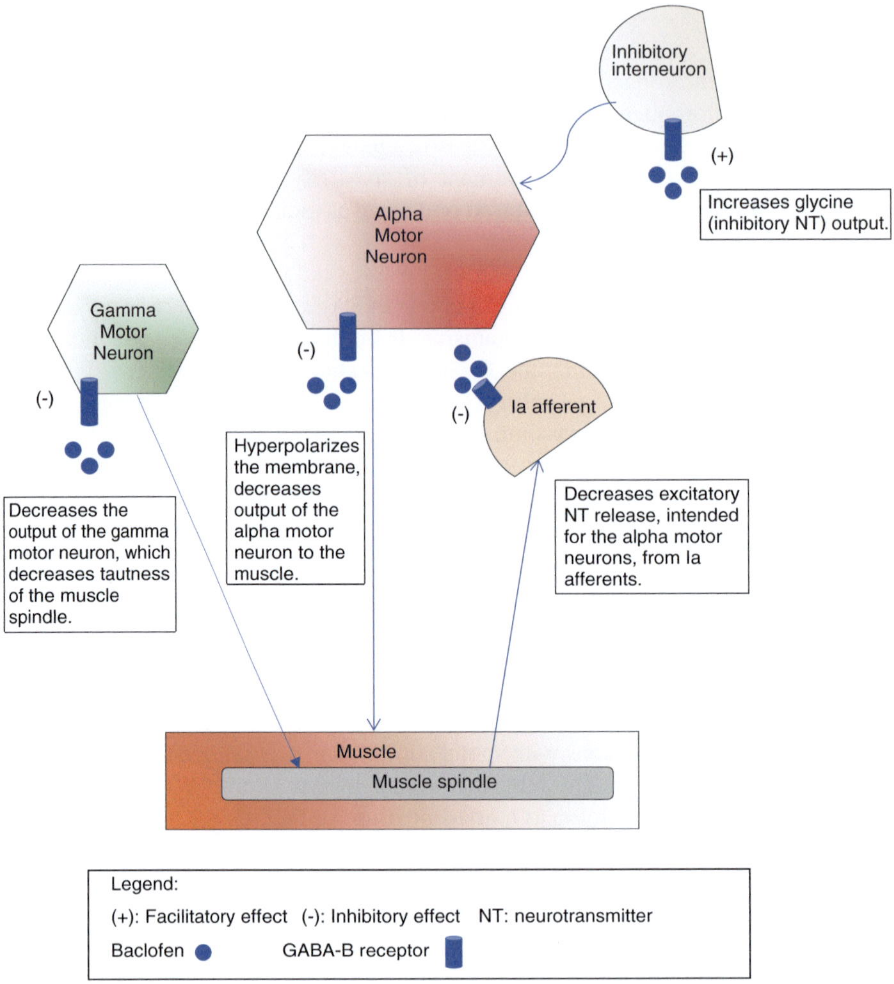

Fig. 10.2 Sites of action of oral baclofen within the muscle stretch reflex arc

The maximum recommended dosage is 80 mg per day, divided into four doses (20 mg four times a day). A total dose of 120 mg/day divided into three to four doses is encountered more frequently when treating spinal cord injured patients. There are reports of improved therapeutic effects at doses as high as 240 mg/day [19]; however, such high doses are not commonly used in practice. The recommendation is to use the lowest dose with the best response, while monitoring constantly for side effects. The medication should be slowly weaned off if beneficial effects are not seen after a reasonable trial.

Side Effect Profile

In a systematic review that included 12 randomized control trials by Montane et al. in 2004, baclofen had a range of adverse events in 25–27% of patients, including sedation, dizziness, and muscle weakness [13]. Neurologic events seemed to be dose-related and tended to resolve when the dose was reduced [21]. Other reported adverse effects include seizures (it lowers the seizure threshold), postural hypotension, memory impairment, urinary incontinence, and blurred vision, among others [10, 19]. Development of adverse effects may be decreased by slower up titration of the medication. Abrupt withdrawal of baclofen can lead to increased spasticity, pruritic symptoms, autonomic instability, hallucinations, central fevers, seizures, and death [10, 19] (also see Chap. 11 on intrathecal baclofen).

Case 1. Initiation of treatment for spasticity poststroke

A 47-year-old man suffered a stroke a year and a half ago with residual left spastic hemiparesis and an abnormal gait. The patient received focal treatment with botulinum toxin injections to which he responded well. However, he also experienced stiffness affecting major muscle groups on the left side, which were not all amenable to treatment with botulinum toxin injections. He declined intrathecal baclofen but was open to a trial of oral baclofen. He was started on 5 mg of oral baclofen at bedtime with plans to increase the dose every 3 days up to 10 mg three times a day. The patient responded favorably to the addition of oral baclofen, with overall reduction in stiffness, including in the proximal muscle groups (hips and shoulders). Further dose titration was limited by the side effect of drowsiness [4, 21].

Key learning: *Baclofen is a common first-line agent for the treatment of spasticity. Slow dose titration will mitigate central side effects.*

Case 2. Withdrawal due to loss of insurance coverage

A 50-year-old woman with a past medical history of chronic paraplegia from a spinal cord injury has been taking oral baclofen, 10 mg every 8 hours, for 2–3 months. She then lost her insurance coverage and was unable to refill her baclofen prescription. She began to notice significant worsening of bilateral lower extremity spasms, primarily in bilateral hip adductors and knee flexors [10, 19]. She went to the emergency room, where she was given oral baclofen. This improved her symptoms. She was given a new prescription for baclofen, and the social worker was able to ensure that she had affordable access to baclofen.

Key learning: *It is important to educate patients regarding the withdrawal symptoms of baclofen and to ensure that there is a long-term plan in place to refill the prescription. This may necessitate involving a social worker as part of the plan of care. Patients need to clearly understand that discontinuing the medication abruptly can place both health and life at risk.*

Case 3. Withdrawal due to change in dose

A 35-year-old woman with incomplete paraplegia from a spinal cord injury took her first vacation since her injury. She usually takes 20 mg of baclofen by mouth every 6 hours. Over the course of her trip, she noticed that the spasms in her leg worsened to the point where she required assistance with transfers and was once almost thrown out of her manual wheelchair due to powerful spasms. It was later discovered that she had mistakenly packed 10 mg tablets of oral baclofen instead of 20 mg tablets. The patient's spasms had worsened due to a sudden decrease in dose [10, 19].

Key learning: *When a patient experiences worsening spasticity, confirm that the medication is being taken as intended/prescribed.*

Case 4. Troubleshooting worsening spasticity
A 68-year-old woman with a history of incomplete tetraplegia from a spinal cord injury two months prior was admitted to an acute rehabilitation hospital. She was noted to have spasticity in all four extremities and was started on oral baclofen at 5 mg three times a day, with significant improvement in symptoms. However, she had sudden increase in lower extremity spasms, accompanied by confusion (previously alert and oriented) and bladder incontinence (bladder had been managed with intermittent catheterization every 6 hours without any incontinence). She was found to have a urinary tract infection (UTI) [22], which can explain the worsening spasms, change in mental status, and the bladder incontinence. Intermittent catheterization is a risk factor for UTI [23]. Management of the UTI should improve spasticity. If the spasms do not improve, it may be appropriate to increase the patient's regular anti-spasticity medication while monitoring for adverse effects until the infection clears and/or the spasms return to baseline levels.

Key learning: *Any infection may cause increased spasms and/or spasticity and must be kept in mind in the differential diagnosis of worsening spasticity* (see Chap. 9).

Benzodiazepines

Benzodiazepines are the oldest class of medication used in the treatment of neural hyperexcitability [24]. They work through GABA-A receptors [25]. This family of medications has a significant side effect profile, which is mediated by supraspinal binding sites that cause depression of neuronal activity in the reticular system. The side effects reported include sedation, reduced attention, memory impairment, and risk of dependence, among others [9]. Benzodiazepines are rarely recommended as a first- or second-line agent in the treatment of spasticity in the brain-injured population [10, 19, 24, 26].

Mechanism of Action

GABA-A receptors are located in the pre-synaptic terminals of the primary afferent fibers in the spinal cord and on post-synaptic sites on interneurons and motor neurons [11]. The drug binds near GABA-A receptors and reduces neuronal excitability by facilitating sodium conductance and enhancing the pre-synaptic inhibition of the polysynaptic and monosynaptic reflexes [10, 19, 24, 25]. It also enhances the pre-synaptic release of GABA, increases the GABA receptor site affinity to GABA, and may depress the post-synaptic excitatory response to glutamate [11, 26]. Benzodiazepines also increase chloride conductance, which in turn decreases the excitatory drive of the motor neuron pool (Fig. 10.3) [11].

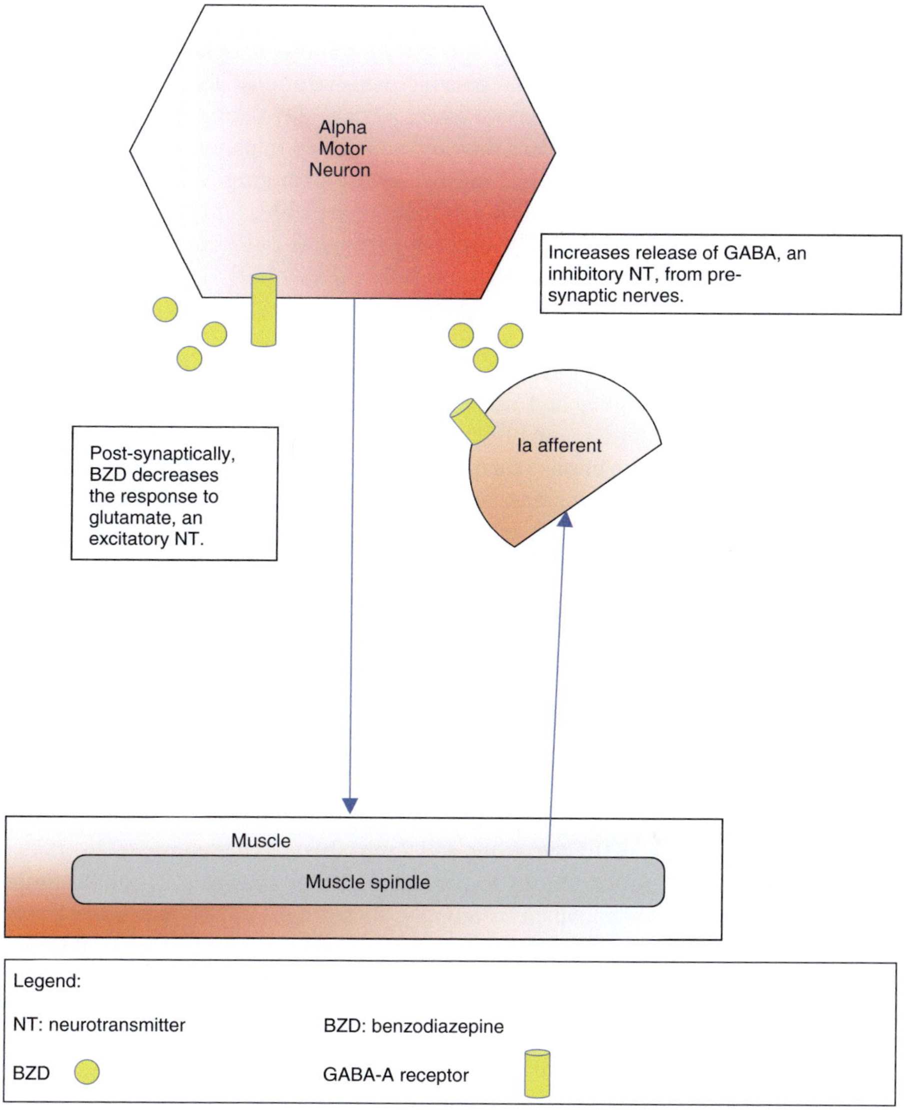

Fig. 10.3 Sites of action of benzodiazepines within the muscle stretch reflex arc

Diazepam

Diazepam is the most widely used benzodiazepine for the treatment of spasticity [17, 24, 25]. In a review by Francisco et al. [19], 13 studies showed superiority of diazepam over placebo, but none of the studies showed superiority of diazepam over dantrolene, baclofen, and tizanidine for anti-spastic effects. This medication is used more commonly as an adjunct to baclofen for spasticity management [27].

Dosing
Diazepam is available in 2 mg, 5 mg and 10 mg tablets. It is rapidly and nearly completely (>90%) absorbed. Peak plasma concentrations are reached within 30 min to 1.5 hours, with a delayed and lower peak in the older population [28]. It is metabolized in the liver; thus, care should be exercised in patients with liver dysfunction. The usual starting dose is 2 mg twice a day, titrating as needed until the desired effect is achieved [27]. Some practitioners start with a 5 mg dose at bedtime, for nighttime symptoms [19, 27]. The usual dose range is 2–10 mg per day, divided into three or four doses. The maximum dose is 30 mg/day [29].

Side Effect Profile
A previously published literature review on diazepam showed that side effects such as drowsiness, fatigue, and muscle weakness were noted in 27–72% of patients [21]. Other reported side effects include lightheadedness, weakness, vertigo, ataxia, paradoxical reactions when used long term (such as insomnia, anxiety, hostility, hallucinations, and increase in spasticity), and hypotension [26]. Abrupt withdrawal after prolonged use of high doses (>40 mg day) may cause seizures and other withdrawal symptoms, such as anxiety, agitation, restlessness, irritability, tremor, muscle fasciculations and twitching, nausea, sensory hypersensitivity, insomnia, nightmares, hyperpyrexia, psychosis, and death [12]. Acute over dosing may produce coma and respiratory depression [26].

Clonazepam

Dosing
Clonazepam is available in 0.5 mg, 1 mg, and 2 mg tablets. It has comparable effects to diazepam [30]. It is used primarily to control nighttime spasms [12] and dystonia [30], especially when accompanied by anxiety. This drug is rapidly and completely absorbed after an oral dose. Maximum blood concentrations are reached 1–4 hours after taking by mouth. It is also metabolized by the liver, so exercise caution when using in patients with hepatic impairment. It is commonly prescribed as 0.25–1 mg at bedtime. A low dose of 0.25 mg in the morning can be considered if it does not produce too much sedation [12].

Side Effect Profile
The side effect profile is similar to that of diazepam.

Case 5. Acquired brain injury with anxiety

A 53-year-old woman with a history of anxiety among other medical comorbidities, suffered an ischemic stroke with residual left hemiparesis, spasticity, and gait abnormality. To control her spasticity, an intrathecal baclofen (ITB) pump was placed earlier on in her recovery. This adequately controlled her spasticity. However, in the past year, the patient gradually developed increasing spasms that were distressing and painful, even though the ITB pump and catheter were deemed to be functioning well. Adjustment of ITB dosing led to incomplete relief. The patient's anxiety worsened. She also complained of worsening pain in the left upper extremity and neck. Electromyography and nerve conduction studies by her neurologist showed cervical radiculopathy. MRI of the cervical spine showed impingement of cervical nerve roots. Hence, a referral to neurosurgery was made. The plan was to initiate botulinum toxin injections for focal management of muscle overactivity. A low dose of clonazepam (0.25 mg at bedtime) was started while awaiting insurance approval for the botulinum toxin injections. Significant improvement in painful spasms, spasticity, and in mood was reported within two days of starting the medication. However, she was only able to take clonazepam for a short period due to side effects of drowsiness [21]. A psychiatry referral was made to further manage her anxiety and depression.

Key learning: *A low dose of clonazepam can be a helpful adjunct to intrathecal baclofen and focal botulinum toxin injections, especially when there is underlying anxiety. Titration and length of treatment may be limited by side effects such as drowsiness.*

Tiagabine

Mechanism of Action

Tiagabine is a GABA uptake inhibitor, which acts by binding to receptors that are associated with the GABA reuptake carrier [31]. The medication is a selective inhibitor of the GABA transporter GAT-1 [32–35]. This allows more of the neurotransmitter GABA to bind with receptors in the post-synaptic cells, thus reducing neuronal excitability.

Clinical Use

Tiagabine is FDA-approved as an adjunct for the treatment of partial seizures in patients 12 years and older [31]. It has been studied in spasticity due to its GABA-mimetic effect. In an animal study in 2012 [36], tiagabine was administered systemically in combination with a glutamate decarboxylase (GAD65) upregulation gene, which was injected into specific lumbar spinal segments. The results showed effective control of spasticity in the targeted spinal segments injected with the upregulation gene. A study of oral tiagabine alone in children with cerebral palsy in 2006, however, did not show a significant decrease in spasticity over a mean treatment duration of 7.2 months, and 8 out of the 9 subjects exhibited adverse effects [37].

Dosing

The FDA does not list spasticity as an indication. For seizure treatment, it is available as 2 mg, 4 mg, 12 mg, and 16 mg tablets. It is well absorbed, with a half-life of 7–9 hours [31]. Peak plasma levels are seen 45 min after dosing, and steady state is reached within two days [31]. It is excreted in the feces (63%) and urine (25%). A typical starting dose for seizure treatment is 4 mg daily. The dose is slowly titrated weekly to 24–32 mg/day in two to four divided doses, over a span of 6 weeks.

Side Effect Profile

Tiagabine has been associated with new-onset seizures and status epilepticus, which may be dose related. Use of other medications that can lower the seizure threshold can increase this risk. It can cause mild-to-moderate impairment in thought processes, fatigue, drowsiness, generalized weakness, and serious skin rashes. Withdrawal seizures may occur if the drug is stopped abruptly.

Alpha 2 Agonists

Tizanidine

Mechanism of Action

Tizanidine is an imidazoline derivative, with the chemical name of 5-chloro-4-(2-imidazolin-2-ylamino)-2,1,3-bezothiodiazole hydrochloride. It binds to both alpha 2 (alpha 2a and alpha 2c) adrenergic receptors and imidazoline (I) receptors at both spinal and supraspinal levels. By activation of these receptors, tizanidine inhibits noradrenergic neurotransmitter release at the spinal level when supraspinal descending facilitatory pathways are activated [38, 39]. In addition, supraspinal mechanisms have been implicated in the regulation of spinal facilitation and an imidazoline receptor pathway for tizanidine-mediated inhibition of spinal reflexes has been described [38]. A quantitative study on the effects of a single dose of tizanidine in patients with spinal cord injury showed that it acts to reduce reflex mechanical responses substantially, without inducing comparable changes in intrinsic muscle properties [40] (Fig. 10.4).

Clinical Use

Tizanidine has been shown to be effective in managing spasticity from several neurological conditions including multiple sclerosis, spinal cord injury, stroke, traumatic brain injury, and cerebral palsy [39]. Tizanidine has also shown to improve pain associated with spasticity in patients with stroke and traumatic brain injury, even though the mechanism is not fully understood [41].

Dosing

Due to commonly reported side effects of dizziness and drowsiness, the dose of tizanidine should be gradually titrated up [39]. The recommended starting dose is 1–4 mg at bedtime, increasing by 1–4 mg every 2–4 days according to patient's tolerance and response. The maximum recommended dose of tizanidine is 36 mg daily divided into three doses (every 8 hours) [41].

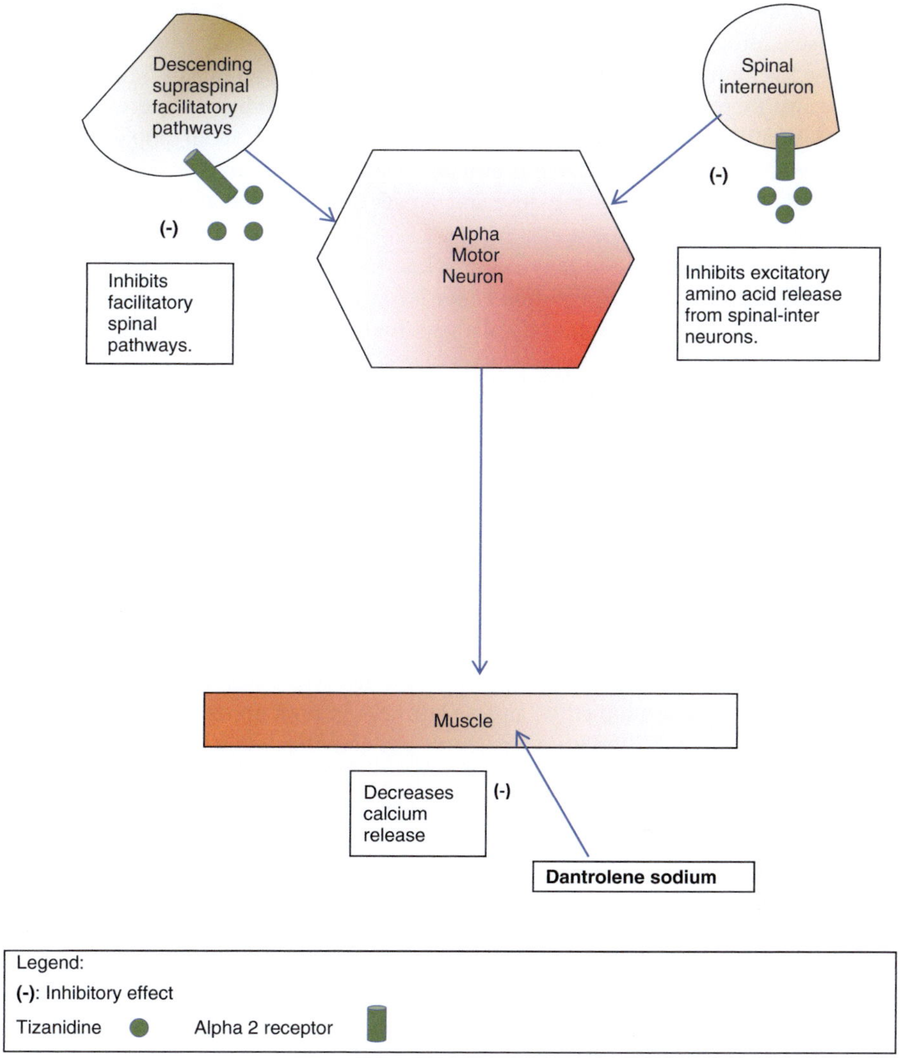

Fig. 10.4 Sites of action of alpha 2 agonists and dantrolene sodium within the muscle stretch reflex arc

Side Effect Profile

Tizanidine is very well tolerated. The most frequent side effects are dry mouth, drowsiness, somnolence, dizziness, weakness, fatigue, and hypotension [38, 39, 41]. Studies comparing tizanidine with other anti-spasticity medications including diazepam and baclofen have shown that tizanidine has a similar clinical efficacy to baclofen and diazepam, but with better tolerability and fewer adverse effects [38, 39]. Patients treated with tizanidine should be monitored for transient elevations in hepatic transaminase levels, which have been reported in approximately 5% of patients. The increase in transaminases does not appear to be dose related, and in most cases, returns to normal after discontinuation of treatment with no sequelae [41]. The liver enzymes should be monitored for the first 6 months of treatment and periodically thereafter. Since approximately 60% of tizanidine is excreted in the urine, it should also be used with caution in patients with renal impairment. In patients with renal or hepatic compromise, a more conservative dosing should be considered using a lower starting dose and slower dose titration with close monitoring for adverse reactions.

Symptomatic hypotension may occur when tizanidine is taken with antihypertensive medications [39, 41]. Caution is needed when a patient is switched between the capsule and tablet formulations of tizanidine. The capsule formulation is not equivalent to the tablet formulation when given with food, and results in a lower maximum concentration and longer times to achieve the maximum concentration [42]. Tizanidine has been shown to be associated with withdrawal symptoms when discontinued abruptly; therefore, gradual taper is recommended.

Case 6. Selection of initial anti-spasticity agent

A 65-year-old man with a past medical history of obesity, obstructive sleep apnea, diabetes mellitus type-2, and chronic kidney disease slipped and fell at his home and hit his head on the floor. This resulted in central cord injury with C5 incomplete tetraplegia. After uncomplicated surgical management and acute inpatient rehabilitation, the patient was discharged home ambulating with a walker. At a subsequent outpatient visit, he complained of muscle stiffness in both upper limbs, proximally and distally, limiting his ability to perform his activities of daily living. He also complained of leg spasms that interfered with his sleep.

Key learning: *The following are some factors that should be considered to guide the selection of the most appropriate oral anti-spasticity medications: the presence of generalized spasticity, functional impact (does spasticity interfere with function or is it assisting it?), comorbidities/medical status, medication review, age, presence and timing of spasms/spasticity. A complete review of history and laboratory work, including renal function tests, is warranted.*

The patient presents with bilateral generalized upper extremity spasticity and muscle stiffness which limits function. It is appropriate to consider starting an oral anti-spasticity medication. The presence of chronic kidney disease should be taken into account in the selection of the medication [4]. *Baclofen is a good first choice, but the dosing plan should include a lower starting dose and a lower maximum dose. This is to avoid medication accumulation and side effects. Tizanidine may also be considered, especially to address the nighttime spasms. Tizanidine may however cause daytime sedation and may also induce hypotension* [6, 43]. *Starting tizanidine at bedtime is appropriate, with gradual increase in frequency to include daytime dosing, as tolerated. It would be appropriate to avoid benzodiazepines given the history of obesity and obstructive sleep apnea, to avoid respiratory depression* [5]. *It is also important to consider that patients with recent trauma and surgery may be using opioid medications for pain management, which may further induce respiratory depression.*

Case 7. Side effects and cross tapering

A 20-year-old man with chronic tetraplegia from a spinal cord injury after trauma was admitted to the rehabilitation unit after his surgeon discontinued his cervical spine precautions. Goals for admission included decreasing the burden of care, and assessment for durable medical equipment to facilitate standing. He takes oral baclofen 10 mg three times a day with acceptable spasticity control. Upon initial assessment, the patient mentioned that he had been experiencing pruritus which he attributes to the use of baclofen. Hence, the patient's baclofen was cross-tapered with tizanidine [38, 39]. Over the course of 1 week, he was weaned off oral baclofen while tizanidine was initiated and titrated up to a dose of 6 mg three times a day with improved spasticity control and resolution of pruritus. Prior to starting the patient's cross taper, his liver function tests were obtained and were found to be within the normal range.

Key learning: *Cross tapering can avoid side effects of withdrawal but must be performed gradually with the patient closely monitored for side effects.*

Case 8. Troubleshooting worsening spasticity

A 25-year-old man with incomplete tetraplegia from a spinal cord injury four months ago developed spasticity approximately 6–8 weeks after his injury, which was managed with range of motion and oral agents, including high doses of oral baclofen (20 mg every 6 hours) [19], followed by tizanidine (12 mg every 8 hours) [41]. However, his spasticity continued to worsen. In addition, he complained of daytime drowsiness which interfered with his ability to participate in outpatient therapy.

Key Learning: *The patient's spasticity seems to follow the natural progression due to his spinal cord injury; however, he is already on the maximum dose of two different oral agents* [19, 41]. *At this point, especially if other contributing factors have been ruled out, it may be appropriate to pursue additional treatment options beyond oral agents (see Chap. 8).*

Clonidine

Mechanism of Action and Clinical Use

Clonidine has similar pharmacology and mechanism of action to tizanidine. It is an alpha 2 receptor agonist with clinical indication for spasticity management. However, it is used less often due to its hypotensive effect.

Dosing

The recommended starting oral dose for clonidine when used for spasticity is 0.1 mg twice a day titrated up to a maximum dose of 0.6 mg daily [44].

Side Effect Profile

The most common side effects of clonidine include dizziness, fatigue, sedation, somnolence, dry mouth, constipation, headaches, orthostatic hypotension, and palpitations. It is very important to gradually titrate down the dose when weaning off clonidine since it may cause rebound hypertension.

Dantrolene Sodium

Mechanism of Action

Dantrolene acts directly on skeletal muscle [45]. It binds to the ryanodine receptor 1 which mediates the release of calcium from the sarcoplasmic reticulum, which is an essential step in muscle contraction. It thus depresses excitation-contraction coupling in skeletal muscle [46, 47]. It is the only peripherally acting medication for spasticity that is approved by the FDA. However, it is only partially absorbed when given orally (35%) [46].

Clinical Use

Dantrolene sodium effectively treats spasticity in conditions such as stroke, traumatic brain injury, spinal cord injury, cerebral palsy, and multiple sclerosis. It is used regularly to control spasms in patients with spinal cord injury [48]. Given its mechanism of action, it has fewer adverse effects in comparison with agents acting on the CNS [49]. It is used to improve function, prevent anticipated functional disability, decrease pain, and improve ease of care [46]. It is also used for reversal of malignant hyperthermia.

Dosing

The current daily recommended dose is 12.5–400 mg (see below).

Side Effect Profile

Dantrolene can cause hepatic dysfunction which can vary from mild elevation in liver enzymes to fatal hepatic injury. The incidence of hepatic dysfunction is reported at 1.8%, whereas the incidence of fatal hepatic injury is 0.35% [50]. Hepatic dysfunction with dantrolene has a dose-response relationship; fatal hepatic injury is reported only when taking more than 200 mg daily [49]. Dosing between 200 and 400 mg per day accounted for approximately 23% of fatal hepatic injuries over 13.8 ± 12.0 months [51]. In a more recent study, fatal hepatic injury was significantly lower attributed to the lower dosing (100 mg or less) in 95.5% of individuals involved in the study [49]. The potential for hepatic injury has limited the use of dantrolene. Hence, it is not used as a first-line agent but deserves consideration as an adjuvant [47]. Baseline liver function tests (LFTs) should be obtained prior to starting dantrolene. The medication is best avoided in patients with known liver disease. LFTs should be monitored approximately every month as some individuals have shown hepatic dysfunction several months after dose adjustment [49]. The use of dantrolene can lead to generalized muscle weakness as it does not act selectively on specific muscles [47].

Dantrolene can potentially worsen severe underlying respiratory disease. Respiratory complications are unusual but include sterile exudative pleural effusion and eosinophilic asymptomatic pleural effusion in patients who use dantrolene chronically. One case has been reported of respiratory failure requiring intubation directly related to the use of oral dantrolene, which resolved shortly after dantrolene was stopped [46]. However, there is limited information regarding dose-related effects of dantrolene on respiration.

Case 9. Multi-drug management in acquired brain injury

A 50-year-old right-handed woman with a past medical history of hypertension, diabetes mellitus, and hypercholesterolemia, sustained a right middle cerebral artery stroke one year ago, with residual left hemiplegia and spasticity involving the proximal and distal muscles. She reports that severe spasticity limits her therapy as passive range of motion leads to pain, and spasms of the limbs occur intermittently. She does not complain of daytime drowsiness and is cognitively intact.

Key Learning: *In this case, several options are available to address the spasticity and spasms. The more conservative options such as therapy, including a home exercise program, positioning, and bracing, are a mainstay and must be continued. Owing to the generalized nature of the spasticity, considering oral medications is appropriate. Baclofen is a popular choice, even though this may not be the first-line agent in managing spasticity for patients with brain injury due to its possible sedating effect. However, baclofen can still be considered for this patient as she is farther away from the stroke, is cognitively intact, and does not suffer from daytime drowsiness. A low dose of 5–10 mg of oral baclofen can be started at night. The frequency can be increased every 3 days as tolerated up to 3–4 times a day. The goal is to use the lowest dose that produces the desired response, or until the occurrence of side effects. Benzodiazepines should be avoided due to a high incidence of sedation. Tizanidine may be an option with monitoring of liver enzymes* [41]. *Monitor blood pressure due to the potential for hypotension* [6], *especially in this patient who is presumably also taking antihypertensive medication. Dantrolene sodium is used commonly in some centers in the brain-injured population. This medication acts peripherally* [46, 47, 49] *and does not have drowsiness as a significant side effect. Careful and regular monitoring of liver function should be instituted* [49]. *However, avoid dantrolene in the presence of underlying severe respiratory disease* [7]. *In patients with concomitant pain, adding gabapentin may augment spasticity control. Focal treatments for muscle overactivity and muscle stiffness may also be considered (see Chap. 8).*

Sodium and/or Calcium Channel Blocking Agents

Mechanism of Action

Voltage-gated ion channel blocking agents act on the pre-synaptic Ia afferents in the spinal cord and are used for their anti-spastic effects. The medications that fall under this mechanism can be broadly classified into drugs that block the voltage-gated sodium channels, those that block voltage-gated calcium channels, and those that block both the sodium and calcium channels.

Anti-epileptic agents that block sodium channels are phenytoin, levetiracetam, carbamazepine, and lamotrigine. Calcium channel blockers include gabapentin and pregabalin. Tolperisone and its derivatives, invented specifically for the treatment of spasticity [52], block both the sodium and calcium channels (Fig. 10.5).

Sodium Channel Blocking Agents

Mechanism of Action

Various subtypes of voltage-gated sodium channels are present throughout the body [53]. Blocking the specific subtypes related to spasticity can decrease the incidence of unwanted effects. However, anti-epileptics are not subtype specific and do not have the same anti-spastic properties because the degree to which they block specific receptor subtypes varies (i.e., selective inactivation of sodium channels that are hyperexcitable) [53]. There is evidence that sodium channel blockade may be enhanced by co-treatment with a selective serotonin reuptake inhibitor (SSRI) due to its indirect effect on sodium channels [54].

Clinical Use/Dosing

The evidence for sodium channel blockers in the treatment of spasticity is as follows:

Phenytoin Starting at a dose of 200–300 mg/day and achieving serum levels of 12–18 mcg/ml in approximately 2 weeks improved spasticity in a case series of patients with acquired brain injury [55].

Oxcarbazepine Two small case series showed that it can reduce spasticity in patients with acquired brain and spinal cord injury [56, 57]. Oxcarbazepine was started at 300 mg daily and was titrated up to a dose that caused side effects, and then was tapered down to a dose that the patient tolerated. A maximum of 1200 mg per day was tried without side effects.

Levetiracetam A case series and an open-label study showed improvement in spasticity in multiple sclerosis [58], improved spasms and spasticity in motor neuron disease [59], and improved spasms and rigidity in stiff person syndrome [60].

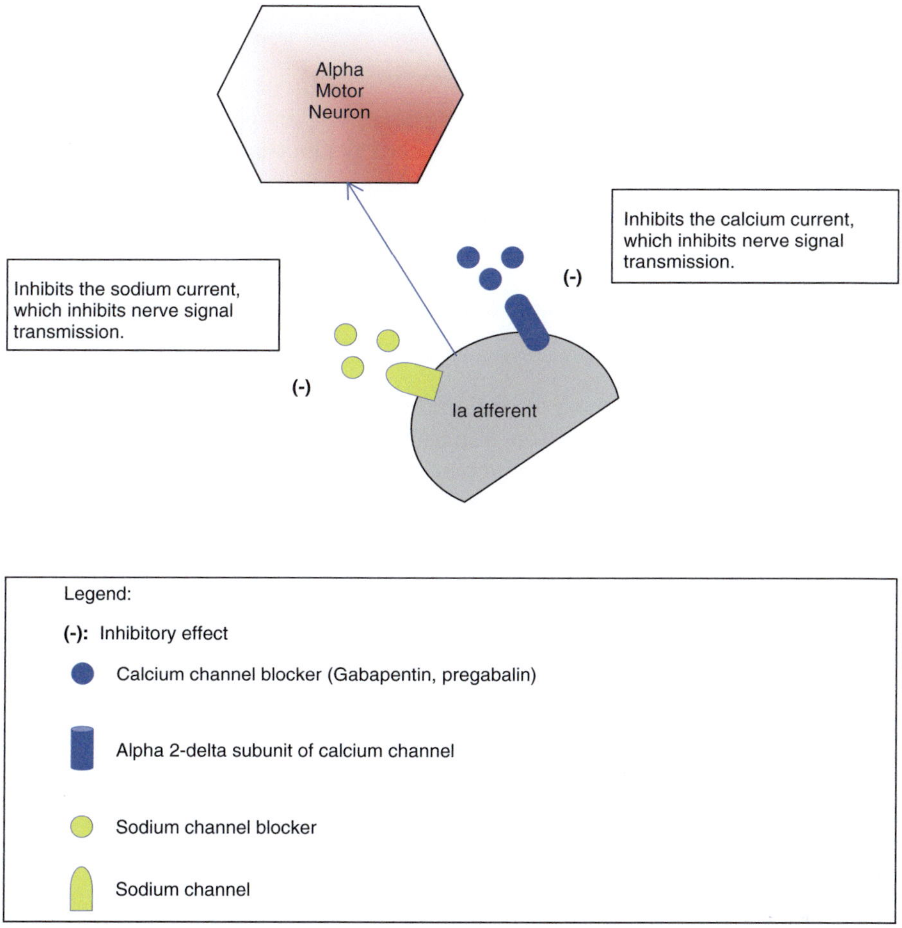

Fig. 10.5 Sites of action of calcium and sodium channel blockers within the muscle stretch reflex arc

However, a randomized, double-blind, placebo-controlled, crossover trial showed no improvement in pain, spasms, or spasticity in patients with spinal cord injury [61]. The dosage used varied, starting from 100 mg daily up to 3000 mg daily. The duration of treatment varied from 1 to 9 months.

Lamotrigine This medication has been widely studied for various pain syndromes, including neurogenic pain [62], with mixed results [63, 64]. No significant human studies have been done on lamotrigine for spasticity. There is some evidence for its use in painful spasms particularly in patients with multiple sclerosis [65]. Dosages of up to 400 mg daily have been used in studies.

Calcium Channel Blocking Agents

Mechanism of Action

Calcium channel blocking agents, such as gabapentin and pregabalin, inhibit presynaptic Ia afferent alpha 2 delta subunits of the calcium channel—the same receptor subtype implicated in neuropathic pain. Hence, they are weak anti-epileptic agents but potent analgesics.

Clinical Use/Dosing

The evidence for calcium channel blockers in the treatment of spasticity is as follows:

Gabapentin It has been found to be useful for spasticity and spasms in multiple sclerosis and spinal cord injury [66–69]. The dosage in these studies varied from 1200 to 2700 mg daily. The duration of treatment ranged from 48 hours to 6 days. There has not been much research conducted in the acquired brain injury population.

Pregabalin This medication has been studied in both acquired brain and spinal cord injury, and has been shown to reduce spasticity in both populations [70, 71]. The maximum dosage after titration was 600 mg daily. Positive responses were seen with higher doses; however, tolerability decreased.

Combination of Sodium and Calcium Channel Blocking Agents

Mechanism of Action

These medications selectively inactivate sodium channels that are hyperexcitable, and also block calcium channels leading to both improved tolerability and efficacy [52].

Clinical Use/Dosing

The evidence for combined sodium and calcium channel blocking agents in the treatment of spasticity is as follows:

Tolperisone It has been extensively studied in acquired brain injury [14, 72], spinal cord injury [14, 73], and cerebral palsy [14]. It has consistently been shown to be efficacious in reducing spasticity and is well tolerated. A comparative study of the clinical efficacy and safety of baclofen versus tolperisone in spasticity caused by spinal cord injury showed that tolperisone was equally effective, better tolerated with fewer side effects, and led to greater functional improvement [73]. The duration of treatment varied from 6 to 12 weeks and the dosage varied between 600 and 900 mg daily.

Eperisone Studies have shown that this medication reduces spasticity in cerebral palsy and is as efficacious as oral baclofen for lower limb spasticity, but is more efficacious than oral baclofen for upper limb spasticity [74, 75]. The dosage was titrated to a maximum of 300 mg daily and was well tolerated. The duration of treatment ranged between 6 and 8 weeks.

Potassium Channel Blocking Agent

4-Aminopyridine

Mechanism of Action

4-Aminopyridine (4-AP, also known as dalfampridine or falpridine in the USA) is a fat-soluble molecule that crosses the blood-brain barrier [76]. In individuals with demyelinating disorders, 4-AP works by blocking potassium channels and promoting the conduction of action potentials along demyelinated axons. The blocking of potassium channels improves synaptic transmission by enhancing pre-synaptic calcium currents and increasing the release of neurotransmitters in synapses and at the neuromuscular junction [76, 77].

Clinical Use

4-AP is FDA-approved for improvement of walking in patients with multiple sclerosis. Several trials have independently found 4-AP to have promising but mixed results in reducing spasticity in persons with multiple sclerosis and spinal cord injury [76, 77]. These studies have also shown mixed results when using different formulations of 4-AP (oral and intravenous) for spasticity measured using the Ashworth Scale, Spasm Frequency Scale, reflex scores, and subjective scores [77, 78].

Dosing

Based on two phase III clinical trials, the FDA-approved dalfampridine (Ampyra) to improve walking in patients with multiple sclerosis at a dosage of 10 mg every 12 hours [79–81]. Although a trend for improvement in spasticity was seen in one of these trials [80], no specific dose recommendations have been established for the treatment of spasticity. In a long-term, controlled trial published in 1999, the administration of 30 mg/day of 4-AP in individuals with chronic spinal cord injury appeared to be safe, relatively free of toxicity, and was associated with decreased spasticity [82]. Two randomized, double-blind, placebo-controlled trials published in 2013 showed similar findings on the safety of a 4-AP sustained-release formulation in chronic spinal cord injury using a dose of 25 mg twice a day. However, no significant differences were observed between treatment groups for the primary end point of spasticity [78].

Side Effect Profile

As a result of its effect on neural membranes, 4-AP can induce seizures in individuals with a lowered threshold for seizure activity. Other published side effects include dizziness, abdominal discomfort, nausea/vomiting, insomnia, paresthesia, anxiety, and generalized pain/discomfort. Most of the side effects tend to be mild, transient, and dose dependent [76, 77].

Serotonergic/Alpha Receptor Antagonist

Cyproheptadine

Mechanism of Action

Research in the 1960s to the early 1980s suggested that 5-hydroxytryptamine (5-HT, serotonin) modulated spinal reflexes [83]. Serotonin regulates calcium currents in the motor neurons, maintaining their excitability [84]. In animals with spinal cord injury, there is an increase in the number of serotonin receptors that are spontaneously active, which facilitates continuous calcium currents without ligand activation or control from the higher centers of the CNS [84]. This may lead to uncontrolled motor neuron activation and hence spasticity and spasms (see also Chap. 1). In some earlier animal studies, cyproheptadine (classified as a serotonin and histamine antagonist) was shown to block the facilitatory effect of administered 5-hydroxytryptophan, a precursor of 5-HT. These and other findings led to studies that investigated cyproheptadine's application in the treatment of spasticity. In more recent publications, it is postulated that activation of the 5-HT_2/alpha 1 constitutive receptors (receptors with basal activity in the absence of ligand activation), below the level of lesion in severe spinal cord injured patients, facilitates muscle spasms. Cyproheptadine is said to block this constitutive activity, as well as the ligand-mediated activation of 5-HT_2/alpha 1 receptors in the spinal motor neuron, acting as an inverse agonist [84, 85]. Older studies and the FDA identify the mechanism of action of cyproheptadine as an antagonist of histamine [86], serotonin [86, 87], and acetylcholine [39].

Clinical Use

The FDA-approved indications are for mild nasal, eye, and skin allergies, cold urticaria, and allergic reactions to blood or plasma. At this time, spasticity is not included in the FDA indications for cyproheptadine. The evidence for cyproheptadine in the treatment of spasticity is as follows:

Several studies evaluated the use of cyproheptadine for spasticity in the spinal cord injury population. The anti-spastic effects of cyproheptadine were found to be similar to that of clonidine and baclofen in this population [39, 88]. A study involving patients with spinal cord injury and multiple sclerosis showed a decrease in ankle clonus [83]. Ankle clonus and frequency of spasms (subjective measure) in six spinal cord injury patients were decreased after at least 6 months of treatment with cyproheptadine [89]. In another study, the long-lasting reflex responses (spasms) in complete spinal cord injury patients were recorded via electromyography. Cyproheptadine given at a dose of 8 mg decreased the spasms [85]. In a recent study on spastic rats with spinal cord injury, the effects of physical rehabilitation and serotonin were investigated in five groups that received the following interventions for two weeks: treadmill training (TMT), TMT with fluoxetine (a selective serotonin reuptake inhibitor), TMT with cyproheptadine, only fluoxetine, or only cyproheptadine. The swimming test was used to quantify the frequency of spastic behaviors. The TMT group and cyproheptadine-treated groups showed decreased spastic behaviors and a reduction in spinal hyperreflexia, whereas the fluoxetine-treated group showed the opposite effect, even with TMT. No additional benefits were noted when TMT and cyproheptadine were combined [90]. In a different study in children with spastic hemiplegia, there was however, no improvement in spasticity in 16 patients (aged 4–18) treated with the medication [91].

Dosing

Cyproheptadine is available in 4 mg tablets. For its FDA-approved indications, the usual starting dose is 4 mg two to three times daily [87]. It is primarily excreted in the urine with a half-life of 1–4 hours. If cyproheptadine is to be used for spasticity, studies suggest dosing the medication at bedtime and increasing the dose every 3–5 days as tolerated [24, 39]. Caution is advised especially in brain-injured patients due to risk of sedation [24]. The maximum dose recommended is 16 mg/day [24].

Side Effect Profile

Cyproheptadine can cause sedation [24, 39, 87], dizziness, confusion, restlessness, tremor, seizures, allergic reactions, blurred vision, diplopia, hypotension, tachycardia, anorexia, nausea, vomiting, diarrhea, urinary retention, and xerostomia, among other side effects [87].

Cannabis

Medical marijuana has received significant attention as a pharmacologic option for the treatment of spasticity recently. There are approximately 60 pharmacologically active compounds in Cannabis Sativa (a.k.a marijuana) called cannabinoids, with delta-9-tetrahydrocannabinol (THC) and cannabidiol (CBD) being the two main active ingredients that modulate the human endocannabinoid system [92–94]. THC is a psychoactive substance that accounts for the therapeutic effects, as well as for some adverse effects of the cannabis extract. CBD is a non-psychoactive substance with its own therapeutic properties and, most importantly, is thought to alleviate the intoxicating effects of THC [94]. There are two known subtypes of cannabinoid receptors (CB1 and CB2). The CB1 receptors are expressed in both the central and peripheral nervous system, whereas the CB2 receptors have been primarily identified on keratinocytes, immune cells, macrophages, and microglia and on spinal cord dorsal horn neurons [93].

The FDA has not yet approved a marketing application for a drug product containing or derived from the whole cannabis plant [95]. It has, however, approved three cannabinoid-based medicines derived from isolated synthetics: Marinol®, Syndros®, and Cesamet®, with indication of anorexia associated with weight loss in patients with AIDS, and nausea and vomiting associated with cancer chemotherapy in patients who have failed to respond adequately to conventional treatment. These synthetic cannabinoids with lower potential for psychotropic side effects have been studied and found to be potentially effective for spasticity and spasticity-related pain [96]. A more recent review of studies in both adult and pediatric populations, including randomized controlled clinical trials, showed that cannabinoids are more effective than placebo in reducing symptoms of spasticity in adults with multiple sclerosis. However, the positive effects were based on patient-rated rather than clinician-rated measures and were modest in size. Pediatric studies of spasticity were inadequate to inform clinical practice [97].

Mechanism of Action

The mechanism of action of cannabinoids in spasticity is not fully understood, but it is thought to be mediated through their action on CB1 receptors. Under normal physiological conditions, the binding of endocannabinoids to pre-synaptic CB1 receptors acts as a signal to inhibit further release of excitatory neurotransmitters such as glutamate, and enhance the effects of the inhibitory neurotransmitter GABA [94].

Clinical Use/Dosing

Routes of administration of medical cannabis include oral administration, sublingual spray, topical ointments, and suppositories [98]. At this time, no specific dosing regimen has been established for spasticity in the USA. In Europe, THC/CBD oromucosal spray is approved as an adjuvant treatment for symptom improvement in adult patients with moderate-to-severe spasticity due to multiple sclerosis. The recommended treatment with THC/CBD oromucosal spray in the UK includes a 14-day self-titration period to reach optimal dose and a 4-week initial trial to identify responders to the treatment [94].

Side Effect Profile

Long-term THC/CBD has not been shown to produce tolerance, and abrupt cessation does not cause withdrawal symptoms in patients with multiple sclerosis [94]. However, a recent review of 16 randomized, double-blind, controlled trials of medical cannabis for the treatment of neuropathic pain consisting of 1750 patients showed that psychiatric disorders occur in 17% of participants using cannabis-based medicines compared with 5% using placebo [99]. The use of THC/CBD is contraindicated in patients with schizophrenia or other psychotic illness, personality disorders, or psychiatric disorders other than depression. Breastfeeding mothers should also avoid the use of THC/CBD since cannabinoids can accumulate in breastmilk [94]. The most common possibly related side effects are short term and include asthenia, balance problems, confusion, dizziness, disorientation, diarrhea, euphoria, drowsiness, dry mouth, fatigue, hallucination, nausea, somnolence, and vomiting [100].

Medications with Unknown Mechanism of Action for Muscle Spasms

Cyclobenzaprine

Mechanism of Action

Cyclobenzaprine is closely related to tricyclic antidepressants (tricyclic amine related to amitriptyline) [101]. The mechanism of action is unclear although it could be related, at least in part, to a sedative effect [102]. It acts at the level of the CNS and functions as a depressant and sedative; it has also been associated with decreasing hyperactivity of the muscle. It influences alpha and gamma motor neurons at the level of the spinal cord and reduces tonic somatic motor activity [101]. It is approved by the FDA as an adjunct treatment for muscle spasms in conjunction with acute, painful musculoskeletal disorders [102, 103].

Clinical Use/Dosing

Cyclobenzaprine is given by mouth and is available as immediate-release tablets (5, 7.5, 10 mg) and extended-release capsules (15 and 30 mg). The maximum dose recommended per day is 30 mg [103]. However, at 60 mg/day it did not show a significant difference compared with placebo in the treatment of spasticity, although one patient who received 150 mg/day showed minimal improvement using objective measurements [101].

Side Effect Profile

Side effects include dizziness, drowsiness, fatigue, headache, nervousness, and confusion. Since it antagonizes muscarinic receptors, it can also lead to xerostomia, ileus, tachycardia, mydriasis, confusion, and hallucinations. It also antagonizes the alpha 1 adrenergic receptors, causing a vasodilatory effect, and may contribute to reflex tachycardia. Most common adverse effects are somnolence, dry mucous membranes, dizziness, and confusion [103].

Cyclobenzaprine is contraindicated in individuals with hyperthyroidism, arrhythmias, heart failure, heart block, or conduction disturbances, as well as in those recovering from an acute myocardial infarction, and those within 14 days of taking a monoamine oxidase inhibitor [103]. It is important to monitor patients for signs and symptoms of serotonin syndrome while taking cyclobenzaprine [103].

Orphenadrine

Mechanism of Action

Orphenadrine is derived from diphenhydramine. The mechanism of action is unclear although it also could be related, at least in part, to a sedative effect [102, 104].

Clinical Use

It is approved for the treatment of muscle spasms that are associated with acute, painful musculoskeletal disorders [102, 104].

Dosing

It is usually taken at a dose of 100 mg by mouth twice per day [104]. It should not be stopped abruptly, and gradual weaning is recommended when taking high doses and/or when used chronically [104].

Side Effect Profile

It has higher anticholinergic effects compared with diphenhydramine. Side effects include xerostomia, nausea, vomiting, constipation, gastric irritation, headache, dizziness, hallucinations, tremor, agitation, tachycardia, palpitation, muscle weakness, urinary hesitancy and retention, blurred vision, increased intraocular pressure, hypersensitivity, pruritus, and very rarely aplastic anemia. The elderly population is at higher risk for side effects [104].

Mexiletine

Mechanism of Action

Mexiletine is classified as a class 1B antiarrhythmic agent and is a sodium channel blocker on cardiac myocytes and neurons [105, 106].

Clinical Use

Although mexiletine is primarily used for the treatment of ventricular arrhythmias, it has also been used in the treatment of muscle pain in myotonic dystrophy and for muscle stiffness in non-dystrophic myotonia [107]. A randomized clinical trial for muscle cramps in amyotrophic lateral sclerosis showed large dose-dependent reductions in muscle cramp frequency and severity [108]. In addition, it is used for the treatment of peripheral neuropathy and chronic pain, although its use is limited by its side effects. It has also been tested in pain in spinal cord injury without significant improvement [109].

Dosing

It is an oral medication that is given one to three times per day depending on the indication. A common dosing regimen is 150–200 mg two to three times per day.

Side Effect Profile

The side effects include irregular heartbeat, chest pain, extreme tiredness, liver injury, jaundice, unusual bleeding or bruising, lack of energy, lightheadedness or dizziness, loss of coordination, numbness or tingling, headache blurred vision, nervousness, difficulty speaking, swelling of the hands, feet, ankles, or lower legs, vomiting, heartburn, changes in appetite, and rash. Cardiac, hepatic, and metabolic monitoring is required when using this medication.

Conclusion

Oral medications are valuable agents for controlling generalized spasticity and spasms in patients with CNS injury. They are frequently used as first-line treatment to control spasticity in persons with spinal cord injury, cerebral palsy, and multiple sclerosis. For individuals with acquired brain injury and in the elderly, the use of oral medications is limited by the negative effects on alertness and cognition. These medications can, however, still be used as adjunct treatments, especially in chronic conditions when cognitive and arousal impairments are no longer a significant concern, and/or when the benefits outweigh the risks. Care must be exercised in choosing the specific medication, as well as in monitoring the treatment response and adverse effects. Many of the more commonly used oral spasmolytics cause significant drowsiness, and withdrawal symptoms if stopped abruptly especially after prolonged use (such as baclofen and benzodiazepines). Baclofen and tizanidine should be used with caution in those with renal function impairment. Liver function monitoring should be kept in mind when choosing dantrolene sodium and tizanidine. In many patient populations, the dictum "start low, go slow" should be applied to improve patient tolerance. To decrease polypharmacy, medication choice should also take into consideration the presence of other conditions, such as neuropathic pain and anxiety as some spasmolytics may be indicated for these diagnoses as well.

References

1. Katz RT, Rymer WZ. Spastic hypertonia: mechanism and measurement. Arch Phys Med Rehabil. 1989;70:144–55.
2. Li S, Kamper DG, Rymer WZ. Effects of changing wrist positions on finger flexor hypertonia in stroke survivors. Muscle Nerve. 2006;33:183–90.
3. Burke D, Wissel J, Donnan GA. Pathophysiology of spasticity in stroke. Neurology. 2013;80(Suppl 2):S20–6.
4. Baclofen – FDA prescribing information, side effects and uses. In: Drugs.com. https://www.drugs.com/pro/baclofen.html. Accessed 22 June 2019.
5. Diazepam – Roche Pharmaceuticals. In: Drugs@FDA: FDA Approved Drugs. https://www.accessdata.fda.gov/drugsatfda_docs/label/2016/013263s094lbl.pdf. Accessed 22 June 2019.
6. Tizanidine – FDA approved labeling. In: Drugs@FDA: FDA Approved Drug Products. https://www.accessdata.fda.gov/drugsatfda_docs/label/2013/021447s011_020397s026lbl.pdf. Accessed 22 June 2019.

7. Dantrium (dantrolene sodium) – FDA approved labeling. In: Drugs@FDA: FDA Approved Drug Products. https://www.accessdata.fda.gov/drugsatfda_docs/label/2012/017443s043s046s048s049lbl.pdf. Accessed 22 June 2019.
8. Olsen R, Li G. GABA. In: Brady ST, Siegel GJ, Albers RW, Price DL, editors. Basic neurochemistry: principles of molecular, cellular, and medical neurobiology. Waltham: Academic Press/Elsevier; 2012. p. 367–76.
9. Francisco G, Li S. Spasticity. In: Cifu DX, Kaelin DL, Braddom RL, editors. Braddoms physical medicine & rehabilitation. Philadelphia: Elsevier; 2016.
10. Meythaler J, Smith R. Pharmacologic management of spasticity: oral medications. In: Brashear A, Elovic E, editors. Spasticity: diagnosis and management. New York: Demos; 2016.
11. Segatore M, Miller M. The pharmacotherapy of spinal spasticity: a decade of progress. II. Therapeutics. SCI Nurs. 1995;12(1):2–7.
12. Nance PW, Young RR. Antispasticity medications. Phys Med Rehabil Clin N Am. 1999;10(2):337–55.
13. Montane E, Vallano A, Laporte JR. Oral antispastic drugs in nonprogressive neurologic diseases: a systematic review. Neurology. 2004;63:1357–63.
14. Agarwal S, Patel T, Shah N, Patel BM. Comparative study of therapeutic response to baclofen vs tolperisone in spasticity. Biomed Pharmacother. 2017;87:628–35. Cited from original article: A. Dario, G. Tomei. A benefit-risk assessment of baclofen in severe spinal spasticity. Drug Saf. 2004;27:799–818.
15. Nair K, Marsden J. The management of spasticity in adults. BMJ. 2014;349:g4737, 1–10.
16. Thibau A, Chatelle C, Ziegler E, Bruno MA, Laureys S, Gosseries O. Spasticity after stroke: physiology, assessment and treatment. Brain Inj. 2013;27(10):1093–105.
17. Al-Shahrani A. Anti-spasticity medication. Saudi Med J. 2003;24(1):19–22.
18. Chang E, Ghosh N, Yanni D, Lee S, Alexandru D, Mozaffar T. A review of spasticity treatments: pharmacological and interventional approaches. Crit Rev Phys Rehabil Med. 2013;25(1–2):11–22.
19. Francisco GE, Kothari S, Huls C. GABA agonists and gabapentin for spastic hypertonia. Phys Med Rehabil Clin N Am. 2001;12(4):875–88.
20. Consensus Development Group. National Collaborating Centre for Chronic Conditions. Multiple sclerosis: national clinical guideline for diagnosis and management in primary and secondary care. London: Royal College of Physicians; 2004.
21. Agarwal S, Kriel R, Cloyd J, Coles L, Scherkenback L, Tobin M, Krach L. A pilot study assessing pharmacokinetics and tolerability of oral and intravenous baclofen in health adult volunteers. J Child Neurol. 2015;30(I):37–41.
22. Kheder A, Nair K. Spasticity: pathophysiology, evaluation and management. Pract Neurol. 2012;12:289–98.
23. Cardenas D, Hooton T. Urinary tract infection in persons with spinal cord injury. Arch Phys Med Rehabil. 1995;76:272–80.
24. Zafonte R, Lombard L, Elovic E. Antispasticity medications uses and limitations of enteral therapy. Am J Phys Med Rehabil. 2004;83:S50–8.
25. Watanabe T. Role of oral medications in spasticity management. Am Acad Phys Med Rehabil. 2009;1:839–41.
26. Young R, Delwaide P. Drug therapy: spasticity. N Engl J Med. 1981;304:96–9.
27. Kita M, Goodkin D. Drugs used to treat spasticity. Drugs. 2000;59(3):487–95.
28. Mandelli M, Tognoni G, Garattini S. Clinical pharmacokinetics of diazepam. Clin Pharmacokinet. 1978;3(1):72–91.
29. Otero-Romero S, Sastre-Garriga J, Comi G, Hartung H, Soelberg SP, Thompson A, Vermersch P, Gold R, Montalban X. Pharmacological management of spasticity in multiple sclerosis: systematic review and consensus paper. Mult Scler J. 2016;22(11):1386–96.
30. Lapeyre E, Kukls JB, Meijler WJ. Spasticity: revisiting the role and the individual value of several pharmacological treatments. NeuroRehabilitation. 2010;27:193–200.

31. Tiagabine – FDA approved labeling. In: Drugs@FDA: FDA approved drug products. https://www.accessdata.fda.gov/drugsatfda_docs/label/2016/020646s021lbl.pdf. Accessed 22 June 2019.
32. Meldrum B, Chapman A. Basic mechanisms of gabitril (tiagabine) and future potential developments. Epilepsia. 1999;40:S2–6.
33. Sałat K, Więckowska A, Więckowski K, Höfner G, Kamiński J, Wanner K, Malawska B, Filipek B, Kulig K. Synthesis and pharmacological properties of new GABA uptake inhibitors. Pharmacol Rep. 2012;64:817–33.
34. Conti F, Minelli A, Melone M. GABA transporters in the mammalian cerebral cortex: localization, development and pathological implications. Brain Res Rev. 2004;45:196–212.
35. Sałat K, Podkowa A, Mogilski S, Zaręba P, Kulig K, Sałat R, Malikowska N, Filipek B. The effect of GABA transporter 1 (GAT1) inhibitor, tiagabine, on scopolamine-induced memory impairments in mice. Pharmacol Rep. 2015;67:1155–62.
36. Kakinohana O, Hefferan M, Miyanohara A, et al. Combinational spinal GAD65 gene delivery and systemic GABA-mimetic treatment for modulation of spasticity. PLoS One. 2012;7:e30561.
37. Chu M, Sala D. The use of tiagabine in pediatric spasticity management. Dev Med Child Neurol. 2006;48:456.
38. Malanga G, Reiter R, Garay E. Update on tizanidine for muscle spasticity and emerging indications. Expert Opin Pharmacother. 2008;9(12):2209–15.
39. Nance P. Alpha adrenergic and serotonergic agents in the treatment of spastic hypertonia. Phys Med Rehabil Clin N Am. 2001;12(4):889–905.
40. Mirbagheri MM, Chen D, Rymer WZ. Quantification of the effects of an alpha-2 adrenergic agonist on reflex properties in spinal cord injury using a system identification technique. J Neuroeng Rehabil. 2010;7:29. https://doi.org/10.1186/1743-0003-7-29. PMID: 20573252; PMCID: PMC2904341.
41. Kamen L, Henney H, Runyan J. A practical overview of tizanidine use for spasticity secondary to multiple sclerosis, stroke, and spinal cord injury. Curr Med Res Opin. 2007;24(2):425–39.
42. Henney H, Shah J. Relative bioavailability of tizanidine 4-mg capsule and tablet formulations after a standardized high-fat meal: a single-dose, randomized, open-label, crossover study in healthy subjects. Clin Ther. 2007;29(4):661–9.
43. Krassioukov A, Eng J, Warburton D, Teasell R, SCIRE Research Team. A systematic review of the management of orthostatic hypotension following spinal cord injury. Arch Phys Med Rehabil. 1995;75:272–80.
44. Kirshblum S, Campagnolo D. Spinal cord medicine. 2nd ed. Philadelphia: Lippincott Williams & Wilkins; 2001.
45. Ellis KO, Butterfield JL, Wessels FL, Carpenter JF. A comparison of skeletal, cardiac, and smooth muscle actions of dantrolene sodium--a skeletal muscle relaxant. Arch Int Pharmacodyn Ther. 1976;224(1):118–32. PMID: 1015907.
46. Javed M, Bodanov A. Oral dantrolene and severe respiratory failure in a patient with chronic spinal cord injury. Anaesthesia. 2010;65:855–6.
47. Chang E, Ghosh N, Yanni D, Lee S, Alexandru D, Moffazar T. A review of spasticity treatments: pharmacological and interventional approaches. Crit Rev Phys Rehabil Med. 2013;25:11–22.
48. Chipman M, Kaul S, Lambie M. Efficacy of dantrolene sodium in the treatment of spasticity. Dis Nerv Syst. 1974;35(9):427–31. PMID: 17894068.
49. Kim J, Chun S, Bang M, Shin H, Lee S. Safety of low-dose oral dantrolene sodium on hepatic function. Arch Phys Med Rehabil. 2011;92:1359–63.
50. Utili R, Boitnott JK, Zimmerman HJ. Dantrolene-associated hepatic injury. Incidence and character. Gastroenterol. 1977;72:610–6.
51. Chan CH. Dantrolene sodium and hepatic injury. Neurol. 1990;40:1427–32.
52. Kocsis P, Farkas S, Fodor L, Bielik N, Thán M, Kolok S, Gere A, Csejtei M, Tarnawa I. Tolperisone-type drugs inhibit spinal reflexes via blockade of voltage- gated sodium and calcium channels. J Pharmacol Exp Ther. 2005;315(3):1237–46.

53. Tarnawa I, Bölcskei H, Kocsis P. Blockers of voltage-gated sodium channels for the treatment of central nervous system diseases. Recent Pat CNS Drug Discov. 2007;2(1):57–78.
54. Thán M, Kocsis P, Tihanyi K, Fodor L, Farkas B, Kovács G, Kis-Varga A, Szombathelyi Z, Tarnawa I. Concerted action of antiepileptic and antidepressant agents to depress spinal neurotransmission: possible use in the therapy of spasticity and chronic pain. Neurochem Int. 2007;50(4):642–52.
55. Cohan SL, Raines A, Panagakos J, Armitage P. Phenytoin and chlorpromazine in the treatment of spasticity. Arch Neurol. 1980;37(6):360–4.
56. Bittencourt PR, Silvado CE. Oxcarbazepine, GP 47779, and spasticity. Lancet. 1985;326:676.
57. Bittencourt PR. Oxcarbazepine and spasticity: further observations. Arq Neuropsiquiatr. 1988;46(4):382–4.
58. Hawker K, Frohman E, Racke M. Levetiracetam for phasic spasticity in multiple sclerosis. Arch Neurol. 2003;60(12):1772–4.
59. Bedlack RS, Pastula DM, Hawes J, Heydt D. Open-label pilot trial of levetiracetam for cramps and spasticity in patients with motor neuron disease. Amyotroph Lateral Scler. 2009;10(4):210–5.
60. Sechi G, Barrocu M, Piluzza MG, Cocco GA, Deiana GA, Sau GF. Levetiracetam in stiff-person syndrome. J Neurol. 2008;255(11):1721–5.
61. Finnerup NB, Grydehøj J, Bing J, Johannesen IL, Biering-Sørensen F, Sindrup SH, Jensen TS. Levetiracetam in spinal cord injury pain: a randomized controlled trial. Spinal Cord. 2009;47(12):861–7.
62. Titlic M, Jukic I, Tonkic A, Josipovic-Jelic Z, Boschi V, Mihalj M, Punda A. Lamotrigine in the treatment of pain syndromes and neuropathic pain. Bratisl Lek Listy. 2008;109(9):421–4.
63. Breuer B, Pappagallo M, Knotkova H, Guleyupoglu N, Wallenstein S, Portenoy RK. A randomized, double-blind, placebo-controlled, two-period, crossover, pilot trial of lamotrigine in patients with central pain due to multiple sclerosis. Clin Ther. 2007;29:2022–30.
64. Silver M, Blum D, Grainger J, Hammer AE, Quessy S. Double-blind, placebo- controlled trial of lamotrigine in combination with other medications for neuropathic pain. J Pain Symptom Manag. 2007;34(4):446–54.
65. Pöllmann W, Feneberg W, Steinbrecher A, Haupts MR, Henze T. Therapy of pain syndromes in multiple sclerosis – an overview with evidence-based recommendations. Fortschr Neurol Psychiatr. 2005;73(5):268–85.
66. Mueller ME, Gruenthal M, Olson WL, Olson WH. Gabapentin for relief of upper motor neuron symptoms in multiple sclerosis. Arch Phys Med Rehabil. 1997;78(5):521–4.
67. Rabchevsky AG, Patel SP, Duale H, Lyttle TS, O'Dell CR, Kitzman PH. Gabapentin for spasticity and autonomic dysreflexia after severe spinal cord injury. Spinal Cord. 2011;49(1):99–105.
68. Cutter NC, Scott DD, Johnson JC, Whiteneck G. Gabapentin effect on spasticity in multiple sclerosis: a placebo- controlled, randomized trial. Arch Phys Med Rehabil. 2000;81(2):164–9.
69. Gruenthal M, Mueller M, Olson WL, Priebe MM, Sherwood AM, Olson WH. Gabapentin for the treatment of spasticity in patients with spinal cord injury. Spinal Cord. 1997;35(10):686–9.
70. Braid JJ, Kirker SG, Baguley IJ. Spasticity increases during pregabalin withdrawal. Brain Inj. 2013;27:120–4.
71. Bradley L, Kirker S. Pregabalin in the treatment of spasticity: a retrospective case series. Disabil Rehabil. 2008;30(16):1230–2.
72. Stamenova P, Koytchev R, Kuhn K, Hansen C, Horvath F, Ramm S, Pongratz D. A randomized, double-blind, placebo-controlled study of the efficacy and safety of tolperisone in spasticity following cerebral stroke. Eur J Neurol. 2005;12(6):453–61.
73. Luo D, Wu G, Ji Y, Zhang Z, He F, Mou X, Zhu Q, Yang B. The comparative study of clinical efficacy and safety of baclofen vs tolperisone in spasticity caused by spinal cord injury. Saudi Pharm J. 2017;25(4):655–9.

74. Bresolin N, Zucca C, Pecori A. Efficacy and tolerability of eperisone and baclofen in spastic palsy: a double- blind randomized trial. Adv Ther. 2009;26(5):563–73.
75. Bresolin N, Zucca C, Pecori A. Efficacy and tolerability of eperisone in patients with spastic palsy: a cross- over, placebo-controlled dose-ranging trial. Eur Rev Med Pharmacol Sci. 2009;13(5):365–70.
76. Jensen HB, Ravnborg M, Dalgas U, Stenager E. 4-Aminopyridine for symptomatic treatment of multiple sclerosis: a systematic review. Ther Adv Neurol Disord. 2014;7(2):97–113.
77. Wiener J, Hsieh J, McIntyre A, Teasell R. Effectiveness of 4-aminopyridine for the management of spasticity in SCI: systematic review. Top Spinal Cord Inj Rehabil. 2018;24(4):353–62.
78. Cardenas DD, Ditunno JF, Graziani V, McLain AB, Lammertse DP, Potter PJ, Alexander MS, Cphen R, Blight AR. Two phase 3, multicenter, randomized, placebo-controlled clinical trials of fampridine-SR for treatment of spasticity in chronic spinal cord injury. Spinal Cord. 2014;52:70–6.
79. Biogen Canada, Inc (2012). Product monograph Fampyra. https://www.biogen.ca/content/dam/corporate/en_CA/pdfs/products/FAMPYRA/FAMPYRA_PM_E.pdf.
80. Goodman AD, Brown TR, Krupp LB, et al. Sustained release of oral fampridine in multiple sclerosis: a randomized, double-blind, controlled trial. Lancet. 2009;373:732–8.
81. Goodman AD, Brown TR, Edwards KR, et al. A phase 3 trial of extended release oral dalfampridine in multiple sclerosis. Ann Neurol. 2010;68:494–502.
82. Segal F, Pathack M, Hernandez J, Himber P, Brunnemann S, Charter R. Safety and efficacy of 4-aminopyridine in humans with spinal cord injury: a long-term, controlled trial. Pharmacotherapy. 1999;19(6):713–23.
83. Barbeau H, Richards C, Bedard P. Action of cyproheptadine in spastic paraparetic patients. J Neurol Neurosurg Psychiatry. 1982;45:923–6.
84. Murray K, Nakae A, Stephens M, et al. Recovery of motoneuron and locomotor function after spinal cord injury depends on constitutive activity in 5-HT2C receptors. Nat Med. 2010;16:694–700.
85. D'Amico J, Murray K, Li Y, Chan K, Finlay M, Bennett D, Gorassini M. Constitutively active 5-HT2/α1 receptors facilitate muscle spasms after human spinal cord injury. J Neurophysiol. 2013;109:1473–84.
86. Domingo A, Al-Yahya A, Asiri Y, Eng J, Lam T, Spinal Cord Injury Rehabil T. A systematic review of the effects of pharmacological agents on walking function in people with spinal cord injury. J Neurotrauma. 2012;29:865–79.
87. Cyproheptadine – FDA approved labeling. In: Drugs@FDA: FDA Approved Drug Products. https://www.accessdata.fda.gov/drugsatfda_docs/label/2009/087056s045lbl.pdf. Accessed 21 June 2019.
88. Nance P. A comparison of clonidine, cyproheptadine and baclofen in spastic spinal cord injured patients. J Am Paraplegia Soc. 1994;17:150–6.
89. Wainberg M, Barbeau H, Gauthier S. The effects of cyproheptadine on locomotion and on spasticity in patients with spinal cord injuries. J Neurol Neurosurg Psychiatry. 1990;53:754–63.
90. Ryu Y, Ogata T, Nagao M, Sawada Y, Nishimura R, Fujita N. Effects of treadmill training combined with serotonergic interventions on spasticity after contusive spinal cord injury. J Neurotrauma. 2018;35:1358–66.
91. Khodadadeh S, Holstein H, Purushothaman S, Patrick J. A study of the effect of cyproheptadine on gait in hemiplegic children. Gait Posture. 1998;8:205–13.
92. Koppel B, Brust J, Fife T, Brinstein J, Youssif S, Gronseth G, Gloss D. Systematic review: efficacy and safety of medical marijuana in selected neurologic disorders. Neurology. 2014;82:1556–63.
93. Karst M, Wippermann S, Ahrens J. Role of cannabinoids in the treatment of pain and (painful) spasticity. Drugs. 2010;70(18):2409–38.
94. Syed Y, McKeage K, Scott L. Delta-9-tetrahydrocannabinol/cannabidiol (Sativex®) a review of its use in patients with moderate to severe spasticity due to multiple sclerosis. Drugs. 2014;74:563–78.

95. Mack A, Joy J. Marijuana as medicine? The science beyond the controversy. Washington, DC: National Academy Press; 2000.
96. Wissel J, Haydn T, Müller J, Brenneis C, Berger T, Poewe W, Schelosky LD. Low dose treatment with the synthetic cannabinoid Nabilone significantly reduces spasticity-related pain: a double-blind placebo-controlled cross-over trial. J Neurol. 2006;253(10):1337–41.
97. Nielsen S, Murnion B, Campbell G, Young H, Hall W. Cannabinoids for the treatment of spasticity. Dev Med Child Neurol. 2019;61(6):631–8. https://doi.org/10.1111/dmcn.14165. Epub 2019 Jan 25. PMID: 30680713.
98. Zajicek J, Fox P, Sanders H, Wright D, Vichery J, Nunn A, Thompson A. Cannabinoids for treatment of spasticity and other symptoms related to multiple sclerosis (CAMS study): multicenter randomised placebo-controlled trial. Lancet. 2003;362:1517–26.
99. Mücke M, Phillips T, Radbruch L, Petzke F, Häuser W. Cannabis-based medicines for chronic neuropathic pain in adults. Cochrane Database Syst Rev. 2018;3(3):CD012182. https://doi.org/10.1002/14651858.CD012182.pub2. PMID: 29513392; PMCID: PMC6494210.
100. Whitting P, Wolff R, Deshpande S, Di Nisio M, Duffy S, Hernandez AV, Keurentjes JC, Lang S, Misso K, Ryder S, Schmidlkofer S, Westwood M, Kleijnen J. Cannabinoids for medical use: a systematic review and meta-analysis. JAMA. 2015;313(24):2456–73.
101. Ashby P, Burke D, Rao S, Jones RF. Assessment of cyclobenzaprine in the treatment of spasticity. J Neurol Neurosurg Psychiatry. 1972;35(5):599–605.
102. Chou R, Peterson K, Helfand M. Comparative efficacy and safety of skeletal muscles relaxants for spasticity and musculoskeletal conditions: a systematic review. J Pain Symptom Manag. 2004;28(2):140–75.
103. Khan I, Kahwaji C. Cyclobenzaprine. Irvine: University of California; 2018. https://www.ncbi.nlm.nih.gov/books/NBK513362.
104. Frydrych V, Oderda G. Skeletal muscle relaxants drug class review. Salt Lake City: University of Utah College of Pharmacy; 2016. p. 1–40.
105. Ginanneschi F, Mignarri A, Lucchiari S, Ulzi G, Comi GP, Rossi A, Dotti MT. Neuromuscular excitability changes produced by sustained voluntary contraction and response to mexiletine in myotonia congenita. Neurophysiol Clin. 2017;47(3):247–52. https://doi.org/10.1016/j.neucli.2017.01.003. Epub 2017 Jan 30. PMID: 28153715.
106. Statland JM, Bundy BN, Wang Y, Rayan DR, Trivedi JR, Sansone VA, Salajegheh MK, Venance SL, Ciafaloni E, Matthews E, Meola G, Herbelin L, Griggs RC, Barohn RJ, Hanna MG, Consortium for Clinical Investigation of Neurologic Channelopathies. Mexiletine for symptoms and signs of myotonia in nondystrophic myotonia: a randomized controlled trial. JAMA. 2012;308(13):1357–65. https://doi.org/10.1001/jama.2012.12607. PMID: 23032552; PMCID: PMC3564227.
107. Stunnenberg BC, Raaphorst J, Groenewoud HM, Statland JM, Griggs RC, Woertman W, Stegeman DF, Timmermans J, Trivedi J, Matthews E, Saris CGJ, Schouwenberg BJ, Drost G, van Engelen BGM, van der Wilt GJ. Effect of mexiletine on muscle stiffness in patients with nondystrophic myotonia evaluated using aggregated N-of-1 trials. JAMA. 2018;320(22):2344–53. https://doi.org/10.1001/jama.2018.18020. PMID: 30535218; PMCID: PMC6583079.
108. Weiss MD, Macklin EA, Simmons Z, Knox AS, Greenblatt DJ, Atassi N, Graves M, Parziale N, Salameh JS, Quinn C, Brown RH Jr, Distad JB, Trivedi J, Shefner JM, Barohn RJ, Pestronk A, Swenson A, Cudkowicz ME, Mexiletine ALS Study Group. A randomized trial of mexiletine in ALS: safety and effects on muscle cramps and progression. Neurology. 2016;86(16):1474–81. https://doi.org/10.1212/WNL.0000000000002507. Epub 2016 Feb 24. PMID: 26911633; PMCID: PMC4836879.
109. Chiou-Tan F, Tuel S, Johnson J, Priebe M, Hirsh D, Strayer J. Effect of mexiletine on spinal cord injury dysesthetic pain. Am J Phys Med Rehabil. 1996;75(2):84–7.

Intrathecal Baclofen Therapy

11

Michael Saulino

Medicine is a science of uncertainty and an art of probability.
– William Osler, The Principles and Practices of Medicine, 1892.

- Intrathecal baclofen (ITB) exerts its therapeutic effect by delivering baclofen directly into the cerebrospinal fluid with rapid distribution to GABA-B-rich neurons in lamina II of the spinal cord.
- It is indicated for poorly-controlled, generalized spasticity despite maximal therapy and/or limited tolerance of other treatment modalities in patients with spasticity of spinal (traumatic spinal cord injury and multiple sclerosis) and cerebral (acquired brain injury, cerebral palsy, and stroke) origin.
- ITB therapy is accomplished through the use of a surgically-implanted, programmable pump that delivers drug at precise flow rates via a catheter introduced into the spinal canal.
- This chapter reviews the components of ITB therapy, patient selection, trial dose, pump implantation and ITB therapy initiation, pump maintenance and chronic therapy, troubleshooting, management of ITB overdose and withdrawal, and pump explantation.
- Successful implementation of ITB therapy requires a robust team structure to manage the routine, urgent, and emergent needs of the patients receiving this treatment.

M. Saulino (✉)
Cooper University Health Care, Camden, NJ, USA

Department of Physical Medicine and Rehabiliation, Cooper Medical School of Rowan University, Camden, NJ, USA
e-mail: saulino-michael@CooperHealth.edu

P. Raghavan (ed.), *Spasticity and Muscle Stiffness*,
https://doi.org/10.1007/978-3-030-96900-4_11

Introduction

Intrathecal baclofen (ITB) therapy was first approved for use by the FDA in 1992. Since then, it has been used successfully in the management of patients with spasticity from a variety of causes including multiple sclerosis, traumatic brain injury, spinal cord injury, cerebral palsy, and stroke. ITB infusion exerts its therapeutic effect by delivering baclofen directly into the cerebrospinal fluid (CSF) with distribution to GABA-B-rich neurons in lamina II of the spinal cord. Intrathecal administration is accomplished through the use of a surgically-implanted, programmable pump that delivers drug at precise flow rates via a catheter introduced into the spinal canal. Until 2020, only one manufacturer (Medtronic) had active FDA approval for chronic intrathecal baclofen infusion in the United States. In 2020, the FDA approved Flowonix Medical's Prometra II Pump System for use with intrathecal baclofen. This chapter focuses on ITB therapy using the Medtronic system. However, the principles of management would likely be similar with other systems with relatively minor differences in technical application [1, 2].

Components of Intrathecal Baclofen Therapy

Intrathecal delivery systems are comprised of a few key components. These include an accessible drug reservoir and a method of propelling the drug out of the pump into a catheter that connects the drug reservoir to the CSF (Fig. 11.1). While

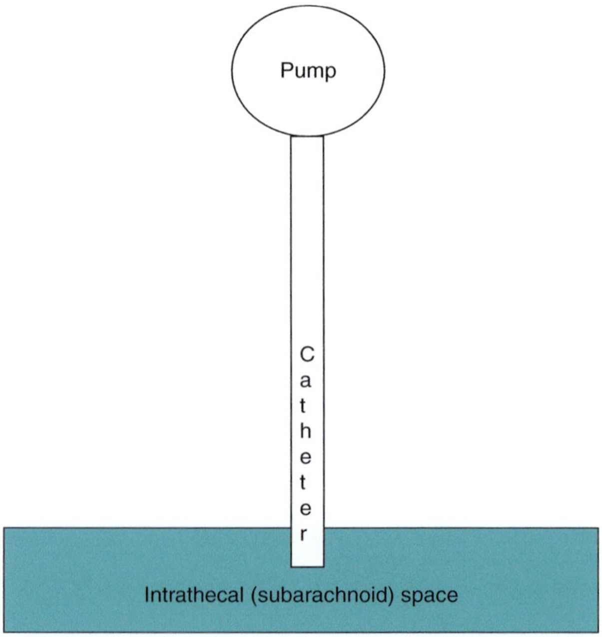

Fig. 11.1 Schematic diagram of an intrathecal delivery system

constant flow systems are available, programmable systems are overwhelmingly preferred due to their adjustability for individual patient needs [3]. Programmable systems require additional components including an external programming device and a communication method between the programmer and the implanted pump. They also require an energy source to support the internal electronic components. In contrast, constant flow pumps can utilize a pneumatic propulsion technique. Future intrathecal baclofen delivery systems may include automated troubleshooting of the system, self-directed patient programming, and integrated sensors to detect patient position and functional activity levels [4, 5].

Patient Selection

Patient selection and education are fundamental to all aspects of medical practice. These principles are of particular importance with interventional procedures involving implantable technology. Patients found to be appropriate candidates for ITB therapy need to be counseled before proceeding with this treatment. They should be apprised of all aspects of the therapy including trialing, pump implantation, postoperative rehabilitation, and chronic maintenance issues [6]. The recognition by the patient that this treatment modality represents a long-term commitment cannot be understated.

Patient Characteristics

In general, patients can be considered candidates for ITB therapy when the following occur:

- Spasticity is poorly controlled despite maximal therapy with other modalities.
- Spasticity is poorly controlled because of limited patient tolerance of other treatment modalities.
- Adjustable spasticity reduction afforded by a programmable, variable-flow pump would be advantageous.

The FDA-approved diagnoses for ITB therapy include spasticity of spinal (spinal cord injury, multiple sclerosis) and cerebral (acquired brain injury, cerebral palsy, and stroke) origin. There is greater experience with spasticity of spinal origin compared to that of cerebral origin since the former indications had earlier FDA approval. ITB therapy has been shown to be efficacious in patients with other degenerative conditions of the brain and spinal cord (amyotrophic lateral sclerosis, hereditary spastic paraparesis) as well [7–9].

To receive ITB therapy, patients should be clinically stable, comprehend the advantages and disadvantages of ITB therapy, be able to return to the clinic for dose titration and pump refills, and have demonstrated a positive response to a test dose of intrathecal baclofen. Caregivers must be involved in the medical decision-making for individuals with cognitive impairment and for children. A reasonable time should have elapsed since the neurological injury to allow natural recovery to occur before considering intrathecal therapy, recognizing however, that early exposure to ITB can be beneficial in selected cases. In patients with multiple sclerosis whose neurologic presentation may vary, patients should not be solely evaluated during an exacerbation. In severe cases, ITB therapy can be considered early in the post-injury recovery period (e.g., <12 months) [10]. ITB therapy generally reduces lower limb spasticity to a greater extent than upper limb spasticity. More cephalad catheter tip placements can potentially improve effects on the upper limb [11], although the response to this strategy is not uniform [12].

Advantages and Disadvantages of Intrathecal Baclofen Therapy

The advantages of ITB therapy include delivery of a higher potency of baclofen with potentially fewer adverse effects compared to oral baclofen, the ability to have a global effect on all affected limbs, and the possibility of dose adjustment with changing needs of the patient and progressive disease. The disadvantages include surgical risks (e.g., bleeding, infection, damage of neural structures), the potential for serious adverse effects including overdose and withdrawal, and the requirement of ongoing follow up with health-care professionals for dose adjustments and pump refills. Ventricular shunting for hydrocephalus is not a contraindication to ITB therapy, but practitioners should be aware of potential effects of the device on CSF flow [13]. Intrathecal baclofen can also be used in patients with seizures with the understanding that this therapy has been occasionally associated with a risk of increased seizures [14–16]. Similarly, prior abdominal or pelvic surgery (e.g., gastrostomy, suprapubic cystotomy) is not a contraindication for intrathecal pump placement but does require some consideration during surgical placement [17, 18]. Patients and caregivers should be fully apprised of these issues to facilitate informed decision-making prior to proceeding with an intrathecal trial.

Intrathecal Baclofen Trial

A successful trial of intrathecal baclofen is necessary to evaluate the risks versus benefits of this invasive treatment. The typical method of ITB trialing is to perform a lumbar puncture and inject a bolus of a baclofen solution into the CSF. A 50 μg dose of baclofen is commonly used for initial screening [19, 20]. The clinical effects from a screening bolus occur within 1–3 hours postinjection, and peak effects are typically observed 4–6 hours postinjection. The effects of the screening bolus are always temporary and routinely last for 6–8 hours [21, 22], although prolonged effects of a single test bolus have been reported [23]. Screening boluses can be repeated if the initial injection is unsuccessful. It is common practice to wait at least 24 hours before repeating a trial to ensure that the patient's neuromuscular status has completely returned to baseline. "Positive" responses are reported in 80–90% of bolus trials [19]. Generally, antibiotic prophylaxis is not needed for a bolus trial. For patients on antiplatelet or anticoagulant therapy, recommendations from the American Society of Regional Anesthesia are followed [24]. Radiologic guidance can assist with needle localization in the intrathecal space since anatomic landmarks for lumbar puncture can be variable [25], and there is a possibility of low CSF flow in this patient population. Several techniques have been described for needle localization using fluoroscopy [26], ultrasound [27], and computed tomography (CT) [28, 29].

An alternative method for conducting an ITB trial involves placement of a temporary intrathecal catheter and monitoring the patient's response to a short-term continuous infusion of baclofen [30]. This technique is more commonly used for evaluating intrathecal therapy in patients with chronic pain. The potential advantages of catheter ITB trials include: (1) avoidance of sequential lumbar punctures, (2) improved approximation of the chronic post-implant intrathecal infusion response compared to single bolus injections, (3) ability to control catheter tip placement, and (4) ability to adjust infusion rates while assessing favorable (and unfavorable) effects of ITB administration. The disadvantages of catheter trials include: (1) increased technical difficulty, (2) increased need for observation, and (3) increased risk of meningitis and structural damage. Fluoroscopic guidance is generally considered mandatory for catheter placement trials. While antibiotic prophylaxis is usually not needed for bolus trials, some degree of antibiotic prophylaxis may be warranted for short duration intrathecal catheter trials. Factors to consider for antibiotic prophylaxis include the duration of the trial, patient immunocompetency, and potential for chronic bacterial colonization. Trial duration is a key risk factor for the development of infectious complications. Thus, the duration of the trial should be just long enough to indicate a potential benefit of chronic ITB therapy [26]. There is no consensus regarding the optimal method of anesthesia for catheter placement. Local anesthesia potentially lowers the risk of inadvertent damage to neural structures. However, if excessive patient movement or severe anxiety is anticipated, deep sedation or general anesthesia may be warranted [31].

Successful Trial

Definitions of "success" for ITB screening trials vary. A liberal description of a successful trial may be any improvement in spasticity that suggests future benefit from chronic long-term infusion. The commonly cited criterion for a successful ITB trial is a 2-point reduction on the Modified Ashworth Scale score [19]. Patients may also demonstrate improvement in joint range of motion, both actively and passively. Sequential assessments every few hours are warranted to evaluate the onset, peak, and resolution of ITB effects. Intrathecal baclofen trials can potentially differentiate range of motion deficits due to severe spasticity, which are potentially reversible without surgery, from fixed contractures. While these assessments are often useful for patients with hypertonia in resting positions, they may be inadequate for prediction of ITB effects during active functional tasks. In functioning patients, excessive tone reduction may impede performance of activities such as transfers and walking (see Chap. 2). Observation of upright posture, transfers, ambulation and wheelchair propulsion during the trial is thus warranted. Objective evaluation techniques may be helpful and include neurophysiologic assessments [32] and instrumented gait analyses [21]. Some individuals may experience excessive spasticity reduction during the peak effect of the ITB bolus. This occurrence is not a contraindication for pump implantation since the infusion system can be used to titrate the dose to the desired effect. However, if excessive or prolonged hypotonia is observed during a screening ITB trial, a repeat trial at a lower dose or a catheter trial may be warranted. Some patients may demonstrate an improvement in resting measures of spasticity (thus qualifying for long-term infusion on the basis of trial "success"), but demonstrate functional worsening during the trial. Post-implant rehabilitation in this subset of patients is particularly important.

Skipping a Trial

Some centers proceed directly to pump implantation without a screening trial. For stroke patients, two justifications for skipping a trial have been proposed: (1) increased risk of spinal hemorrhage in patients who are on anticoagulation or antiplatelet therapy and (2) risk of recurrent stroke if these agents are discontinued. Proceeding directly to implantation without a trial reduces the ability to differentiate fixed contractures from spasticity prior to implantation. While patients may still benefit from pump implantation [33], a full discussion with the patient and caregiver regarding the risks and benefits of a "no trial" approach is warranted.

Adverse Events During a Trial

Adverse effects can occur during intrathecal trialing. Spinal headache or post-lumbar puncture syndrome is a complication of an injection-related dural leak and is not a direct medication effect. Spinal headaches can occur in up to 30% of patients undergoing a lumbar puncture and can vary in severity from mild to incapacitating. The headache typically worsens when the patient sits or stands and decreases in the supine position. These headaches typically begin within two days of the trial but may be delayed for as long as two weeks. Spinal headaches can be accompanied by dizziness, neck or arm pain, cranial nerve palsies, tinnitus, nausea, and distorted vision. Spinal headaches are more common in younger women with a low body mass index and in people who have a history of headaches. The risk of spinal headaches increases with the use of larger bore needles to enter the intrathecal space. The headache resolves spontaneously in most patients. Supportive measures include bed rest, caffeine, theophylline, and abdominal binders [34]. An epidural blood patch is reserved for recalcitrant cases, but this procedure is not without morbidity [35]. A relatively new technique for the management of spinal headaches is a sphenopalatine ganglion block which has fewer adverse effects [36]. Other trial procedure-related complications include bacterial and aseptic meningitis. Adverse effects that are more likely related to the pharmacological effect of baclofen include nausea/vomiting, urinary retention, hypotension, seizures, drowsiness/sedation, respiratory depression, and coma. Nausea/vomiting and drowsiness/sedation are the most common adverse effects observed during an ITB trial with a reported incidence of 2–3% [19].

While the procedural component of the trial should take place in a setting where injection sterility is assured, it can be performed in outpatient clinics, ambulatory surgical centers, inpatient hospitals, and inpatient rehabilitation facilities. It is helpful to use practice protocols or clinical pathways to facilitate consistent assessment of key trial response indicators and to reduce the risk of complications. Sequential evaluation of tone, range of motion, and strength are required. For patients who are functional, sequential evaluation of posture, transfers, and gait should be undertaken. Protocols for management of adverse events should be in place for spinal headache, bowel and bladder changes, seizures, and respiratory depression. Since the effect of the ITB trial may be prolonged, the practice setting should have the capacity for extended observation. Many experienced practitioners of ITB therapy believe that an inpatient rehabilitation facility is an optimal setting for ITB trials since these locations offer the resources to assess functional changes and potentially manage adverse effects [37].

Pump Implantation

Once a patient has had a successful ITB trial, one can proceed to implantation of the intrathecal delivery system. Some centers proceed immediately to implantation following the trial dose, while others have patients undergo a more extensive preadmission testing for permanent implantation after the screening trial. While the implantation procedure might be considered relatively minor surgery, the patient population served by ITB therapy can be quite fragile. Special attention should be paid to the cardiac, pulmonary, and nutritional status of the patient preoperatively. Patients should be clinically stable prior to surgery to minimize perioperative complications. Preoperative antibiotics are typically utilized with careful attention to potential bacterial colonization due to neurogenic bladder or decubitus ulcers. Patients on chronic anticoagulation will need to discontinue anticoagulation in the days preceding the procedure [24]. The risks of permanent pump implantation and infusion are the same as for the screening trial with the additional risks of drug overdose, drug withdrawal, and device-related complications.

Pump Options

Various options for pump and catheter placement should be considered prior to the procedure. The size of the pump to be implanted should be determined based on the patient's body habitus and anticipated intrathecal dosing. Smaller and thinner individuals may prefer a smaller pump size, either for aesthetic reasons or to prevent erosion of the pump through the skin and subcutaneous tissue. The pump can also be placed under the abdominal fascia to make it less conspicuous [38]. Patients who are likely to require high intrathecal baclofen doses or who reside at a great distance from the follow-up clinic will benefit from a larger pump with a larger drug reservoir to accommodate longer refill intervals. The tip of the intrathecal catheter is routinely placed in the mid-to-lower thoracic region, particularly if reduction of lower extremity spasticity is the primary goal. More rostral tip placement can be attempted to improve upper limb spasticity [11, 39], although this is not a consistent observation [12] and is subject to debate.

Initiation of ITB Therapy

The goal of chronic ITB therapy is to reduce the negative consequences of spasticity and provide functional spasticity control as quickly and safely as feasible. Since optimization of therapy will require multiple, graded dose adjustments, a baclofen solution is typically placed in the reservoir intraoperatively with immediate commencement of intrathecal infusion. While there are three commercially available concentrations of baclofen (500 mcg/ml, 1000 mcg/ml, and 2000 mcg/ml), it is generally recommended that therapy be initiated with the 500 mcg/ml concentration to provide maximum flexibility for dosing in the lower range without having to dilute the drug. Occasionally, clinical factors such as the tenuous medical status of a patient may warrant a delay in therapy initiation. In those rare circumstances, the pump can be filled with a baclofen solution at the time of implant and therapy can be initiated at a minimum rate; the dose may be increased once the patient's medical status is stable.

The initial dose of intrathecal baclofen is often determined by the patient's response to the test dose during the trial. A reasonable starting dose is 100–200% of the bolus dose given at the trial divided over 24 hours. If a patient demonstrated prolonged or excessive hypotonia during the screening trial, it may be prudent to start at 50% of the bolus dose divided over 24 hours. Occasionally, it may be appropriate to start at an even lower dose. It is imperative for the implanting physician or surgeon to have a close relationship with the trialing physician to determine the appropriate starting dose. Once therapy has been initiated, patients should be appropriately monitored until they demonstrate stable neurological, respiratory, and cardiac function. The typical duration of acute hospitalization for pump implantation is 1–2 days [27, 40]. Dose adjustments can commence immediately after pump implantation. In general, 24 hours is a reasonable time to wait between each dosing adjustment to allow for the full effect of the dose to be observed. Dose modifications are performed by "interrogating" the pump with a handheld programmer, programming the needed adjustments, and then updating the pump's dosing schedule. The programmer communicates with the pump via radiotelemetry.

Modes of Dose Delivery

Various modes of dosing can be programmed and are represented diagrammatically in Fig. 11.2. In the example, the total daily dose for the three modes of delivery is the same, but the timing of the dose is different. The modes include the following:

- Simple continuous – A single dose is delivered continuously throughout the 24 hour cycle.
- Complex continuous – The dose can be varied for different times of the day during the 24 hour cycle.
- Periodic bolus – Regularly scheduled boluses are delivered within a 24 hour cycle.
- Single bolus/simple continuous delivery – Two different dosing levels are delivered automatically during specific time periods during the 24 hour cycle.
- Patient-controlled delivery.

The complex continuous dosing mode allows for differential dosing over the course of the day. For example, a patient may find it beneficial to be on a lower dose during the day to minimize weakness and maximize functional mobility, and on a higher dose at night to minimize spontaneous nocturnal spasms. Periodic bolus dosing delivers several boluses rapidly over a few minutes with a relatively low rate of delivery between the boluses. This mode of delivery allows for greater distribution of the drug during the boluses with enhanced access to more cephalad spinal levels. This mode of delivery may be particularly beneficial for addressing upper limb spasticity. The periodic bolus delivery mode places a patient at a higher risk of overdose theoretically, although this has not been observed clinically. Both the complex continuous and periodic bolus modes of delivery are thought to be beneficial for the management of pharmacologic tolerance [41, 42]. When a clinician is unsure if a dosing adjustment is warranted, a single bolus at a given dose per day can be

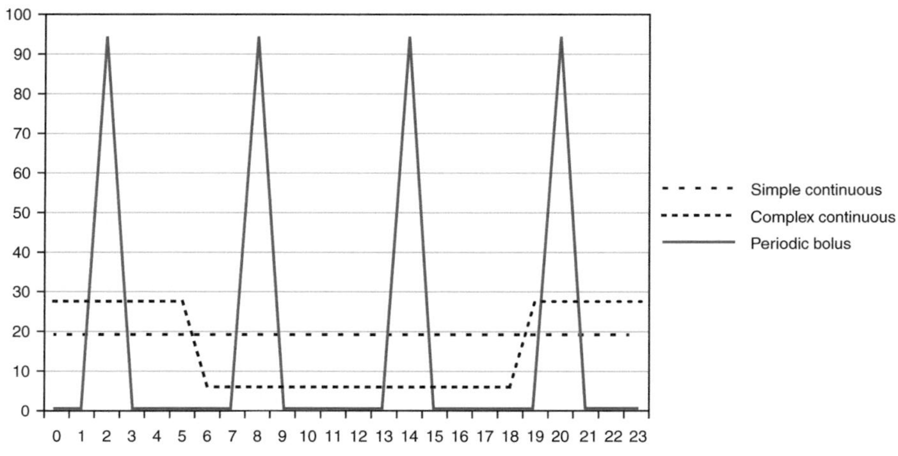

Fig. 11.2 Various modes of programmable intrathecal drug delivery

programmed for several days followed by an automatic return to the baseline dose. This mode of delivery is called single bolus/simple continuous delivery and allows a patient to be exposed to two different dosing levels automatically without the need for a visit to the physician. This mode of delivery can also be used for stepwise titration of intrathecal delivery.

More recently, a handheld accessory for intrathecal delivery has become available that allows for patient-controlled preprogrammed boluses of intrathecal drug delivery. The amount, frequency, and lockout period for these boluses are set by the physician. At present, this device is only FDA approved for intrathecal drug delivery for pain control [43]. While this device may allow the patient to adjust their intrathecal dosing to address the variability in their spasticity and/or functional needs, it does have the theoretical risk of masking ongoing or progressive noxious stimuli that could be driving the increase in spasticity. In the neurologic patient, increased spasticity may be the only sign of a potentially serious medical condition, such as urolithiasis or appendicitis. See Chap. 9 for details on medical conditions that may exacerbate spasticity. Hence, the use of the handheld patient activation device could potentially delay seeking medical attention. The patient activation device could also be utilized as a tool for guiding intrathecal titration. Further investigation is warranted into the safety and efficacy of the use of patient-controlled intrathecal baclofen delivery. The programming options described above, both alone and in combination, allow for an extraordinarily wide range of options for intrathecal drug delivery. The programmability and precise drug delivery of the intrathecal delivery system cannot be obtained with any other method of spasticity management.

Until recently, relatively little attention was paid to the mode of drug delivery, the concentration of the baclofen solution, and the flow rate of intrathecal delivery. These components of ITB therapy influence the effectiveness of ITB therapy. It is reasonable to postulate that lower drug concentrations and higher flow rates can potentially distribute the dose over a larger volume within the intrathecal space compared to a highly concentrated solution at slower flow rates [44, 45]. This hypothesis may be especially pertinent in the management of spasticity as CSF flow can be dramatically altered in the presence of neurologic disease, and should be considered in the management of patients receiving ITB therapy.

Dose Titration

During the titration phase of ITB therapy, patients are usually weaned off their oral antispasticity medications, and the intrathecal dose is increased depending on patient tolerability. Nonambulatory patients may tolerate dose titrations of 20% of total daily dose, whereas others, especially ambulatory patients, will require lower increments (5–10%). Adverse effects that may be seen during this phase of therapy include excessive hypotonia, changes in bowel [46, 47] and bladder status

[48], and increased risk of thromboembolic events [49, 50]. The frequency and size of dosing titrations should be individualized based on the patient's response to prior changes. Some patients tolerate rapid daily dose titrations, while others may require longer periods of observation and accommodation prior to making further adjustments. While there is no ideal titration frequency, an adjustment one or twice a week until optimal dose is achieved is reasonable and practical. Some patients may also benefit from a low dose of oral medications to address breakthrough spasms or to address upper limb spasticity that is not addressed by ITB therapy. The titration phase of therapy could last 6–9 months after implantation. It is advisable for patients to always have oral baclofen available in case they experience symptoms of withdrawal.

Post-implant Rehabilitation

Since ITB therapy has the capacity to affect a patient's active functional status, a rehabilitation program after pump implantation is appropriate. Post-implant rehabilitation may also be needed for caregiver training. The setting, scope, and complexity of the rehabilitation program will vary depending upon the patient's individual goals as well as the availability of these services in each region. Potential disciplines involved in the rehabilitation process include physiatry/neurorehabilitation physician, physical therapy, occupational therapy, and rehabilitation nursing. Issues that require attention during this phase of therapy include incision care, medical management for spinal headache, pain control, medication adjustment, and dosing changes, mobility, self-care ability, and bowel/bladder function. Patients, especially ambulatory individuals, should be thoroughly counseled on the need for post-implant rehabilitation to maximize the benefits of ITB therapy [27]. The timing of rehabilitation is subject to some debate. Some centers defer therapy for a few weeks after the pump is implanted due to concerns of catheter fracture or incisional dehiscence, whereas others favor immediate post-implant rehabilitation. Some implanters limit thoracolumbar flexion and/or twisting of the spine for a few weeks to minimize potential complications such as catheter migration and incisional dehiscence. However, there have been no reports of incisional or catheter difficulties related to specific activities. Rapid initiation of therapy may place the patient at a higher risk of thromboembolic phenomena in the postoperative phase. Both lower extremity venous thrombosis and secondary pulmonary embolism have been reported in the postoperative phase of ITB therapy [49, 50]. Consideration of mechanical and/or chemical prophylaxis for venous thromboembolism is therefore warranted. The use of anticoagulation to prevent thromboembolic complications must be balanced against the risk of spinal hemorrhage and incisional hematoma. There is no standard of care for the length or type of preventive measure, and each clinician must make decisions based on the individual patient's risk factor profile.

Patient and Caregiver Education

Patient and caregiver education on the risks of ITB therapy is a key aspect of therapy initiation. Patients should be educated to avoid sudden, excessive, repeated movements like bending, twisting, bouncing, or stretching. These movements can damage the pump system, may dislodge, kink, or block the catheter and stop drug delivery causing serious baclofen withdrawal. Dose titrations may lead to drowsiness due to a sudden increase in dose, making certain activities like driving risky. Hot tubs, steam rooms, saunas and tanning beds, and other facilities with temperatures higher than 102 °F (39 °C) should be avoided as the flow rate of the pump increases as body temperature rises, and can lead to an inadvertent overdose. Diving below 33 feet (10 m) and high-pressure environments such as hyperbaric chambers can damage the pump and lead to changes in pump flow as the pressure increases. The pump may set off the alarm in security devices and metal detectors, and patients should be advised to keep their device ID card handy to show to security personnel. Not all medical centers have teams to handle baclofen pump emergencies and refills. Patients must be informed of their medical options both locally and when they travel. Common procedures such as an MRI can cause the pump to temporarily stop, which will suspend drug delivery during the MRI. The pump usually resumes normal operation immediately after but may require interrogation to confirm that it is working properly. Patients and caregivers should be directed to information from the manufacturer to supplement their education and training (https://www.medtronic.com/us-en/patients/treatments-therapies/drug-pump-severe-spasticity/living-with-itb-therapy/cautions-activities-procedures.html).

Pump Refill and Therapy Maintenance

A pump reservoir refill is a sterile, office-based procedure that is needed every few weeks or months for the duration of ITB treatment. The baclofen solution is stable in the pump reservoir for up to six months. Therefore, a refill is needed at least every six months but often more frequently especially at the beginning of ITB therapy, before the residual volume of drug solution in the pump reaches the low reservoir volume. The low reservoir volume is the lowest volume of drug solution in the pump that supports stable flow through the catheter. The refill interval is the time required for the pump to dispense the volume of solution from a full reservoir to the low reservoir volume. The refill interval depends on the baclofen concentration used and the daily dose dispensed by the pump.

Refill Appointments

It is imperative to schedule pump refills in sufficient advance of the low residual volume alarm date to avoid "low reservoir syndrome" and associated symptoms of ITB withdrawal [51]. This requires an organized system of care where the alarm dates are carefully monitored by members of the team to ensure that "alarm dates" are not inadvertently missed due to missed appointments, travel, inclement weather, and staff vacations.

Refill Procedure

Pump refills are typically accomplished by palpating the pump in the abdomen, and using a template to guide a needle through the abdomen into the reservoir chamber of the pump. In challenging situations, such as when a patient is morbidly obese, or when the position of the pump is unusual or at an angle, fluoroscopy or ultrasound can be used to assist in guiding the needle through the access port into the pump reservoir chamber [52, 53]. The baclofen solution remaining from the previous refill is aspirated and measured and should correspond with the residual volume calculated and displayed during interrogation of the pump by the programmer. The new baclofen solution is then instilled through the same needle. The needle tip must be reliably determined to be within the reservoir chamber. Inadvertent injection of an intrathecal solution into the subcutaneous tissue can result in serious adverse events [54], such as swelling around the pump and baclofen withdrawal. Some patients require large ITB daily doses with a subsequent increase in refill frequency. Under these circumstances, a higher concentration of baclofen solution will extend the refill interval. When changing drug concentrations, it is imperative to program the pump correctly by incorporating a bridge bolus to compensate for the difference in baclofen concentration of the residual baclofen solution in the pump and catheter [55]. Failure to compensate for this residual solution can result in serious under- or overdosing. The therapeutic effect of intrathecal baclofen is closely linked to the dose administered.

Baclofen Withdrawal

Abrupt reduction or cessation of ITB delivery can result in withdrawal syndrome that can have serious, and even fatal, consequences. The severity of ITB withdrawal syndrome is not consistently related to dosing levels. The most common symptomatic presentation of ITB withdrawal syndrome is the return of the patient's "baseline" degree of spasticity. Additional characteristics of this syndrome can include pruritus, seizures, hallucinations, and autonomic dysreflexia. Some patients will demonstrate a life-threatening syndrome exemplified by exaggerated/rebound spasticity (i.e., greater than the baseline degree of spasticity), fever, hemodynamic instability, and altered mental status. If not treated aggressively, this syndrome may progress over 24–72 hours leading to rhabdomyolysis and elevated liver function tests that may cause renal and hepatic failure, disseminated intravascular coagulation, multi-organ system failure, and rarely death [56]. It is imperative that patients and caregivers are educated about recognizing the signs and symptoms of ITB withdrawal syndrome, and are provided with instructions regarding what they should do if they notice any symptoms. Backup oral baclofen tablets should always be available. Typically, the withdrawal symptoms will abate in several days with treatment, although there are reports of prolonged ITB withdrawal syndrome [57]. Following recognition of ITB withdrawal, initial treatment includes urgent replacement with oral baclofen, supportive care, careful observation, and restoration of intrathecal drug delivery [27]. At present, there is no intravenous form of baclofen available although this may be a possibility in the future [58]. There are no guidelines for the conversion of an intrathecal dose to an oral dose or vice versa. Thus, the dosing of oral baclofen may require frequent modification to attenuate the symptoms of withdrawal. Adjunctive pharmacotherapy can also include the administration of benzodiazepines (enteral or intravenous), tizanidine, dantrolene, or cyproheptadine [27]. The management of withdrawal should be executed in an urgent, if not emergent, fashion and should precede diagnostic investigation into the cause of the malfunction of the ITB delivery system. Once the patient is no longer experiencing symptoms of withdrawal, begin troubleshooting to identify and correct the delivery system malfunction.

Baclofen Overdose

In contrast to ITB withdrawal, which can occur despite vigilant attention, ITB overdose is generally due to human miscalculation during dosing adjustments or drug concentration changes [59]. Mechanical pump malfunction as a cause of ITB overdosing is rare. Subdural encapsulation of the intrathecal catheter with subsequent rupture of the subdural pocket could lead to inadvertent exposure to excessive baclofen [60]. There are rare reports of inadvertent injection of a refill solution into the catheter access port (CAP) during catheter patency investigations resulting in a massive overdose [61]. Overinfusion by the pump itself can rarely occur, and is more likely with off-label drug concentrations or compounded agents infused via the pump than with commercially available baclofen solutions [61, 62]. While off-label drug concentrations can result in an overdose, they can also result in withdrawal since the predicted low reservoir alarm date will not correlate with the actual low reservoir alarm date resulting in the pump running out of medication early. Additionally, if a catheter disruption is detected and the patient is undergoing restoration of intrathecal delivery, overdosing can occur if intrathecal delivery is resumed at the prior dosing level. In this clinical scenario, intrathecal delivery should be restarted at the low dose used at the initiation of ITB therapy [27]. Symptoms of baclofen overdose include profound hypotonia or flaccidity, hyporeflexia, respiratory depression, apnea, seizures, coma, autonomic instability, hallucinations, hypothermia, and cardiac rhythm abnormalities. Plasma and CSF levels of baclofen can be obtained, but the results may be misleading since there is no direct correlation between the programmed intrathecal dose and CSF baclofen levels [63]. Initial management of overdose is supportive and includes maintenance of airway, respiration, and circulation. Intubation and ventilatory support may be necessary. Secondary measures include reduction or temporary interruption of intrathecal delivery by pump reprogramming, as well as cessation of concomitant medications that could contribute to CNS depression. Optional measures for management of ITB overdose include CSF drainage via catheter access port aspiration or lumbar puncture and the administration of an "antidote." While not true antidotes, both physostigmine and flumazenil have been reported to reduce the effects of baclofen on the CNS, such as somnolence and respiratory depression. Physostigmine is the more commonly used agent, but may produce adverse effects such as bradycardia, seizures, and increased respiratory secretions. Patients who are treated for baclofen overdose must be watched closely for rebound withdrawal once the pump is stopped and the drug load is decreased [64].

Troubleshooting

While ITB therapy is a reliable treatment for severe spasticity, the possibility of suboptimal therapy must always be considered in the management of patients. Troubleshooting is a means of optimizing ITB therapy. ITB therapy may be suboptimal in patients who present with hypertonia, as well as in those who appear hypotonic, and troubleshooting should be considered in either of these two scenarios. While this section will focus on difficulties with drug delivery systems, it is important to recognize that some problems may be related to the patient's underlying condition and the correct diagnosis of spasticity versus muscle stiffness (see Chaps. 4, 6, 8, and 13). For patients with chronic, nonprogressive neurologic conditions (e.g., spinal cord injury, stroke), the ITB dose should stay relatively stable during the maintenance phase of therapy [42, 65]. Individuals with progressive disease (e.g., amyotrophic lateral sclerosis or multiple sclerosis) may require frequent evaluation and dose adjustments [66, 67]. Comorbidities of neurological disease can serve as noxious stimuli that act as triggers for increased spasticity (e.g., urinary tract infection, bladder distention, urolithiasis, etc.) [68]. See Chap. 9 for details regarding medical exacerbation of spasticity. Additionally, several disorders may mimic ITB underdosing/withdrawal, including sepsis, autonomic dysreflexia, neuroleptic malignant syndrome, and malignant hyperthermia [56]. If no patient-related cause for the increased spasticity is discovered, an investigation into potential malfunction of the intrathecal delivery system should be undertaken.

Diagnosis of Pump Catheter Malfunction

Two initial techniques for investigation of potential pump malfunction include pump interrogation and checking the pump residual reservoir volume. The pump's active dosing parameters on interrogation should match the previously prescribed dosing parameters. If a programming error is detected, reversion to the appropriate dosing level may result in symptom reversal. The presence of an audible pump alarm or an electronic alarm during pump interrogation, or discovery of unexpected "extra" residual volume in the reservoir, suggests pump-related malfunction. Alarm conditions generally occur either due to a low battery or a low reservoir volume. A low battery alarm will sound when the battery has discharged significantly, for example at the end of the pump's battery life, in the sixth year. A low reservoir alarm will indicate that the pump has delivered nearly all the contents of the reservoir and that the patient needs an immediate refill. Exposure of the Medtronic intrathecal delivery system to high magnetic fields, such as during an MRI scan, will result in a temporary cessation of drug delivery. Rarely, there is a delayed restart of drug delivery that may be associated with ITB underdosing/withdrawal. A rotor stall and restart can be detected by inspection of the system's internal logs during interrogation [69]. It is pertinent to note that intrathecal delivery systems from manufacturers other than Medtronic have different MRI recommendations. Additionally, there are rare cases of rotor stall in the absence of magnetic field exposure [2].

Bolus Dosing

A combined diagnostic and therapeutic maneuver for troubleshooting is bolus dosing. A single intrathecal baclofen bolus dose comparable to or higher than a trial or test dose (usually 50–100 mcg) can be programmed over 5 min followed by sequential evaluation of spasticity over the following 4-6 hours. An alternative method of bolus dosing is bolus administration (single or multiple boluses) via lumbar puncture. Attainment of adequate spasticity control with ITB boluses administered by lumbar puncture in the absence of radiographic findings suggests the possibility of microtears in the catheter. Patients who show improved spasticity control with bolus dosing can be programmed to receive scheduled bolus doses to allay their symptoms until further workup is completed and the catheter is changed [27].

Residual Volume Mismatch

Checking the residual volume within the pump reservoir is an important step in troubleshooting. The low reservoir alarm is based on calculation from the programmed settings, and is not a true measure of the actual residual volume. Therefore, premature emptying of the pump reservoir will not trigger a low reservoir alarm. There are rare reports of overinfusion, manifested by symptoms of overdosing, and a lower-than-expected residual reservoir volume [70, 71]. Similarly, an increase in residual reservoir volume may suggest an abnormality of the pump rotor or a severely kinked catheter, resulting in underdosing or withdrawal. If there are any concerns about the content of the reservoir solution, such as drug concentration, then the residual volume in the pump should be withdrawn and the pump should be refilled with a new solution. Similarly, if a low reservoir alarm is detected, a timely refill should be undertaken. The presence of a permanent rotor stall, unexplained rotor stalls, overinfusion, or low battery should prompt urgent replacement of the pump.

Catheter Access Port Aspiration

Catheter access port (CAP) aspiration can be used to diagnose catheter patency or malfunction. Figure 11.3 illustrates the potential sites of catheter disruption.

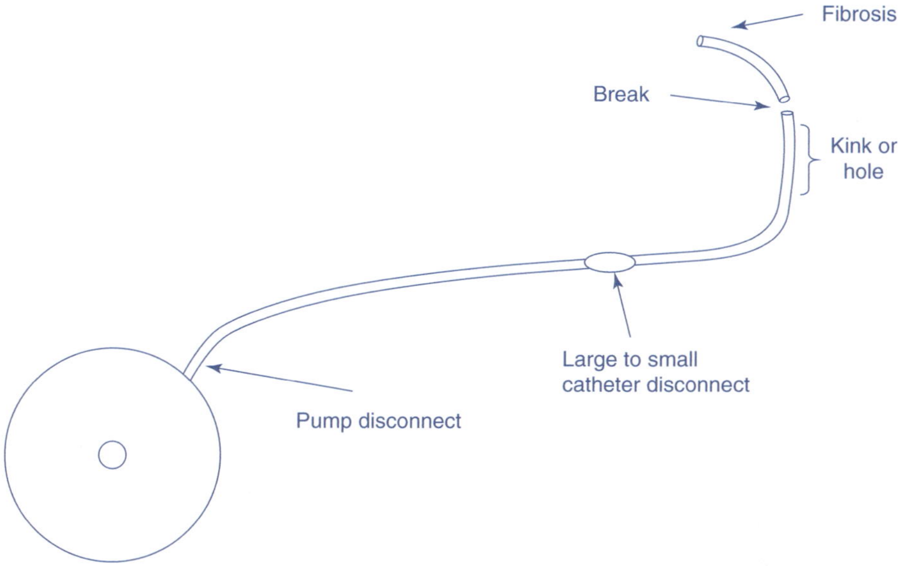

Fig. 11.3 Potential catheter disruptions

Diagnostic CAP aspiration may be performed after the pump is confirmed to be functioning through interrogation and pump reservoir volume verification. The CAP aspiration procedure involves accessing a port on the pump that is in direct continuity with the catheter, and different from the port used to access the pump reservoir for refills. If the distal end of the catheter lies within the subarachnoid space, then CSF should be readily withdrawn through the CAP. Aspiration of only 2–3 ml of CSF is sufficient to suggest that the catheter is patent, since the volume in the catheter is typically less than 0.25 ml. Failure to aspirate CSF during CAP aspiration strongly suggests catheter disruption or occlusion. If the catheter is partially occluded, aspiration may be difficult. If the catheter is completely kinked/occluded, minimal fluid would be obtained from CAP aspiration. If CSF cannot be aspirated, a catheter revision or replacement is likely to be needed. Further diagnostic workup with scintigraphy may be necessary. If the catheter cannot be aspirated, consider the risks of overdose from drug in the catheter before proceeding with a catheter contrast study. A priming bolus must be programmed after a successful CAP aspiration to avoid subsequent baclofen underdosing and acute withdrawal.

Imaging

Imaging evaluation of the catheter typically begins with plain X-rays, although some catheters are radiolucent [53]. A flat anteroposterior (AP) X-ray of the abdomen and lateral lumbar and thoracic spine series should be obtained to visualize all tubing, connectors, and the entrance of the catheter into the spinal canal. A contrast study can be used to visualize the catheter and verify the location of the catheter tip. Once CSF is aspirated from the CAP, contrast medium may be injected through the catheter, and the flow of the contrast through the catheter can be visualized fluoroscopically or with computed tomography (CT). If a CT study is undertaken, all portions of the pump and catheter should be visualized, which usually requires examination of the abdomen, lumbar spine, and thoracic spine. Extravasation of contrast out of the catheter can diagnose catheter breaks, catheter tip loculations, and catheter migration into the subdural or epidural spaces [72, 73]. Contrast should not be injected if 2–3 ml of CSF cannot be easily aspirated, since this can potentially expose the patient to an ITB overdose from infusion of drug remaining in the catheter [60]. A CT myelogram also has the advantage of providing structural information regarding other organs that may reveal the underlying problem.

Other imaging techniques for diagnosis of catheter malfunction include radionuclide scintigraphy and MRI. Indium-111 DTPA is used for radionuclide scintigraphy and can be injected into the pump reservoir and used as a tracer to determine the patency of the infusion system. After injection, serial sequential scanning occurs every 24 hours for 2–3 days. Demonstration of an intact catheter and full ventriculogram indicates a normal study. Radionuclide scintigraphy can detect catheter occlusions, pump malfunction, and large leaks. The disadvantages of radionuclide scintigraphy include cost, limited availability and access to the technology, the need for sequential imaging to confirm the abnormality, limited anatomic resolution, and a potentially high false-negative rate. Careful calculations are required to determine the proper timing of imaging to avoid a false-negative study. Indium-111 DTPA has also not been tested or approved for delivery through intrathecal pumps [74].

MRI of the thoracic spine can demonstrate spinal hemorrhage, abscess, and other soft tissue abnormalities near the catheter tip. Rarely, granulomas can develop at the catheter tip, but these have only been pathologically confirmed with intrathecal opiate therapy for chronic pain. While rare, granulomas have the potential to cause serious neurologic injury from spinal cord compression. MRI of the catheter tip with gadolinium contrast is the diagnostic test of choice for granuloma detection [75].

Pump Replacement and Explantation

Elective pump replacement is required when the pump is nearing the end of its battery life. Current systems have an alarm indicating the end of pump battery life. It is imperative that the pump is replaced prior to its stopping to avoid withdrawal syndrome. A pump replacement need not be accompanied by a catheter replacement if there is no reason to suspect catheter damage or malfunction. Other reasons for pump replacement are pump stall or failure, infection, and failed ITB therapy. Infection requires explantation of the pump, treatment of the infection, and potential reimplantation. Explantation requires gradual dose reduction while increasing oral baclofen and/or supplementing with other treatments to prevent withdrawal. Simultaneous explantation of an infected pump and concurrent implantation of a new pump has also been described [76].

Conclusion

The efficacy of ITB therapy has been demonstrated for over three decades. Initially, nonambulatory patients with severe spasticity who demonstrated difficulties with passive function, such as positioning, maintenance of hygiene, etc., were referred for this therapy. More recently, ambulatory patients have benefitted from ITB therapy. Both groups are best served by a dedicated medical, surgical, and rehabilitation team that is well organized and capable of systematically managing all aspects of the therapy. As the sophistication of intrathecal delivery systems increases and newer delivery systems become available, the requirement for a team-based approach will become even more paramount. Clinicians interested in providing ITB therapy should develop a robust team structure to manage the routine, urgent, and emergent needs of patients needing this treatment.

References

1. Meng E, Hoang T. MEMS-enabled implantable drug infusion pumps for laboratory animal research, preclinical, and clinical applications. Adv Drug Deliv Rev. 2012;64(14):1628–38.
2. Pope JE. Intrathecal drug delivery: available technologies. In: Pope JE, Deer TR, editors. Treatment of chronic pain conditions: a comprehensive handbook. New York: Springer New York; 2017. p. 191–3.
3. Ethans KD, Schryvers OI, Nance PW, Casey AR. Intrathecal drug therapy using the Codman Model 3000 constant flow implantable infusion pumps: experience with 17 cases. Spinal Cord. 2005;43(4):214–8.
4. Czernicki M, Sinovich G, Mihaylov I, Nejad B, Kunnumpurath S, Kodumudi G, et al. Intrathecal drug delivery for chronic pain management-scope, limitations and future. J Clin Monit Comput. 2015;29(2):241–9.
5. Saulino M, Turner M, Miesel K, Cochran FR, Stromberg K, Fehrmann E, et al. Can cerebrospinal fluid pressure detect catheter complications in patients who experience loss of effectiveness with intrathecal baclofen therapy? Neuromodulation. 2017;20(2):187–97.
6. Saulino M, Ivanhoe CB, McGuire JR, Ridley B, Shilt JS, Boster AL. Best practices for intrathecal baclofen therapy: patient selection. Neuromodulation. 2016;19(6):607–15.
7. Francisco GE, Yablon SA, Schiess MC, Wiggs L, Cavalier S, Grissom S. Consensus panel guidelines for the use of intrathecal baclofen therapy in poststroke spastic hypertonia. Top Stroke Rehabil. 2006;13(4):74–85.
8. Sadiq SA, Wang GC. Long-term intrathecal baclofen therapy in ambulatory patients with spasticity. J Neurol. 2006;253(5):563–9.
9. Francisco GE. The role of intrathecal baclofen therapy in the upper motor neuron syndrome. Eura Medicophys. 2004;40(2):131–43.
10. Francisco GE, Hu MM, Boake C, Ivanhoe CB. Efficacy of early use of intrathecal baclofen therapy for treating spastic hypertonia due to acquired brain injury. Brain Inj. 2005;19(5):359–64.
11. Burns AS, Meythaler JM. Intrathecal baclofen in tetraplegia of spinal origin: efficacy for upper extremity hypertonia. Spinal Cord. 2001;39(8):413–9.
12. Sivakumar G, Yap Y, Tsegaye M, Vloeberghs M. Intrathecal baclofen therapy for spasticity of cerebral origin-does the position of the intrathecal catheter matter? Childs Nerv Syst. 2010;26(8):1097–102.
13. Fulkerson DH, Boaz JC, Luerssen TG. Interaction of ventriculoperitoneal shunt and baclofen pump. Childs Nerv Syst. 2007;23(7):733–8.

14. Buonaguro V, Scelsa B, Curci D, Monforte S, Iuorno T, Motta F. Epilepsy and intrathecal baclofen therapy in children with cerebral palsy. Pediatr Neurol. 2005;33(2):110–3.
15. Schuele SU, Kellinghaus C, Shook SJ, Boulis N, Bethoux FA, Loddenkemper T. Incidence of seizures in patients with multiple sclerosis treated with intrathecal baclofen. Neurology. 2005;64(6):1086–7.
16. Solaro C. Incidence of seizures in patients with multiple sclerosis treated with intrathecal baclofen. Neurology. 2006;66(5):784–5; author reply 784–5.
17. Toh Yoon EW, Kobayashi M. Percutaneous endoscopic gastrostomy in a patient with continuous intrathecal baclofen infusion therapy. Gastroenterology Res. 2017;10(2):132–4.
18. Martens FM, Somford DM, van Kuppevelt DH, van den Burg MJ, Heesakkers JP. Retraction of an intrathecal baclofen infusion catheter following suprapubic cystotomy: a case report. J Rehabil Med. 2009;41(1):90–1.
19. Stempien L, Tsai T. Intrathecal baclofen pump use for spasticity: a clinical survey. Am J Phys Med Rehabil. 2000;79(6):536–41.
20. Hoving MA, van Raak EP, Spincemaille GH, Palmans LJ, Sleypen FA, Vles JS, et al. Intrathecal baclofen in children with spastic cerebral palsy: a double-blind, randomized, placebo-controlled, dose-finding study. Dev Med Child Neurol. 2007;49(9):654–9.
21. Horn TS, Yablon SA, Stokic DS. Effect of intrathecal baclofen bolus injection on temporospatial gait characteristics in patients with acquired brain injury. Arch Phys Med Rehabil. 2005;86(6):1127–33.
22. Stokic DS, Yablon SA, Hayes A. Comparison of clinical and neurophysiologic responses to intrathecal baclofen bolus administration in moderate-to-severe spasticity after acquired brain injury. Arch Phys Med Rehabil. 2005;86(9):1801–6.
23. Baguley IJ, Bailey KM, Slewa-Younan S. Prolonged anti-spasticity effects of bolus intrathecal baclofen. Brain Inj. 2005;19(7):545–8.
24. Narouze S, Benzon HT, Provenzano DA, Buvanendran A, De Andres J, Deer TR, et al. Interventional spine and pain procedures in patients on antiplatelet and anticoagulant medications: guidelines from the American Society of Regional Anesthesia and Pain Medicine, the European Society of Regional Anaesthesia and Pain Therapy, the American Academy of Pain Medicine, the International Neuromodulation Society, the North American Neuromodulation Society, and the World Institute of Pain. Reg Anesth Pain Med. 2015;40(3):182–212.
25. Snider KT, Kribs JW, Snider EJ, Degenhardt BF, Bukowski A, Johnson JC. Reliability of Tuffier's line as an anatomic landmark. Spine (Phila Pa 1976). 2008;33(6):E161–5.
26. Pierce DB, Shivaram G, Koo KSH, Shaw DWW, Meyer KF, Monroe EJ. Ultrasound-guided lumbar puncture in pediatric patients: technical success and safety. Pediatr Radiol. 2018;48(6):875–81.
27. Saulino M, Anderson DJ, Doble J, Farid R, Gul F, Konrad P, et al. Best practices for intrathecal baclofen therapy: troubleshooting. Neuromodulation. 2016;19(6):632–41.
28. Weaver JJ, Natarajan N, Shaw DWW, Apkon SD, Koo KSH, Shivaram GM, et al. Transforaminal intrathecal delivery of nusinersen using cone-beam computed tomography for children with spinal muscular atrophy and extensive surgical instrumentation: early results of technical success and safety. Pediatr Radiol. 2018;48(3):392–7.
29. Brook AD, Burns J, Dauer E, Schoendfeld AH, Miller TS. Comparison of CT and fluoroscopic guidance for lumbar puncture in an obese population with prior failed unguided attempt. J Neurointerv Surg. 2014;6(4):324–8.
30. Phillips MM, Miljkovic N, Ramos-Lamboy M, Moossy JJ, Horton J, Buhari AM, et al. Clinical experience with continuous intrathecal baclofen trials prior to pump implantation. PM R. 2015;7(10):1052–8.
31. Staats PS. Complications of intrathecal therapy. Pain Med. 2008;9(S1):S102–7.
32. Yablon SA, Stokic DS. Neurophysiologic evaluation of spastic hypertonia: implications for management of the patient with the intrathecal baclofen pump. Am J Phys Med Rehabil. 2004;83(10 Suppl):S10–8.
33. Gwartz BL. Intrathecal baclofen for spasticity caused by thrombotic stroke. Am J Phys Med Rehabil. 2001;80(5):383–7.

34. Ahmed SV, Jayawarna C, Jude E. Post lumbar puncture headache: diagnosis and management. Postgrad Med J. 2006;82(973):713–6.
35. Riley CA, Spiegel JE. Complications following large-volume epidural blood patches for postdural puncture headache. Lumbar subdural hematoma and arachnoiditis: initial cause or final effect? J Clin Anesth. 2009;21(5):355–9.
36. Kent S, Mehaffey G. Transnasal sphenopalatine ganglion block for the treatment of postdural puncture headache in obstetric patients. J Clin Anesth. 2016;34:194–6.
37. Boster AL, Bennett SE, Bilsky GS, Gudesblatt M, Koelbel SF, McManus M, et al. Best practices for intrathecal baclofen therapy: screening test. Neuromodulation. 2016;19(6):616–22.
38. Kopell BH, Sala D, Doyle WK, Feldman DS, Wisoff JH, Weiner HL. Subfascial implantation of intrathecal baclofen pumps in children: technical note. Neurosurgery. 2001;49(3):753–6; discussion 756–7.
39. Motta F, Stignani C, Antonello CE. Upper limb function after intrathecal baclofen treatment in children with cerebral palsy. J Pediatr Orthop. 2008;28(1):91–6.
40. Penn RD. Intrathecal medication delivery. Neurosurg Clin N Am. 2003;14(3):381–7.
41. Heetla HW, Staal MJ, van Laar T. Tolerance to continuous intrathecal baclofen infusion can be reversed by pulsatile bolus infusion. Spinal Cord. 2010;48(6):483–6.
42. Heetla HW, Staal MJ, Kliphuis C, van Laar T. The incidence and management of tolerance in intrathecal baclofen therapy. Spinal Cord. 2009;47(10):751–6.
43. Ilias W, le Polain B, Buchser E, Demartini L, oPTiMa study group. Patient-controlled analgesia in chronic pain patients: experience with a new device designed to be used with implanted programmable pumps. Pain Pract. 2008;8(3):164–70.
44. Flack SH, Bernards CM. Cerebrospinal fluid and spinal cord distribution of hyperbaric bupivacaine and baclofen during slow intrathecal infusion in pigs. Anesthesiology. 2010;112(1):165–73.
45. Heetla HW, Proost JH, Molmans BH, Staal MJ, van Laar T. A pharmacokinetic-pharmacodynamic model for intrathecal baclofen in patients with severe spasticity. Br J Clin Pharmacol. 2016;81(1):101–12.
46. Kofler M, Matzak H, Saltuari L. The impact of intrathecal baclofen on gastrointestinal function. Brain Inj. 2002;16(9):825–36.
47. Morant A, Noe E, Boyer J, Escamilla B, Trenor C, Ferri J, et al. Paralytic ileus: a complication after intrathecal baclofen therapy. Brain Inj. 2006;20(13–14):1451–4.
48. Vaidyanathan S, Soni BM, Oo T, Hughes PL, Singh G, Watt JW, et al. Bladder stones – red herring for resurgence of spasticity in a spinal cord injury patient with implantation of Medtronic Synchromed pump for intrathecal delivery of baclofen – a case report. BMC Urol. 2003;3:3.
49. Carda S, Cazzaniga M, Taiana C, Pozzi R. Intrathecal baclofen bolus complicated by deep vein thrombosis and pulmonary embolism. A case report. Eur J Phys Rehabil Med. 2008;44(1):87–8.
50. Murphy NA. Deep venous thrombosis as a result of hypotonia secondary to intrathecal baclofen therapy: a case report. Arch Phys Med Rehabil. 2002;83(9):1311–2.
51. Rigoli G, Terrini G, Cordioli Z. Intrathecal baclofen withdrawal syndrome caused by low residual volume in the pump reservoir: a report of 2 cases. Arch Phys Med Rehabil. 2004;85(12):2064–6.
52. Maneyapanda MB, Chang Chien GC, Mattie R, Amorapanth P, Reger C, McCormick ZL. Ultrasound guidance for technically challenging intrathecal baclofen pump refill: three cases and procedure description. Am J Phys Med Rehabil. 2016;95(9):692–7.
53. Miracle AC, Fox MA, Ayyangar RN, Vyas A, Mukherji SK, Quint DJ. Imaging evaluation of intrathecal baclofen pump-catheter systems. AJNR Am J Neuroradiol. 2011;32(7):1158–64.
54. Coyne PJ, Hansen LA, Laird J, Buster P, Smith TJ. Massive hydromorphone dose delivered subcutaneously instead of intrathecally: guidelines for prevention and management of opioid, local anesthetic, and clonidine overdose. J Pain Symptom Manag. 2004;28(3):273–6.
55. Elovic E, Kirshblum SC. Managing spasticity in spinal cord injury: safe administration of bridge boluses during intrathecal baclofen pump refills. J Spinal Cord Med. 2003;26(1):2–4.

56. Coffey RJ, Edgar TS, Francisco GE, Graziani V, Meythaler JM, Ridgely PM, et al. Abrupt withdrawal from intrathecal baclofen: recognition and management of a potentially life-threatening syndrome. Arch Phys Med Rehabil. 2002;83(6):735–41.
57. Hansen CR, Gooch JL, Such-Neibar T. Prolonged, severe intrathecal baclofen withdrawal syndrome: a case report. Arch Phys Med Rehabil. 2007;88(11):1468–71.
58. Agarwal SK, Kriel RL, Cloyd JC, Coles LD, Scherkenbach LA, Tobin MH, et al. A pilot study assessing pharmacokinetics and tolerability of oral and intravenous baclofen in healthy adult volunteers. J Child Neurol. 2015;30(1):37–41.
59. Dalton C, Keenan E, Stevenson V. A novel cause of intrathecal baclofen overdosage: lessons to be learnt. Clin Rehabil. 2008;22(2):188–90.
60. Lew SM, Psaty EL, Abbott R. An unusual cause of overdose after baclofen pump implantation: case report. Neurosurgery. 2005;56(3):E624; discussion E624.
61. Sauter K, Kaufman HH, Bloomfield SM, Cline S, Banks D. Treatment of high-dose intrathecal morphine overdose. Case report. J Neurosurg. 1994;81(1):143–6.
62. Sgouros S, Charalambides C, Matsota P, Tsangaris I, Kostopanagiotou G. Malfunction of SynchroMed II baclofen pump delivers a near-lethal baclofen overdose. Pediatr Neurosurg. 2010;46(1):62–5.
63. Albright AL, Thompson K, Carlos S, Minnigh MB. Cerebrospinal fluid baclofen concentrations in patients undergoing continuous intrathecal baclofen therapy. Dev Med Child Neurol. 2007;49(6):423–5.
64. Shirley KW, Kothare S, Piatt JH Jr, Adirim TA. Intrathecal baclofen overdose and withdrawal. Pediatr Emerg Care. 2006;22(4):258–61.
65. Penn RD, Savoy SM, Corcos D, Latash M, Gottlieb G, Parke B, et al. Intrathecal baclofen for severe spinal spasticity. N Engl J Med. 1989;320(23):1517–21.
66. Bethoux F, Boulis N, McClelland S 3rd, Willis MA, Hussain M, Machado A, et al. Use of intrathecal baclofen for treatment of severe spasticity in selected patients with motor neuron disease. Neurorehabil Neural Repair. 2013;27(9):828–33.
67. Erwin A, Gudesblatt M, Bethoux F, Bennett SE, Koelbel S, Plunkett R, et al. Intrathecal baclofen in multiple sclerosis: too little, too late? Mult Scler. 2011;17(5):623–9.
68. Vaidyanathan S, Soni BM, Oo T, Hughes PL, Singh G, Mansour P. Delayed complications of discontinuation of intrathecal baclofen therapy: resurgence of dyssynergic voiding, which triggered off autonomic dysreflexia and hydronephrosis. Spinal Cord. 2004;42(10):598–602.
69. Kosturakis A, Gebhardt R. SynchroMed II intrathecal pump memory errors due to repeated magnetic resonance imaging. Pain Physician. 2012;15(6):475–7.
70. Maino P, Koetsier E, Perez RS. Fentanyl overdose caused by malfunction of SynchroMed II intrathecal pump: two case reports. Reg Anesth Pain Med. 2014;39(5):434–7.
71. Wesemann K, Coffey RJ, Wallace MS, Tan Y, Broste S, Buvanendran A. Clinical accuracy and safety using the SynchroMed II intrathecal drug infusion pump. Reg Anesth Pain Med. 2014;39(4):341–6.
72. Pasquier Y, Cahana A, Schnider A. Subdural catheter migration may lead to baclofen pump dysfunction. Spinal Cord. 2003;41(12):700–2.
73. Sorokin A, Annabi E, Yang WC, Kaplan R. Subdural intrathecal catheter placement: experience with two cases. Pain Physician. 2008;11(5):677–80.
74. Stinchon JF, Shah NP, Ordia J, Oates E. Scintigraphic evaluation of intrathecal infusion systems: selection of patients for surgical or medical management. Clin Nucl Med. 2006;31(1):1–4.
75. Deer TR, Prager J, Levy R, Rathmell J, Buchser E, Burton A, et al. Polyanalgesic Consensus Conference--2012: consensus on diagnosis, detection, and treatment of catheter-tip granulomas (inflammatory masses). Neuromodulation. 2012;15(5):483–95; discussion 496.
76. Leibold AT, Weyhenmeyer J, Lee A. Simultaneous explantation and implantation of intrathecal pumps: a case series. J Neurosurg. 2020;132(5):1398–404.

12 Treatment of Focal Muscle Overactivity Using Botulinum Toxin Injections

Elina Zakin, Yaowaree Leavell, and David M. Simpson

Each muscle has its own peculiar purpose, and it obeys the decree of the composite sense.
– Avicenna, Canon of Medicine, 1025.

- Botulinum toxin, a neurotoxin produced by the bacteria *Clostridium botulinum*, has been used in the management of neurologic disorders. There are currently four formulations of toxin available for use in the United States: onabotulinumtoxinA (Botox®), abobotulinumtoxinA (Dysport®), incobotulinumtoxinA (Xeomin®), and rimabotulinumtoxinB (Myobloc®).
- This chapter describes the mechanism of action, pharmacology, guidelines for use, and techniques for administration of botulinum toxin in the management of adult upper and lower limb muscle overactivity in the context of spasticity.
- Additionally, it discusses the importance of goal attainment scales and optimization of the clinical response.
- The clinician must remember that botulinum toxin has only been shown to be efficacious in the symptomatic control of muscle overactivity, without a proven role in disease modification. Rehabilitation therapy, in addition to the administration of botulinum toxin, is necessary to improve functional outcomes.

E. Zakin (✉)
Department of Neurology, Division of Neuromuscular Medicine, NYU Grossman School of Medicine, New York, NY, USA
e-mail: elina.zakin@nyulangone.org

Y. Leavell
Department of Neurology, Division of Neuromuscular Medicine, Oregon Health and Science University, New York, NY, USA
e-mail: Leavell@ohsu.edu

D. M. Simpson
Department of Neurology, Icahn School of Medicine at Mount Sinai, New York, NY, USA
e-mail: david.simpson@mssm.edu

P. Raghavan (ed.), *Spasticity and Muscle Stiffness*,
https://doi.org/10.1007/978-3-030-96900-4_12

Introduction

Widely considered as one of the most toxic substances known to man, botulinum toxin (BoNT) is an elegant example of how science can reveal the dual nature of naturally occurring compounds. The German physician-poet Joseph Kerner first characterized the clinical syndrome of autonomic dysfunction, diplopia, mydriasis, and skeletal muscle paralysis in a series of monographs published between 1817 and 1822. He attributed these findings to what he termed "sausage poison" or "fatty acid," on account of its presence in the fat of undercooked sausages consumed by victims of several outbreaks in Wurttemberg at the end of the eighteenth century [1–3]. In 1897, Emile Pierre-Marie van Ermengem was able to isolate the anaerobic bacteria we now know as *Clostridium botulinum* in the viscera of outbreak victims during autopsy. Beginning in 1928, the first stable toxin precipitates were isolated, and it was subsequently demonstrated that localized atrophy of chicken embryo leg muscles could be produced without undesired effects on the cardiovascular or central nervous systems [4]. This paved the way for the groundbreaking research of ophthalmologist Dr. Alan Scott in the late 1970s in which he was able to successfully treat strabismus with BoNT injection [5]. Since then, there has been a rapidly expanding body of research characterizing BoNT as remarkably safe and effective for the treatment of myriad medical conditions in multiple subspecialties including dermatology, urology, gastroenterology, physical medicine and rehabilitation, and neurology [6]. The goal of this chapter is to focus on the application of BoNT for the treatment of muscle overactivity in patients with spasticity.

Structure

Botulinum toxin is a metalloprotease produced by neurotoxigenic strains of *C. botulinum*. There are seven known serotypes designated A–G, six of which have known subtypes, some with recently discovered mosaic recombinations such as CD or DC. In its initial form, it is synthesized as a 150 kD polypeptide which is then cleaved by host or clostridial proteases, resulting in a mature form consisting of a 100 kD heavy chain (HC) and a 50 kD light chain (LC) attached by a disulfide bridge [7–9]. The HC mediates specific binding and endocytosis at the presynaptic membrane, and the LC contains the toxic moiety responsible for cleavage of the SNARE (SNAP REceptor) protein and subsequent failure of exocytosis of acetylcholine at the axon terminal. The toxin is usually found as a heterodimer along with the nontoxic non-hemagglutinin protein (NHTA), which is encoded by a neighboring gene. The heterodimer interacts with larger hemagglutinin complexes, forming what is referred to as the progenitor toxin complex (PTC). The exact role of these associated proteins is not fully characterized, but it is thought that they may protect the toxin from being denatured in local and gastric environments and facilitate transepithelial migration [6–8, 10]. This structural complex becomes pharmacologically significant in that most available formulations include the inactive proteins found in the PTC, whereas incobotulinum toxin does not [6, 8, 9].

Mechanism of Action

For BoNT to cause paralysis, it must first reach the cytosol of the presynaptic neuron by means of a multistep process, which includes binding, internalization, translocation, and cleavage.

Binding

Botulinum toxin demonstrates a highly specific binding process mediated by the Hcc (heavy chain carboxy terminus), polysialogangloside (PSG) receptors, and one of two protein receptors integral to the vesicular membrane (Syt, SV2). As it is located on the presynaptic membrane, the PSG receptor is exposed to the extracellular environment – this is the first interaction between the BoNT complex and the neuronal membrane.

Internalization

Once a vesicle has fused with the presynaptic membrane, the Syt and SV2 proteins become exposed and bound to the BoNT Hcc, allowing it to take advantage of the neuron's innate vesicular recycling process and gain entry into the presynaptic neuron via endocytosis.

Translocation

The mechanism of LC translocation from the synaptic vesicle into the cytosol is yet to be fully characterized, but is known to be dependent on the relatively acidic environment created by the active vesicle membrane proton pump. The change in pH triggers the creation of a membrane channel involving both the chains, which allows LC entry into the cytosol. At this point the disulfide bridge is reduced by the redox system NADPH-thioredoxin reductase (TrxR)-thioredoxin (Trx), resulting in the release of the toxic metalloprotease LC into the cytosol.

Cleavage

Having reached the cytosolic compartment, the LC now has access to its target – the SNARE protein complex. SNAP (soluble N-ethylmaleimide-sensitive factor attachment protein) receptor protein complexes are assembled from several membrane-associated proteins including syntaxin, SNAP25, and VAMP, which mediate the docking and fusion of synaptic vesicles with the presynaptic cell membrane. The LC is able to cleave these isolated cytosolic SNARE proteins with a high degree of specificity, rendering them unable to complex with each other and thus preventing the release of the neurotransmitter acetylcholine at peripheral nerve terminals. Without the ability to release acetylcholine at the neuromuscular junction and at autonomic nerve terminals, the neuron is effectively silenced, unable to activate its companion muscle unit or parasympathetic organ, resulting in the clinical syndrome of paralysis, dry mouth, mydriasis, and symptoms of autonomic dysfunction [6, 7, 9–11].

Pharmacology

There are currently four trademarked BoNT formulations that are branded and used in the United States. Three of these are serotype A1 (onabotulinumtoxinA, Botox®; abobotulinumtoxinA, Dysport®; incobotulinumtoxinA, Xeomin®), and the fourth is serotype B (rimabotulinumtoxinB, Neurobloc/Myobloc®). There are several other brands produced mainly in China and Korea and distributed primarily in Asia including Botulax®, Neuronox®, Prosigne®, PurTox®, and Nabota®, a few of which have additional trade names [5, 6, 12–14].

OnabotulinumtoxinA (onaBoNT-A) and AbobotulinumtoxinA (aboBoNT-A) preparations consist of purified precursor toxin complexes (PTC), which are composed of both the active 150 kD BoNT and several HA/NHTA proteins discussed above. IncobotulinumtoxinA (incoBoNT-A) contains only the purified botulinum A1 toxin and thus carries the lowest foreign protein load. All three of the BoNT-A1 toxins are either frozen or vacuum dried for reconstitution with sterile saline, yielding a solution with pH of around 7.4. RimabotulinumtoxinB (rimaBoNT-B), like onaBoNT-A and aboBoNT-A, contains both the BoNT and the PTC and is unique in its preparation in that it is shipped as an injectable solution with a pH of about 5.6. The lower pH may contribute to mildly increased patient discomfort at the site of injection as compared to the other BoNT-A formulations. Due to a single amino acid substitution at the toxin binding site, it has a lower affinity than the BoNT-A toxins for synaptogogin. This results in a shorter duration of action and higher dose requirements to achieve the same clinical effect on skeletal muscles; however, it has similar efficacy at autonomic nerve terminals [6].

Little is known about the pharmacokinetics of BoNT at currently used therapeutic doses. Even at the high doses required for the treatment of muscle overactivity in large muscle groups, the total protein content amounts to only a few nanograms, rendering pharmacokinetic studies very difficult. It is clinically important to note that the toxin binds quickly, locally, and irreversibly with little effect distal to the site, which is why higher dilutions are recommended for larger muscle groups. There are no known blocking agents, and the paralytic effect does not wear off until the natural activity of the toxin has stopped. The duration of action at skeletal nerve terminals on in vitro cultured neurons is about 3–4 months [6]; however, in vivo, there are complex remodeling processes, including axon sprouting and acetylcholine receptor spreading across the sarcolemma, which can significantly shorten the toxin's clinical effect.

While potency is described in terms of the LD50 (the quantity required to kill 50% of a test population) of a mouse assay, it is difficult to standardize dosing equivalents and potencies between different toxin formulations. This is due to differences between the bioassays used by each producer, including the strain of mouse used, variations in times of the day of injection, and other diluents present in the injection. Furthermore, it is unclear how generalizable this animal data is to the human population [6, 10, 13].

Review of AAN Guidelines for the Utility of BoNT in Spasticity

The American Academy of Neurology (AAN) first published guidelines for use of BoNT to treat spasticity in 2008, with a companion update in 2016. Recommendations are provided for adult upper limb, adult lower limb, and child spasticity in the context of cerebral palsy. The strength of the evidence for each recommendation is delineated using the GRADE EBM scale [14].

Adult Upper Limb Spasticity

Based on multiple Class I studies, aboBoNT-A, incoBoNT-A, and onaBoNT-A are considered safe and effective for the reduction of adult upper limb spasticity and improvement of passive function (Level A). One Class I study was able to demonstrate superiority of onaBoNT-A over tizanidine for improving wrist flexor tone, with a notably lower incidence of adverse events; therefore, it is recommended that onaBoNT-A should be offered before tizanidine for this indication (Level B). To date, there has been only one Class I study of rimaBoNT-B for this indication, and so it is considered probably safe and effective (Level B). There is insufficient evidence for the use of BoNT in the improvement of active function at this time.

Adult Lower Limb Spasticity

At the time of publication of the AAN 2016 Guideline Update, there was sufficient Class I evidence to recommend aboBoNT-A and onaBoNT-A for the reduction of adult lower limb spasticity (Level A); however, there was insufficient evidence to recommend incoBoNT-A or rimaBoNT-B. Again, as in the case of upper limb spasticity, there is insufficient evidence to demonstrate efficacy of BoNT administration for the improvement of active function in the lower limb, such as for walking.

Techniques for optimization of treatment response There are two Class I studies demonstrating that high-volume, low-potency injection and end plate targeting using onaBoNT-A enhanced tone reduction in adult spasticity (Level B). There is only one Class II study with inconsistent outcomes comparing manual needle placement, electrical stimulation, and ultrasound guidance techniques. At this time, while guidance techniques improve the accuracy of needle placement in the muscle, no single technique has demonstrated superiority in outcomes of treatment.

Cerebral Palsy

Evidence for use of BoNT in children with cerebral palsy were reviewed in the 2008 Guidelines for the treatment of equinus varus, hamstring, adductor, and calf spasticity. There was sufficient evidence to recommend that BoNT should be offered for treatment of equinus varus (Level A) and that it should be considered for treatment of adductor spasticity and pain control for children undergoing adductor lengthening surgery and as a treatment option for upper extremity spasticity in children (Level B) [14].

Emerging Evidence

Given the favorable side effect profile and effectiveness in reducing spasticity, it is not surprising that there has been a robust proliferation of toxin formulations and an accompanying body of literature to support their clinical utility. There have been several randomized controlled trials for Chinese and Korean toxin preparations. Neuronox®, Botulax®, and Nabota® each have one large multicenter randomized controlled trial, demonstrating non-inferiority to Botox® for the treatment of post-stroke upper limb spasticity [15–17]. In 2013, Guarany et al. published a double-blind, randomized crossover trial comparing Prosigne® to Botox® for spasticity of several etiologies, which found no significant difference in adverse events or Modified Ashworth Scale (MAS) scores in each group at 4 and 12 weeks [18]. There are currently several studies underway which have the potential to result in updated recommendations and answer some of the many questions which still surround BoNT, both in the laboratory and in clinical practice.

Review of Dose Recommendations

There is much controversy regarding the increase in motor function relative to the improvement in spasticity using BoNT. The AAN, as well as several European consensus statements, have supported the use of BoNT-A as a first-choice therapy for focal upper and lower extremity spasticity [19]. Current guidelines suggest doses of up to 600 units (U) of onaBoNT-A or up to 1500 U of aboBoNT-A per injection session to treat spasticity after stroke. Several studies suggest no difference in potency between onaBoNT-A and incoBoNT-A, further supporting a dose ratio of 1:1 for incoBoNT-A and onaBoNT-A [20]. However, FDA labels indicate that dose conversions between formulations of BoNT are not possible. Initial treatment with BoNT-A sometimes fails to produce an adequate response, although with subsequent injections, the desired clinical effect may be achieved with modification of dosing and muscle selection.

Reduced or nonresponse to BoNT-A injection may be due to the following:

1. Inappropriate selection of muscles for treatment
2. Inaccurate placement of injections

3. Spread beyond targeted muscles
4. Insufficient doses
5. Lack of specific goals or outcome measures
6. Handling errors during drug storage or preparation [21]

Upper Limb Spasticity

Upper limb spasticity should be evaluated in terms of active and passive disability (see Chaps. 3 and 8 for details on assessment). Active disability in the proximal upper limb is associated with restricted ability to reach for objects in the environment or on the body. Distally, there may be impairment of hand orientation and difficulties with grasping and/or manipulating fine objects. Passive disability leads to difficulty with dressing, washing, and bathing. In the hand, reduced access to the palm for washing and nail cutting may occur due to passive disability. Disabilities involving the upper limb are detailed in Chap. 7. The neurotoxin dosages for selected muscles in upper limb spasticity are shown in Table 12.1.

Lower Limb Spasticity

Lower limb spasticity should also be evaluated in terms of active and passive disability (see Chaps. 3 and 8 for details on assessment). Active disability in the distal

Table 12.1 Neurotoxin dosages for selected muscles in upper limb spasticity

	Recommended dose: total dose, number of sites		
Muscle	AboBoNT-A[a]	IncoBoNT-A[b]	OnaBoNT-A[c]
Flexor digitorum superficialis	100–200 U, 1–2 sites	25–100 U, 2 sites	30–50 U, 1 site
Flexor digitorum profundus	100–200 U, 1–2 sites	25–100 U, 2 sites	30–50 U, 1 site
Flexor carpi radialis	100–200 U, 1–2 sites	25–100 U, 1–2 sites	12.5–50 U, 1 site
Flexor carpi ulnaris	100–200 U, 1–2 sites	20–100 U, 1–2 sites	12.5–50 U, 1 site
Brachioradialis	100–200 U, 1–2 sites	25–100 U, 1–3 sites	
Biceps brachii	200-400 U, 1–2 sites	50–200 U, 1–4 sites	100–200 U, 4 sites
Brachialis	200–400 U, 1–2 sites	25–100 U, 1–2 sites	
Pronator quadratus		10–50 U, 1 site	
Pronator teres	100–200 U, 1 site	25–75 U, 1–2 sites	
Adductor pollicis		5–30 U, 1 site	20 U, 1 site
Flexor pollicis brevis		5–30 U, 1 site	
Opponens pollicis		5–30 U, 1 site	
Flexor pollicis longus		10–50 U, 1 site	20 U, 1 site

[a]DYSPORT [Prescribing information]. Basking Ridge, NJ: Ipsen Biopharmaceuticals, Inc.; 12/2016
[b]XEOMIN. [Prescribing information]. Raleigh, NC: Merz Pharmaceuticals, LLC; 12/2015
[c]BOTOX [Prescribing information]. Irvine, CA: Allergan; 10/2017

Table 12.2 Neurotoxin dosages for selected muscles in lower limb spasticity

Muscle	Recommended dose: total dose, number of sites OnaBoNT-A
Gastrocnemius, medial head	75 U, 3 sites
Gastrocnemius, lateral head	75 U, 3 sites
Soleus	75 U, 3 sites
Tibialis posterior	75 U, 3 sites
Flexor halluces longus	50 U, 2 sites
Flexor digitorum longus	50 U, 2 sites

[a]BOTOX [Prescribing information]. Irvine, CA: Allergan; April 2017

lower extremity interferes with maintenance of comfort with ambulation, as well as balance and limb advancement. Distally, in the ankle and foot, walking discomfort can be alleviated with the use of BoNT-A. Scissoring of gait that interferes with standing and walking is another example of active disability, most prominently involving the thigh muscles. Proximally, in the muscles of the hip girdle, active disability interferes with sexual intimacy, as well as gait. Passive disability leads to difficulty with dressing, perineal care, transfers, and positioning in the chair and in bed. Disabilities involving the lower limb are detailed in Chap. 7. The neurotoxin dosages for selected muscles in lower limb spasticity are shown in Table 12.2.

Patient and Muscle Selection for Treatment

Patient and muscle selection is fundamental in planning treatment with BoNT-A. The clinician must consider the predominant active muscles in relation to the intended goals for treatment.

The Preinjection Consultation

There are several critical aspects of the preinjection evaluation that must be discussed with the patient, including goals of the treatment, explanation of the treatment and subsequent therapy, and informed consent.

Patients and family members often have high expectations for functional gain. Prior to treatment with BoNT, the treatment goals and the expected outcomes should be discussed and agreed upon with the patient and family. The literature suggests that goal attainment scaling provides a responsive measure for evaluating focal intervention with BoNT and helps identify outcomes of importance to the patient and/or caregiver [22]. Examples of attainable treatment goals include relief of pain, ability to dress more easily, and hand opening to prevent fingernails from digging into the palm.

A thorough explanation of the treatment must be provided by the clinician to the patient and family regarding what the treatment will entail, which muscles will be injected, the number of injections, and the potential benefits and side effects. Finally, informed consent must be obtained from the patient or caregiver after careful discussion of the potential for adverse events, including excess bleeding, infection, focal weakness, generalized weakness, diaphragmatic paresis, and even death.

Planning the Injection

Several localization techniques are available for the identification of target muscles. Examples include anatomic localization using surface anatomy, electromyography, electrical stimulation, and ultrasound guidance. The clinician's experience with injection of BoNT is vital in muscle targeting. Selection of the appropriate muscles for injection requires clear treatment goals as well as a thorough physical and neurologic examination. Since controlled data are limited, there are variations in clinical practice concerning dilutions and volumes of BoNT, the number of injection sites per muscle, and the total dose injected.

Localization of Muscles

Anatomic localization The physician identifies anatomic landmarks by way of palpation to delineate target muscles. Many atlases and guides to electromyography (EMG) are available for this purpose. The clinician must examine and palpate the spastic muscle in individuals who are unable to voluntarily activate the muscle. Passive movement to initiate a stretch in the target muscle may be performed to identify the muscle belly. For patients who can voluntarily contract the muscle, the physician may ask the patient to perform the desired movement for muscle belly identification [23].

The advantages of this technique include the lack of need for additional equipment, the possibility of using a smaller gauge needle for injection (equating to reduced patient discomfort), and rapid injection technique (which may be favorable in children or individuals with fear of needles). The disadvantages include difficulty targeting deeper and smaller muscles. Additionally, muscle and end plate localization in hypertrophied muscles of patients with spasticity may be different, making BoNT injection targeting more difficult. A cadaveric study in 2012 evaluated the accuracy of using palpation and surface landmarks to guide injections into the gastrocnemius muscle of 30 cadavers [24]. The study found that only 43% of the injections were successfully placed within the gastrocnemius muscle, whereas 57% were placed outside the muscle, either in the soft tissue (19.8%) or deep to the gastrocnemius in the soleus muscle (37.2%). Finally, anatomic landmarks may be challenging based on the difficult positioning of spastic limbs in this patient population, and as a result, there is a higher potential for inadvertent injection into nontarget muscles, with suboptimal BoNT localization. In this event, patients may experience unanticipated weakness with incomplete relief of spasticity in the muscles of interest.

Electromyographic guidance This technique requires the use of an EMG auditory signal amplifier or an EMG machine with a needle electrode. Initially, anatomic localization is used and EMG guidance is employed as support for more precise localization. With needle insertion into the spastic muscle of interest, the physician will hear (and see) the involuntary motor unit action potentials (MUAPs) that become sharper as the needle tip is advanced closer to the motor end plate. To ensure that the needle tip is within the target muscle, the physician may ask the patient with some voluntary muscle control to activate the muscle, while listening (and looking) for increased firing of motor unit action potentials (MUAPs). If the patient is unable to voluntarily contract the muscle, the physician may perform passive range of motion to initiate a stretch of the target muscle, which will result in depolarization bursts due to reflex spastic motor unit recruitment [25] (also see Chap. 4).

There are several advantages to using this technique for muscle localization. EMG is widely available and familiar to many physicians who inject BoNT. A simple auditory EMG device is inexpensive, and more accurate muscle targeting can be achieved using EMG along with anatomic localization. Listening for crisp MUAPs, the clinician can better target BoNT injection to the muscle motor end plate. There are also disadvantages in using this technique: in individuals who are unable to voluntarily contract the muscle, needle localization cannot be confirmed, and the clinician risks inadvertently injecting BoNT into an adjacent muscle. Proper localization of the motor end plate may require more time, and possibly additional needle manipulation, making this a more painful procedure. The costs of the EMG amplifier or machine and the insulated EMG needle must also be considered.

Electrical stimulation Electrical stimulation is a technique in which an insulated needle is connected to an electrical stimulation machine. Again, anatomic landmarks are initially used to delineate the muscle of interest, and the needle is inserted. Once the needle is positioned in the muscle, electrical stimulation is delivered through the needle electrode to activate the muscle, usually using low levels of electrical current. The physician then observes for movement across the joint(s) of interest due to electrical activation of the muscle. For example, when targeting the flexor digitorum superficialis muscle, the clinician observes for flexion of the proximal interphalangeal joints.

The advantage of electrical stimulation is that it affords accuracy of muscle localization with visual feedback of movement. With finer targeting, less current may be needed to achieve muscle contraction and lower doses of BoNT may need to be injected, thus reducing the costs of the toxin. There are, however, several disadvantages. This technique is more time-consuming and requires that a trained clinician performs the injections. Additionally, there is more discomfort to the patient, from both the needle and the delivery of electrical stimulation through it. Furthermore, in patients with severe spasticity and marked limitation of range of motion, it may be difficult to appreciate the contraction of individual muscles and verify the joint movement. Lastly, there is also the consideration of cost for both the electrical stimulation machine and the needle electrodes.

Neuromuscular ultrasound The use of neuromuscular ultrasound was first reported by Schiano et al. in injecting BoNT for achalasia [26]. The ultrasound machine consists of various parts, including a transducer which contains transducing crystals which allow for sound transmission, a central processing unit, which receives data from the transducer, and a monitor, which displays the data from the tissue being evaluated. Ultrasound uses high-frequency sound waves that are emitted by the transducer and penetrate the soft tissues, with some portion of the sound waves reflected back to the transducer, to produce the images. The higher the frequency of the transducer, the better the resolution and quality of the image. Tissue density and depth of structures of interest also determine the characteristics of the reflected sound waves. This allows for direct visualization of the target muscles for BoNT administration.

The advantages of using ultrasound include real-time visualization of needle advancement into the muscle(s) of interest, allowing the clinician the opportunity to not only confirm the target muscle but also avoid certain structures (i.e., nerves and blood vessels) as the needle approaches the target. Techniques to verify needle placement, such as voluntary muscle contraction with either EMG or electrical stimulation guidance, along with the visualization of joint movement, further increase the accuracy of needle localization when combined with ultrasound. The procedure is relatively quick, and with direct muscle visualization there can be less pain with the use of a smaller gauge needle. There is also the possibility that with more exact targeting, there would be less spread of BoNT and greater delivery of the BoNT dose into the muscle of interest. The disadvantages of this technique are that it is largely operator dependent and requires a degree of proficiency with using ultrasound prior to incorporation into practice. Additionally, handling both the transducer and the syringe/needle may require the aid of an assistant. If both electrical stimulation and ultrasound are employed, an assistant must be present in the procedure room. The cost of the ultrasound machine and transducer must also be considered.

Comparison of techniques A systematic review of the various injection-guiding techniques performed in 2015 revealed that instrumented guidance using ultrasonography, electrical stimulation, and/or EMG was more effective than manual needle placement using anatomic landmarks alone in the treatment of upper limb spasticity and spastic equinus in patients with stroke, as well as in spastic equinus in children with cerebral palsy (Level A evidence). This review also reported Level A evidence of similar effectiveness of ultrasound and electrical stimulation guidance for the treatment of upper and lower limb spasticity in patients with stroke, with poor evidence for EMG guidance alone [27]. We are currently performing a head-to-head study comparing ultrasound and electrical stimulation guidance techniques in the treatment of upper limb spasticity and dystonia.

After Injection

After injection of BoNT, the clinician and team must provide the patient with postinjection care instructions including stretching the weakened muscles, assessing the need for orthotics and/or splinting, and therapy to increase muscle strength of the antagonist muscle groups, if indicated. It is helpful to assess the patient 2–4 weeks after the injection, once the clinical effect of muscle weakness is noted, to determine if BoNT dosing and muscle selection should be adjusted for future injections. Measurement of outcomes, reassessment of therapy needs, and review of goal achievement, which should have been carefully discussed at the preinjection visit, should once again be addressed during the postinjection visit. Continuation of therapy in addition to BoNT administration has been shown to be more effective than toxin injection alone. A 24-week multicenter trial of 31 patients with poststroke upper limb spasticity who were treated with onaBoNT-A showed significant improvement in upper extremity motor function when combined with upper limb rehabilitation as compared to without rehabilitation, using the upper extremity Fugl-Meyer score which measures motor function, sensation, range of motion, coordination, and speed [28].

Measuring Outcomes

Standardized measures before and after treatment are integral components of the assessment process. Measures should focus on impairment, activity limitation, and participation, as well as achievement of the patient's own goals, using goal attainment scales [29].

Goal Attainment

Goal attainment measures are used to evaluate active function, passive function, and symptom relief. Typically, active function is measured by assessing gait pattern and gait efficiency for improved mobility. Timed walking tests and videos for gait analysis are suggested outcome measures. Passive function can be assessed by the degree of improvement in caregiving or self-care by the patient. Some outcome measures include the ease of application of splints/orthoses, ease of maintenance of hygiene, and ease of dressing and improvement in seated posture. Improvements in passive function may be measured by the amount of time it takes the patient or a caregiver to complete the task. Additionally, it is important to ask the patient about symptom relief and reduction of pain. Rating scales for pain relief may include a verbal scale (no pain, mild pain, moderate pain, or severe pain), a numeric rating scale (from 0, no pain, to 10, for severe pain), or pictorial pain rating scales (e.g., the visual analog scale).

Measures of Spasticity

The Modified Ashworth Scale (MAS) is widely-accepted as a reliable measure of spasticity [30]. Although it is commonly used as an outcome measure in many studies of BoNT use in spasticity management, it has been most reliably validated for assessing resistance to passive movement rather than spasticity per se. The Tardieu Scale, which was initially developed for use in children with cerebral palsy, is considered more reliable than the MAS for measuring spasticity. These scales are discussed in detail in Chaps. 3 and 4.

Caregiver Burden and Quality of Life

Several studies in the past two decades have revealed that individuals with spasticity who underwent BoNT injection had improvements in quality of life, as well as reduced caregiver burden. Lam et al. in 2012 performed a double-blind, placebo-controlled trial over a 24-week period, where they randomized 55 individuals with upper limb spasticity to BoNT versus saline injections. The 30 patients who received BoNT had a significant reduction in caregiver burden with marked improvements in goal attainment and MAS scores [31]. Another double-blind, randomized, sham-controlled trial that evaluated BoNT-A in non-ambulant children with cerebral palsy revealed improvement in ease of care and comfort in the toxin group as compared to the saline group, using the Canadian Occupational Performance Measure at 4 and 16 weeks postinjection [32].

Conclusion

Botulinum toxin is a neurotoxin with a very long history, which is now used widely in various neurologic indications. There are four available toxin formulations that are FDA-approved and available for use in the United States: onabotulinumtoxinA (Botox®), abobotulinumtoxinA (Dysport®), incobotulinumtoxinA (Xeomin®), and rimabotulinumtoxinB (Myobloc®). The available evidence suggests that these toxin formulations can improve passive, but not active function, in the management of adult upper and lower limb spasticity. Incorporation of rehabilitation therapy after BoNT administration in this patient population results in improved outcomes in caregiver burden, goal attainment, and quality of life. It is vital for the clinician to understand that BoNT is indicated for use in symptomatic control of muscle overactivity in patients with spasticity and, at this time, has not been shown to play a role in disease modification.

References

1. Ali FR, Al-Niaimi F. Justinus Kerner and sausage poisoning: the birth of botulinum toxin. Int J Dermatol. 2016;55(11):1295–6.

2. Erbguth FJ, Naumann M. Historical aspects of botulinum toxin: Justinus Kerner (1786–1862) and the "sausage poison". Neurology. 1999;53(8):1850–3.
3. Erbguth FJ. Historical notes on botulism, Clostridium botulinum, botulinum toxin, and the idea of the therapeutic use of the toxin. Mov Disord. 2004;19(Suppl 8):S2–6.
4. Pellett S. Learning from the past: historical aspects of bacterial toxins as pharmaceuticals. Curr Opin Microbiol. 2012;15(3):292–9.
5. Dressler D. Botulinum toxin drugs: brief history and outlook. J Neural Transm (Vienna). 2016;123(3):277–9.
6. Pirazzini M, Rossetto O, Eleopra R, Montecucco C. Botulinum neurotoxins: biology, pharmacology, and toxicology. Pharmacol Rev. 2017;69(2):200–35.
7. Rossetto O, Pirazzini M, Montecucco C. Botulinum neurotoxins: genetic, structural and mechanistic insights. Nat Rev Microbiol. 2014;12(8):535–49.
8. Humeau Y, Doussau F, Grant NJ, Poulain B. How botulinum and tetanus neurotoxins block neurotransmitter release. Biochimie. 2000;82(5):427–46.
9. Tighe AP, Schiavo G. Botulinum neurotoxins: mechanism of action. Toxicon. 2013;67:87–93.
10. Simpson L. The life history of a botulinum toxin molecule. Toxicon. 2013;68:40–59.
11. Pantano S, Montecucco C. The blockade of the neurotransmitter release apparatus by botulinum neurotoxins. Cell Mol Life Sci. 2014;71(5):793–811.
12. Cocco A, Albanese A. Recent developments in clinical trials of botulinum neurotoxins. Toxicon. 2018;147:77–83.
13. Simpson DM, Gracies JM, Graham HK, Miyasaki JM, Naumann M, Russman B, et al. Assessment: botulinum neurotoxin for the treatment of spasticity (an evidence-based review): report of the Therapeutics and Technology Assessment Subcommittee of the American Academy of Neurology. Neurology. 2008;70(19):1691–8.
14. Simpson DM, Hallett M, Ashman EJ, Comella CL, Green MW, Gronseth GS, et al. Practice guideline update summary: botulinum neurotoxin for the treatment of blepharospasm, cervical dystonia, adult spasticity, and headache: report of the Guideline Development Subcommittee of the American Academy of Neurology. Neurology. 2016;86(19):1818–26.
15. Seo HG, Paik NJ, Lee SU, Oh BM, Chun MH, Kwon BS, et al. Neuronox versus BOTOX in the treatment of post-stroke upper limb spasticity: a multicenter randomized controlled trial. PLoS One. 2015;10(6):e0128633.
16. Nam HS, Park YG, Paik NJ, Oh BM, Chun MH, Yang HE, et al. Efficacy and safety of NABOTA in post-stroke upper limb spasticity: a phase 3 multicenter, double-blinded, randomized controlled trial. J Neurol Sci. 2015;357(1–2):192–7.
17. Do KH, Chun MH, Paik NJ, Park YG, Lee SU, Kim MW, et al. Safety and efficacy of letibotulinumtoxinA(BOTULAX®) in treatment of post stroke upper limb spasticity: a randomized, double blind, multi-center, phase III clinical trial. Clin Rehabil. 2017;31(9):1179–88.
18. Guarany FC, Picon PD, Guarany NR, dos Santos AC, Chiella BP, Barone CR, et al. A double-blind, randomised, crossover trial of two botulinum toxin type a in patients with spasticity. PLoS One. 2013;8(2):e56479.
19. Esquenazi A, Albanese A, Chancellor MB, et al. Evidence-based review and assessment of botulinum neurotoxin for the treatment of adult spasticity in the upper motor neuron syndrome. Toxicon. 2013;67:115–28.
20. Jost WH, Kohl A, Brinkmann S, Comes G. Efficacy and tolerability of a botulinum toxin type A free of complexing proteins (NT 201) compared with commercially available botulinum toxin type A (BOTOX) in healthy volunteers. J Neural Transm (Vienna). 2005;112:905–13.
21. Sheean GL. Botulinum treatment of spasticity: why is it so difficult to show a functional benefit? Curr Opin Neurol. 2001;14:771–6.
22. Turner-Stokes L, Baguley IJ, De Graaff S, et al. Goal attainment scaling in the evaluation of treatment of upper limb spasticity with botulinum toxin: a secondary analysis from a double blind placebo-controlled randomized clinical trial. J Rehabil Med. 2010;42(1):81–9.
23. Walker HW, Yee MY, Bahroo LB. Botulinum toxin injection techniques for the management of adult spasticity. PMR. 2015;7:417–27.

24. Schnitzler A, Roche N, Denormandie P, Lautridou C, Parratte B, Genet F. Manual needle placement: accuracy of botulinum toxin A injections. Muscle Nerve. 2012;46(4):531–4.
25. O'Brien CF. Injection techniques for botulinum toxin using electromyography and electrical stimulation. Muscle Nerve Suppl. 1997;6:S176–80.
26. Schiano TD, Fisher RS, Parkman HP, et al. Use of high-resolution endoscopic ultrasonography to assess esophageal wall damage after pneumatic dilation and botulinum toxin injection to treat achalasia. Gastrointest Endosc. 1996;44:151–7.
27. Grigoriu AI, Dinomais M, Remy-Neris O, et al. Impact of injection-guiding techniques on the effectiveness of botulinum toxin for the treatment of focal spasticity and dystonia: a systematic review. Arch Phys Med Rehabil. 2015;96:2067–78.
28. Devier D, Harnar J, Lopez L, Brashear A, Graham G. Rehabilitation plus OnabotulinumtoxinA improves motor function over onabotulinumtoxinA alone in post-stroke upper limb spasticity: a single-blind, randomized trial. Toxins (Basel).2007;9(7). pii: E216. https://doi.org/10.3390/toxins9070216.
29. Ashford S, Turner-Stokes L. Goal attainment for spasticity management using botulinum toxin. Physiother Res Int. 2006;11:24–34.
30. Bohannon RW, Smith MB. Interrater reliability of a modified Ashworth scale of muscle spasticity. Phys Ther. 1987;67(2):206–7.
31. Lam K, Lau KK, So KK, Tam CK, Wu YM, Cheung G, et al. Can Botulinum toxin decrease carer burden in long term care residents with upper limb spasticity? A randomized controlled study. J Am Med Dir Assoc. 2012;13(5):477–84.
32. Copeland L, Edwards P, Thorley M, Donaghey S, Gascoigne-Pees L, Kentish M, Cert G, et al. Botulinum toxin A for nonambulatory children with cerebral palsy: a double blind randomized controlled trial. J Pediatr. 2014;165(1):140–6.

Treatment of Focal Muscle Stiffness with Hyaluronidase Injections

13

Preeti Raghavan, Alexandra Gordon, Ryan Roemmich, and Antonio Stecco

...the beauty and strength of the mechanical construction lie not in one part or in another, but in the harmonious concatenation which all the parts, soft and hard, rigid and flexible, tension bearing and pressure bearing, make up together.
—D'Arcy Thompson, On Growth and Form, 1917.

- Spasticity develops because of injury to the central nervous system. However, secondary changes within the connective tissue of the muscle also contribute to muscle stiffness.
- The hyaluronan hypothesis postulates that the accumulation and biophysical alteration of hyaluronan, a high molecular weight glycosaminoglycan that normally acts as a lubricant within the extracellular matrix of muscles, promotes the development of muscle stiffness and progression to fibrosis and muscle contracture.

The original version of this chapter was revised. Affiliation of Alexandra Gordon has been updated. The correction to this chapter can be found at https://doi.org/10.1007/978-3-030-96900-4_15

P. Raghavan
Departments of Physical Medicine and Rehabilitation and Neurology, The Johns Hopkins University School of Medicine, Baltimore, MD, USA
e-mail: praghavan@jhmi.edu

A. Gordon
Albert Einstein College of Medicine, Bronx, NY, USA
e-mail: alexandra.gordon@einsteinmed.edu

R. Roemmich
Department of Physical Medicine and Rehabilitation, Johns Hopkins University School of Medicine, Baltimore, MD, USA
e-mail: rroemmi1@jhu.edu

A. Stecco (✉)
Rusk Rehabilitation, NYU Grossman School of Medicine, New York, NY, USA
e-mail: Antonio.stecco@nyulangone.org

P. Raghavan (ed.), *Spasticity and Muscle Stiffness*,
https://doi.org/10.1007/978-3-030-96900-4_13

- Intramuscular injections of the enzyme hyaluronidase, which catabolizes the altered hyaluronan polymer, were shown to reduce muscle stiffness and increase passive and active range of motion in patients with spasticity.
- This chapter discusses the preliminary evidence for the emerging treatment of muscle stiffness using the enzyme hyaluronidase and its potential to prevent fibrosis and contracture.

Introduction

Hyaluronidases are a group of enzymes distributed throughout the animal kingdom that regulate the metabolism of hyaluronic acid (hyaluronan, HA). The hyaluronan hypothesis of muscle stiffness postulates that the accumulation and biophysical alteration of HA in the extracellular matrix (ECM) of muscle leads to the development of muscle stiffness [1, 2]. Chapter 6 describes the evidence for the role of altered HA metabolism in the development of increased passive resistance to movement. HA is a non-sulfated high molecular weight glycosaminoglycan (GAG) and a major component of the endomysium, perimysium, and epimysium which together constitute the ECM of the muscle [3]. In the healthy state, HA in the ECM acts as a lubricant to facilitate sliding and myofascial force transmission within and between muscles [4, 5]. However, disruption in the homeostasis of HA due to reduced clearance and/or increased production, for example, because of paresis and immobility [6] as well as muscle overactivity and compensatory overuse [7, 8], can lead to the accumulation of HA and an alteration in its physiological properties leading to muscle stiffness and increased resistance during passive movement [9, 10] (Fig. 13.1).

GAGs and specifically HA, the largest GAG, can self-organize into diverse supramolecular complexes that determine the physical properties of the tissue [11]. Figure 13.2 shows the various ways in which GAGs can self-organize and form

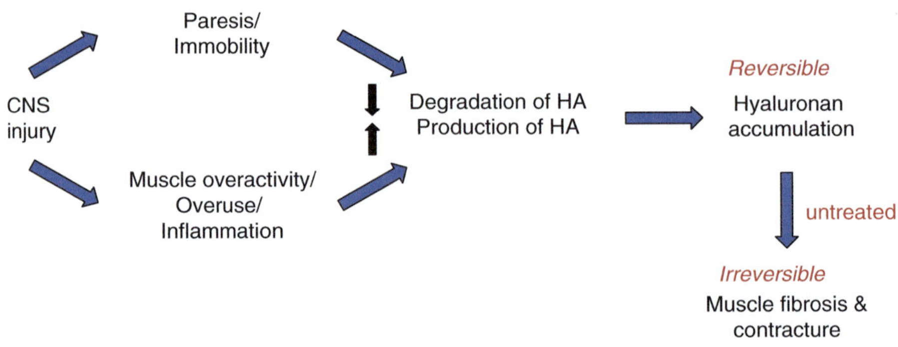

Fig. 13.1 Paresis and immobility after CNS injury can lead to reduced degradation of hyaluronan (HA), whereas muscle overactivity, overuse of compensating muscles, and/or inflammation can lead to increased production of HA. If HA accumulation is untreated, it may contribute to irreversible muscle fibrosis and contracture

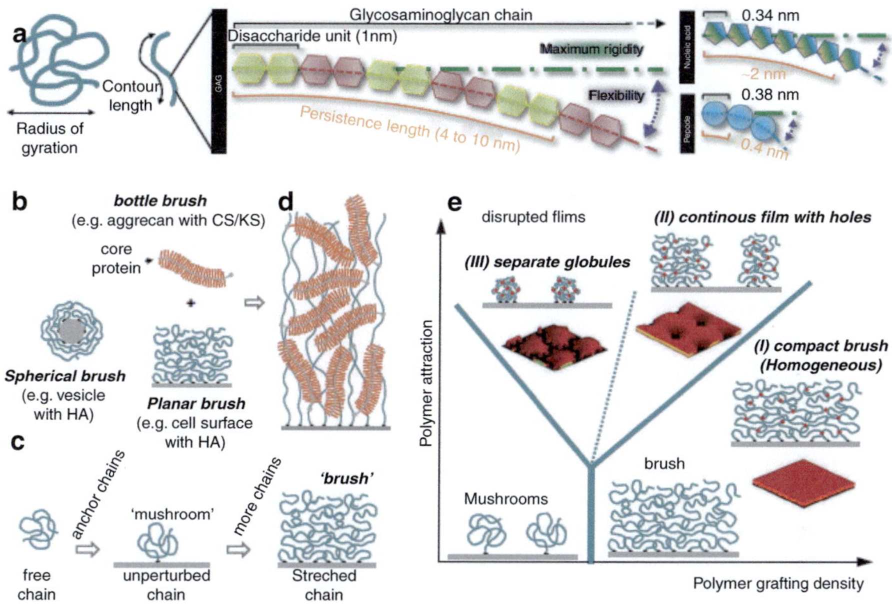

Fig. 13.2 Schematic diagrams illustrating the self-organization of glycosaminoglycans (GAGs), and specifically hyaluronan (HA), from a soft matter physics perspective. (**a**) The radius of gyration and the contour length of polymer chains, and the sizes of the building blocks and persistence lengths for GAGs relative to nucleic acids and (poly)peptides. (**b**) Polymer brushes: a bottle brush forms upon anchorage of chondroitin sulfate (CS) and keratan sulfate (KS) at high density to a core protein (e.g., aggrecan); HA, when retained via attachment to hyaluronan synthases (HASs), can form a planar brush on the cell surface, spherical brushes around extracellular vesicles and cylindrical brushes around cell membrane protrusions. (**c**) Brushes form when the flexible GAG chains are anchored at high density to a substrate. (**d**) Assemblies of GAGs and GAG-rich proteoglycans are intrinsically mechanically soft and swollen owing to the mutual repulsion of GAGs and the high negative charge, providing an osmotic swelling pressure due to associated counter ions. The schematic shows how aggrecan swells and extends HA brushes. (**e**) Crosslinking of GAGs with proteins causes compaction, phase separation, and rigidification. As the attraction between polymers increases (in the case of GAGs by crosslinking with proteins), the film becomes more compact and rigid, and a homogeneous brush (I) can phase separate into heterogeneous films of distinct morphology: a continuous film with holes (II) or separate globules (III). Boundaries between phases are drawn qualitatively and three-dimensional views (red) illustrate the gross morphology of phases I, II, and III. (Modified from Richter RP (2018), with permission)

rigid structures. The aggregation and self-organization of HA polymers is highly dependent on HA concentration, temperature, and pH, which together affect the viscoelasticity of the ECM [5, 12, 13]. The compliant nature of the HA aggregations may explain how physical modalities, such as the application of heat and cold, and physical manipulation, such as stretching and massage, affect the resistance to passive movement in individuals with muscle stiffness with or without spasticity [14, 15]. For example, it has been shown that passive resistance to stretching at slow speeds, which is thought to reflect non-neural muscle stiffness, is increased with the application of a cold stimulus, whereas it is decreased with the application of a warm stimulus in individuals with spasticity [16]. Repetitive static stretching can lead to a temporary reduction in viscoelastic stress relaxation in individuals with and without spasticity [17, 18]. Increased GAG content is seen in non-spastic myofascial pain and muscle stiffness [19, 20], and deep friction massage has been shown to reduce GAG content as measured by muscle imaging [8]. Taken together, these studies suggest that the alteration in the biophysical properties of HA can affect muscle stiffness. Since hyaluronidases catabolize HA, they could play a critical role in the clearance of HA, particularly in individuals with severe muscle stiffness.

The potential role of HA and hyaluronidase in spasticity may be surmised from a study that demonstrated the presence of HA in the capsular space of the cat muscle spindle, which was responsible for the transcapsular potential across the sensory terminal membrane that makes the sensory nerve ending sensitive to mechanical stimuli. The diffusion of hyaluronidase into the capsular space reduced both resting and stretch-induced impulses in the muscle spindle [21]. HA is also abundant around the nerve endings in the perimysium (see Chap. 6, Fig. 6.9). Excessive amounts of HA in the muscle spindle and around the nerves in the perimysium may affect the stretch reflex response. Furthermore, HA is also a key component of perineuronal nets (PNNs), which refer to the ECM around neurons in the central nervous system (CNS) and are shown to be crucial in the control of neuronal plasticity both during development and after CNS injury – the formation of mature PNNs signals the closure of neuronal plasticity [22, 23]. PNN removal after spinal cord injury enhances plasticity, for example, by allowing de novo sprouting of axons and the formation of new synapses for the recovery of function [24, 25]. Thus, excessive HA accumulation in the ECM of muscle increases its viscoelasticity and the resistance to passive movement and may also increase the sensitivity of the muscles spindles and exacerbate spasticity. In addition, it may disrupt peripheral plasticity which may be crucial for recovery of movement and function.

Catabolism of Hyaluronan by Hyaluronidases

Hyaluronidases were first described by Duran-Reynals who observed that extracts of mammalian testis and other tissues contain a “spreading factor” which could facilitate the diffusion of dyes and antiviral vaccines injected subcutaneously [26, 27]. The term “hyaluronidase” was introduced by Karl Meyer in 1971 to denote that the enzymes degrade HA. Meyer classified hyaluronidases based on biochemical analysis and the end products generated into mammalian hyaluronidases, leech hyaluronidase, and microbial hyaluronidases [28]. The initial degradation of HA is accomplished by hyaluronidase, which cleaves the linkage between glucuronic acid and N-acetyl glucosamine and generates oligosaccharides of different chain lengths which are the substrates for two other exoglycosidases [29] (Fig. 13.3a).

The human genome contains six hyaluronidase-like genes which share about 40% of their identity with one another, suggesting that they evolved by gene duplication, although the expression of each gene has a unique tissue distribution. The

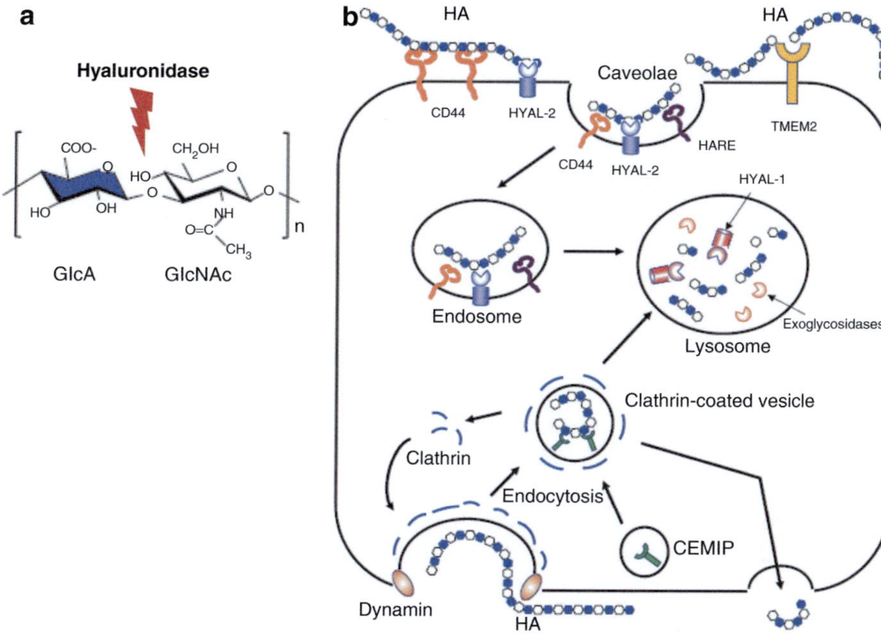

Fig. 13.3 Schematic illustration of mechanisms of hyaluronan (HA) degradation. (**a**) The initial degradation of HA is accomplished by hyaluronidase (HYAL), which cleaves the linkage between glucuronic acid and N-acetyl glucosamine and generates oligosaccharides of different chain lengths. (**b**) In HYAL-mediated HA degradation (top), high molecular weight HA is tethered to the cell surface by CD44 and GPI-anchored HYAL2 into caveolin-rich lipid rafts and then cleaved into approximately 2×10^4 Da fragments. The HA fragments are subsequently delivered to endo-lysosome compartments and degraded into smaller oligosaccharides by HYAL1 and monosaccharides by exoglycosidases. In the proposed model of CEMIP-mediated HA degradation (bottom), high-molecular-weight HA is endocytosed into clathrin-coated vesicles and cleaved into lower-molecular-weight HA fragments by the action of CEMIP, which is localized in the peripheral vesicles of the cell. The fragmented HA is then depolymerized in endo-lysosome compartments or released extracellularly without intracytoplasmic accumulation. TMEM2 is expressed on the cell surface in a type II transmembrane topology and degrades high molecular weight HA into approximately 5×10^3 Da fragments. (From Kobayashi T (2020), with permission)

genes HYAL1, HYAL2, and HYAL3 are located on chromosome 3p21.3, whereas HYAL4, PHYAL1 (a pseudogene), and sperm adhesion molecule 1 (SPAM1, also known as PH20) are clustered on chromosome 7p31.3. HYAL1 and HYAL2 are the major hyaluronidases expressed in human somatic tissues and are both needed for catabolism of tissue HA [30, 31]. HYAL1 plays an important role in HA degradation within the liver, whereas HYAL2 is required for clearance of high molecular weight HA in lymph nodes and plasma and for HA endocytosis by liver non-parenchymal cells [32].

In a recently proposed model of HA catabolism (Fig. 13.3b), the glycosylphosphatidylinositol (GPI)-anchored cell surface hyaluronidase HYAL2 cleaves high molecular weight HA into approximately 2×10^4 Da fragments at the cell surface with the HA receptor CD44 [33]. The partially fragmented HA is internalized by binding to the HA receptors [34] and is then further degraded by HYAL1 and exoglycosidases in the lysosomal system. Interestingly, HYAL2 appears to favor an acidic pH for its hyaluronidase activities [35]. More recently, two novel molecules, the cell migration inducing protein (CEMIP/KIAA1199) and transmembrane protein 2 (TMEM2), have been identified that contribute to digesting extracellular high molecular weight HA into smaller fragments [36–38]. As the fragmented HA in the ECM is usually internalized by cells through receptors, HA receptors have roles not only in intracellular signaling but also in HA clearance [39–43].

Pharmacology and Uses of Exogenous Hyaluronidases

The interstitial connective tissue matrix is a complex three-dimensional dynamic structure comprised of numerous structural macromolecules including collagens, elastin, and fibronectin, in which GAGs such as HA and proteoglycans form a hydrated gel-like substance that allows the ECM to resist compressive forces. Collagens are the predominant fibers that hold tissues in place and maintain tissue integrity. HA acts as a barrier to bulk fluid flow through the interstitial collagenous matrix due to its hydration and viscosity [44]. While the concentration of HA is only 1% of the concentration of collagen in the skin, it occupies a fluid exclusion volume tenfold higher than that of collagen on a mL H_2O/mg basis [45]. In contrast to collagen, which has a half-life approaching 15 years [46], HA is rapidly turned over in the body with a half-life of 15–20 hours in the skin [47, 48]. Thus, HA in the skin and subcutaneous interstitial connective tissue matrix forms an effective dermal barrier.

"Spreading agents" derived from animal testes extracts containing interstitial matrix-degrading enzymes have been used clinically for over 50 years to facilitate the dispersion and absorption of other drugs through the skin and subcutaneous tissue, including procaine for patients with spasticity [28, 49]. SPAM1 or PH20 is the predominant hyaluronidase in mammalian testes and is the only neutral pH-active hyaluronidase that degrades GAGs under physiologic conditions. Thus, PH20 is used therapeutically to increase the speed of absorption of drugs, to promote resorption of excess fluids, to increase the effectiveness of local anesthesia, and to diminish tissue destruction by subcutaneous and intramuscular injection of fluids [50, 51]. While animal testes-derived hyaluronidase extracts have been used extensively in the clinic to disperse other injected drugs, they have generally been limited by both immunogenicity and impurity profiles, typically comprising less than 1% enzyme per mg total protein. Such preparations are frequently contaminated with proteases, immunoglobulin, and factors that increase capillary permeability and can also give rise to IgE-mediated allergic reactions upon repeat administration [52, 53].

The human PH20 enzyme is a 509 amino acid glycoprotein anchored to the plasma membrane through a GPI moiety that facilitates penetration of spermatozoa through the cumulus cells to enable fertilization [54]. A purified soluble recombinant human hyaluronidase (rHuPH20) lacking the GPI membrane attachment, containing 447 amino acids with an approximate molecular weight of 61 kDa, is produced by genetically engineered Chinese hamster ovary (CHO) cells containing a DNA plasmid encoding for a soluble fragment of human hyaluronidase (PH20). Recombinant human hyaluronidase (Hylenex®, Halozyme Therapeutics, San Diego, California) enhances the infusion rates and penetration of molecules up to 200 nm in diameter up to 20-fold without eliciting inflammation, vascular permeability, and immunogenic or allergic reactions [55]. This product was FDA approved in 2005.

Recombinant human hyaluronidase is supplied as a sterile, clear, colorless, non-preserved, ready-for-use solution with an approximate pH of 7.0 and an osmolality of 280–340 mOsm/kg. It is indicated as an adjuvant in subcutaneous fluid administration for achieving hydration, to increase the dispersion and absorption of other injected drugs [56], and in subcutaneous urography for improving resorption of radiopaque agents. It is approved for infiltration use, interstitial use, intramuscular use, intraocular use, retrobulbar use, soft tissue use, and subcutaneous use. Hyaluronidase is antigenic; repeated injections of relatively large amounts of hyaluronidase preparations may result in the formation of neutralizing antibodies. However, allergic reactions have been reported in less than 0.1% of patients. Anaphylactic-like reactions following retrobulbar block or intravenous injections have occurred rarely. The most frequently reported adverse reactions have been mild local injection site reactions, such as erythema and pain. The long-term effects of hyaluronidase on fertility are unknown. It also has several off-label uses in dermatology, plastic surgery, ophthalmology, and surgery [56–61]. The use of hyaluronidase for the treatment of muscle stiffness is a novel off-label application at present.

Novel Off-Label Use of Hyaluronidase for Treatment of Muscle Stiffness

Upper Limb Muscle Stiffness

Safety and Preliminary Efficacy of a Single Injection Treatment

In an initial retrospective case series [1], 20 patients with unilateral upper limb spastic-muscle stiffness of cerebral origin received off-label injections of recombinant human hyaluronidase in combination with preservative-free normal saline into 6–8 upper limb muscles at a single visit. All patients (mean age 41 ± 22 years and mean time since injury 40.6 ± 38.9 months) had moderately severe unilateral upper limb spasticity across more than one joint, defined by a Modified Ashworth Scale (MAS) score ≥2. The dose ranged from 450 to 600 units of hyaluronidase diluted with normal saline which was distributed in multiple synergistically acting muscles.

There were no clinically significant adverse effects related to the treatment. Resistance to passive movement was assessed clinically using the MAS (see Chaps. 3 and 4). The percentage of joints with MAS = 3 decreased by 38.5% and those with MAS = 0 increased by 46.9% within 3 days to 2 weeks postinjection, suggesting a clear effect of the injections (Fig. 13.4). Passive range of motion

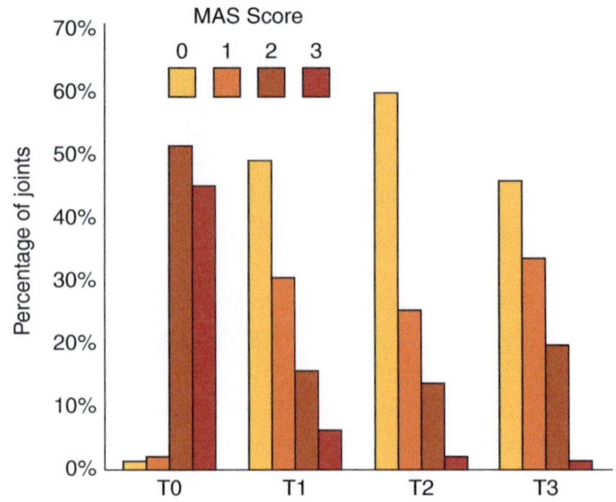

Fig. 13.4 Modified Ashworth Scale (MAS) score across upper limb joints at T0 = preinjection, T1 = within 2 weeks post hyaluronidase injection, T2 = within 4–6 weeks post hyaluronidase injection, and T3 = within 3–5 months post hyaluronidase injection. (Data from Raghavan P (2016), with permission)

(PROM) and active range of motion (AROM) were evaluated pre- and postinjection to assess clinical response to treatment. PROM at all joints and AROM at most joints increased within 2 weeks postinjection (T1) and persisted at 4–6 weeks postinjection (T2) and 3–5 months postinjection (T3) (Fig. 13.5). There was a delayed increase in active elbow extension and forearm pronation, which was unexpected, suggesting a possible effect on plasticity. The results persisted for at least 3 months. Most importantly, there were no side effects of muscle weakness or sedation. These results provide preliminary evidence that intramuscular hyaluronidase injections can reduce muscle stiffness and increase passive and active movement in multiple upper limb joints of patients with chronic muscle stiffness secondary to spasticity.

Safety and Dose-Response of Multiple Injection Treatments

In a follow-up retrospective study of 30 patients with moderate-to-severe muscle stiffness (approved by the New York University School of Medicine Institutional Review Board), the safety of multiple off-label hyaluronidase injections was assessed by examining the percentage of patients who had immediate or delayed hypersensitivity reactions or reported any adverse effects such as prolonged muscle soreness. The maximum total dose used in this cohort was 1575 IU, with a maximum of 300 IU injected into a single site at once, which is well below the threshold of toxicity of hyaluronidase [62]. Of the 30 subjects, 5 subjects had only one injection visit during the study period. The remaining subjects had multiple injection visits (range 2–10). The average time between injection visits was 17.7 weeks (range 4.2–57.5), and an average of 11.3 muscles (range 3.8–20.0) were injected per visit. The average volume injected per session was 14.1 ml (range 4.0–25.3), which equated to an average dose of 1054.4 units (range 300–1575) (unpublished data).

None of the subjects in this retrospective cohort demonstrated evidence of immediate hypersensitivity on intradermal testing, i.e., no erythema, itching, or wheal

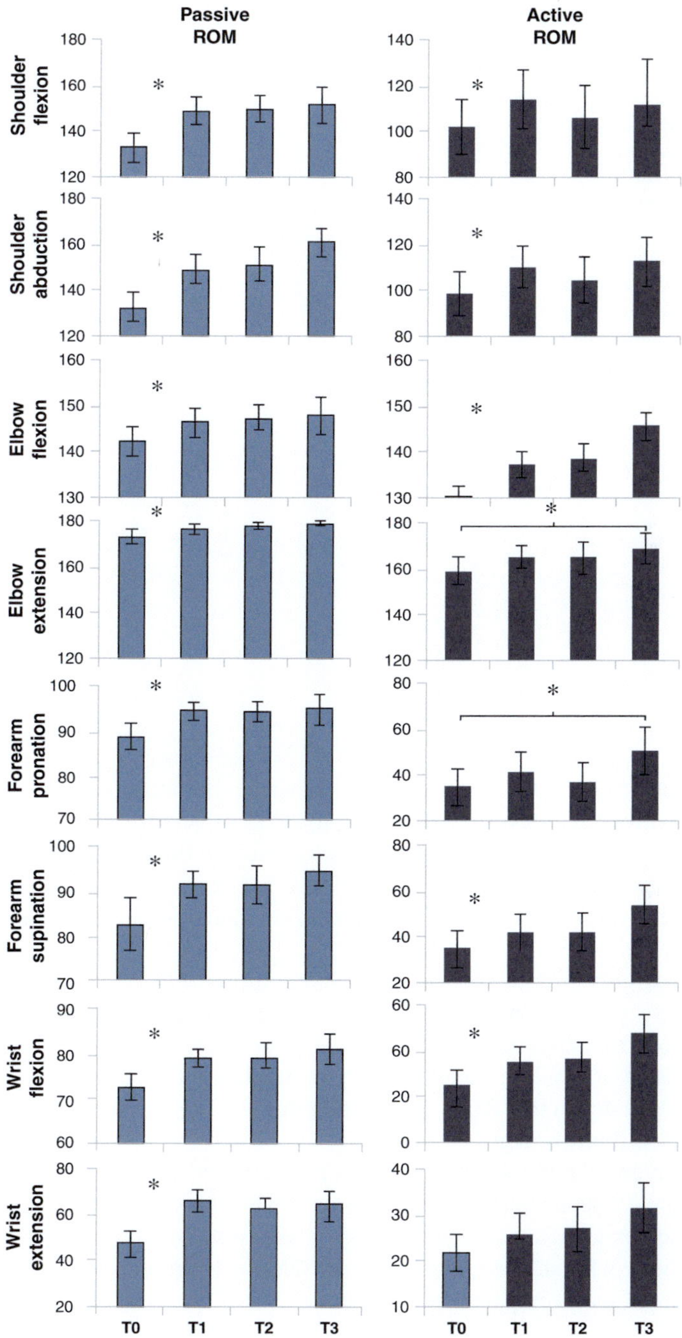

Fig. 13.5 Passive and active range of motion across upper limb joints (in degrees) at T0 = preinjection, T1 = within 2 weeks post hyaluronidase injection, T2 = within 4–6 weeks post hyaluronidase injection, and T3 = within 3–5 months post hyaluronidase injection. * statistically significant differences at $p < 0.05$. (Data from Raghavan P (2016), with permission)

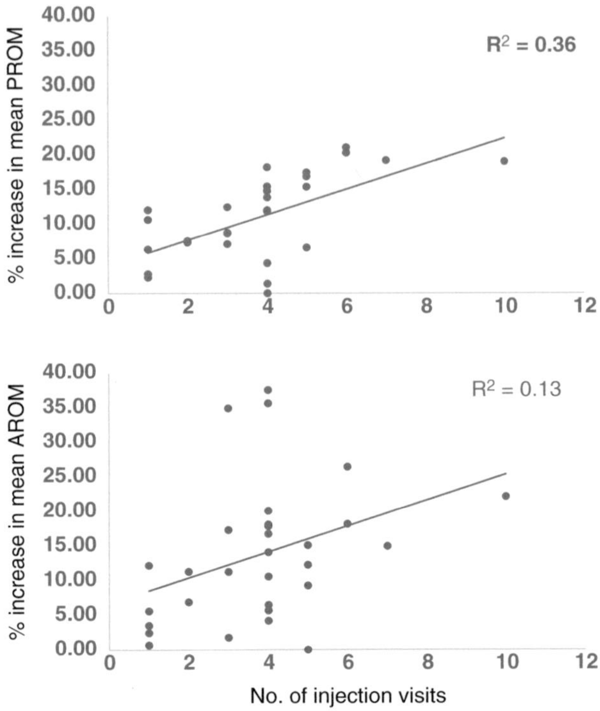

Fig. 13.6 Relationship between percentage change in average passive (PROM) and active range of motion (AROM) across the upper limb joints (shoulder abduction, shoulder flexion, elbow extension, elbow flexion, forearm supination, forearm pronation, wrist extension and wrist flexion) and the number of injection visits

was noted in or around the injection site prior to the intramuscular injections. None of them experienced delayed hypersensitivity. One subject had pain in the shoulder girdle which persisted after the injections and resolved once the statin that she was taking was discontinued. The subject continued to tolerate repeated injections without prolonged muscle soreness thereafter. No injection-related adverse effects were noted.

There was greater than 15% increase in maximum PROM from baseline in at least one joint in 87% (26/30) of subjects, and greater than 15% increase in maximum AROM from baseline in at least one joint in 70% (21/30) of subjects. As expected, ROM at baseline was negatively correlated with the percentage improvement in passive and active ROM, suggesting that the higher the baseline ROM, the less room for improvement. Across all joints, the improvements in PROM and AROM were correlated with the number of injection visits, suggesting an additive effect of repeat injections (Fig. 13.6). Subjects who showed little change in PROM showed changes in AROM and had lower levels of motor impairment at baseline, where as those who showed changes in PROM with little change in AROM had higher levels of motor impairment at baseline.

Lower Limb Muscle Stiffness

Preliminary Efficacy of a Single Injection Treatment

Off-label hyaluronidase has also been used clinically in the lower limb in several patients. Here, we present the changes in gait parameters in one patient who presented for instrumented gait analysis before and after the injections as part of an observational study (approved by the Johns Hopkins University Institutional Review Board). The patient, a 64-year-old woman, sustained left spastic hemiparesis and presented with muscle stiffness that affected her ability to walk. She was referred for off-label hyaluronidase injections by her neurologist to treat the muscle stiffness in her lower limbs. She underwent instrumented gait analysis prior to one set of injections and subsequently received 1500 units of human recombinant hyaluronidase distributed over 14 lower limb muscles, mostly on the left side at a single visit. Approximately two months postinjection, she underwent follow-up gait analysis. Note marked increases in the patient's gait speed (Table 13.1). Both her preferred and fastest comfortable walking speeds increased by nearly 20% (preferred, 1.05 m/s preinjection to 1.22 m/s postinjection; fastest comfortable, 1.20 m/s preinjection to 1.42 m/s postinjection). These improvements exceed reported minimal clinically important difference thresholds for persons with neurologic damage or disease. Instrumented gait analysis recorded lower extremity joint kinematics and ground reaction forces. The most noticeable changes in the patient's kinematics were observed in her left hip and knee, as extension in both joints improved by nearly 5 degrees following the injections (Fig. 13.7; note that the increased flexion in the right knee throughout the gait cycle was due to a previous orthopedic issue). These improvements in leg extension led to a 14% increase in the forward propulsion force generated by her left leg, which likely facilitated the observed increases

Table 13.1 Results of gait analysis pre- and postinjection

Gait parameters	Preinjection		Postinjection	
Ankle kinematics	Right	Left	Right	Left
Peak dorsiflexion (deg)	1.7	1.8	2.1	4.1
Peak plantarflexion (deg)	−31.6	−24.1	−31.8	−22.1
Knee kinematics				
Peak flexion (deg)	62.5	57.5	65.1	59.9
Peak extension (deg)	12.5	2.6	13.4	−2.7
Hip kinematics				
Peak flexion (deg)	25.3	23.6	27.9	25.8
Peak extension (deg)	−10.6	−17.0	−14.5	−21.8
Ground reaction forces				
Peak propulsion (N/kg)	0.17	0.14	0.19	0.16
Peak braking (N/kg)	−0.19	−0.15	−0.16	−0.24
Walking speeds				
Preferred (m/s)	1.05		1.22	
Fastest (m/s)	1.20		1.42	

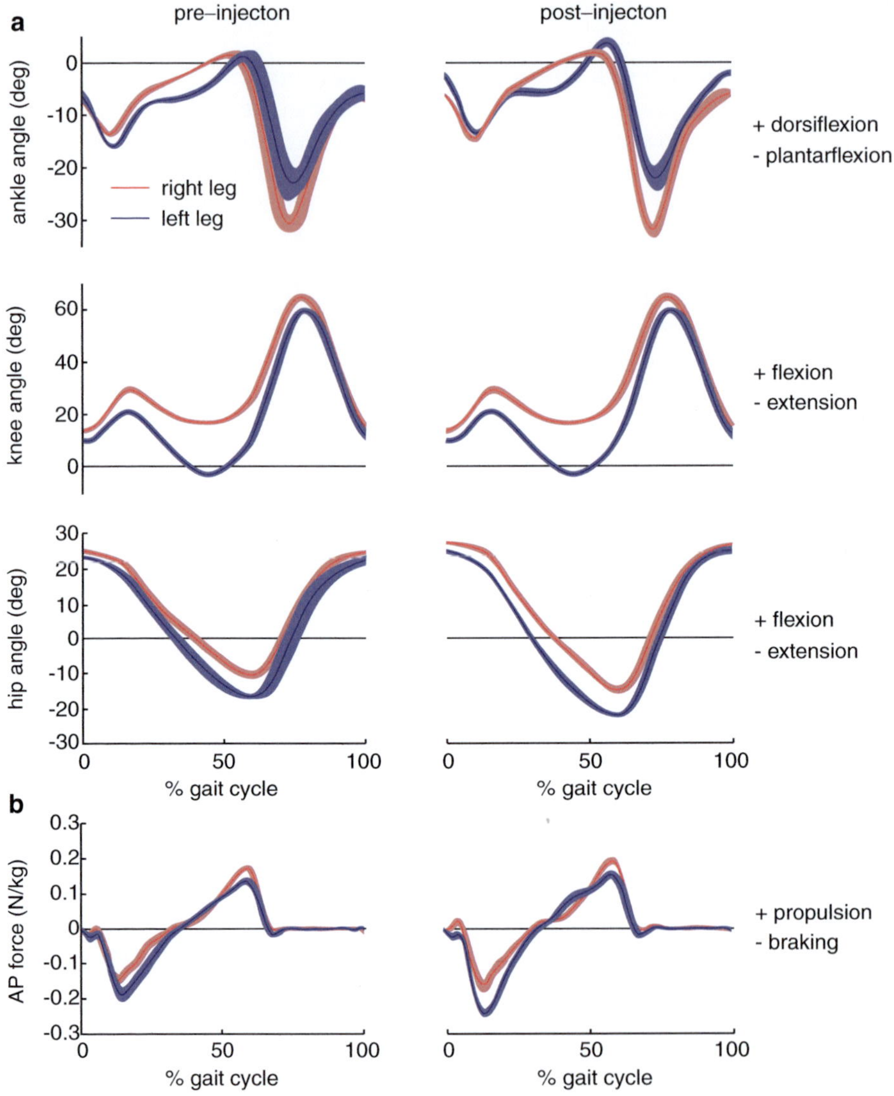

Fig. 13.7 Changes in gait parameters pre-post hyaluronidase injections to the lower limb muscles. (**a**) In joint kinematics. (**b**) In anteroposterior (AP) ground reaction forces

in gait speed. Importantly, these improvements were noticeable to the patient, as she perceived her gait to be smoother and more normal following the injections.

The clinical data presented above for the upper and lower limbs provides indirect evidence for the hyaluronan hypothesis, since HA content was not quantified. The results suggest that use of the enzyme hyaluronidase is a possible solution for the treatment of muscle stiffness associated with spasticity after neurological injury that does not cause muscle weakness [63, 64]. These results need to be confirmed in randomized controlled trials, one of which is currently ongoing (NCT03306615).

Imaging Quantification of Hyaluronan Content in Patients with Muscle Stiffness

T1rho (T1ρ) magnetic resonance imaging (MRI) mapping has been used to quantify GAG content in cartilage [65, 66], muscle [67–69], and intervertebral discs [70, 71]. T1ρ contrast is an endogenous noninvasive MRI contrast mechanism that refers to the spin lattice relaxation time constant in the rotating magnetic field and measures the transverse magnetization decay in the presence of a spin-lock radiofrequency (RF) field [72]. T1ρ contrast is sensitive to low energy interactions related to the chemical exchange between extracellular water and macromolecules and is well suited to characterize proteoglycan content [66, 73]. Hence, 3D-T1ρ MR mapping of the upper arm muscles was used to quantify intramuscular GAG content before and after hyaluronidase injection treatment [74]. Figure 13.8 shows representative mono-exponential T1ρ maps of the upper arm in controls and patients with post-stroke muscle stiffness before and after hyaluronidase injection treatment. Note the increased T1ρ relaxation times before the injections (middle panel, red) in the biceps and triceps muscles, reflecting increased intramuscular GAG content in patients with poststroke muscle stiffness. All three patients showed significant improvement in the T1ρ relaxation time of the biceps muscle within two weeks after treatment with hyaluronidase, approaching that of control values. The triceps muscle also showed increased GAG content but was not consistently targeted with the injections and therefore did not show a significant change given the small sample size. These results suggest that T1ρ mapping can be used to quantify GAG content in the muscles of patients with poststroke muscle stiffness noninvasively and that muscle HA content is increased in stiff muscles compared with controls, providing imaging corroboration for the hyaluronan hypothesis of muscle stiffness [74].

Accumulated Hyaluronan Traps Intramuscular Free Water in Stiff Muscles

In contrast to mono-exponential T1ρ mapping described above, bi-exponential T1ρ mapping can provide a more detailed characterization of the changes in the extracellular microenvironment (e.g., chemical exchange rate of protons, pH, GAG concentration, viscosity, and presence of free water) that contribute to the net increase observed in the mono-exponential T1ρ values shown in Fig. 13.8. The bi-exponential modeling uses a two-compartment model that breaks down the observed mono-exponential decay into its constituent parts, a short component that relaxes quickly and a long component that relaxes slowly. Increased GAG accumulation can increase the chemical exchange of the negatively charged GAGs with the protons of the water molecules, increasing the fraction of the short component. However, a more significant consequence is the aggregation of the GAGs into macromolecular spheres that trap free water in the ECM and increase the duration of the long component, T1ρl.

In patients with muscle stiffness, bi-exponential T1ρ mapping showed that the relaxation time of the short component was relatively unchanged, but the fraction of

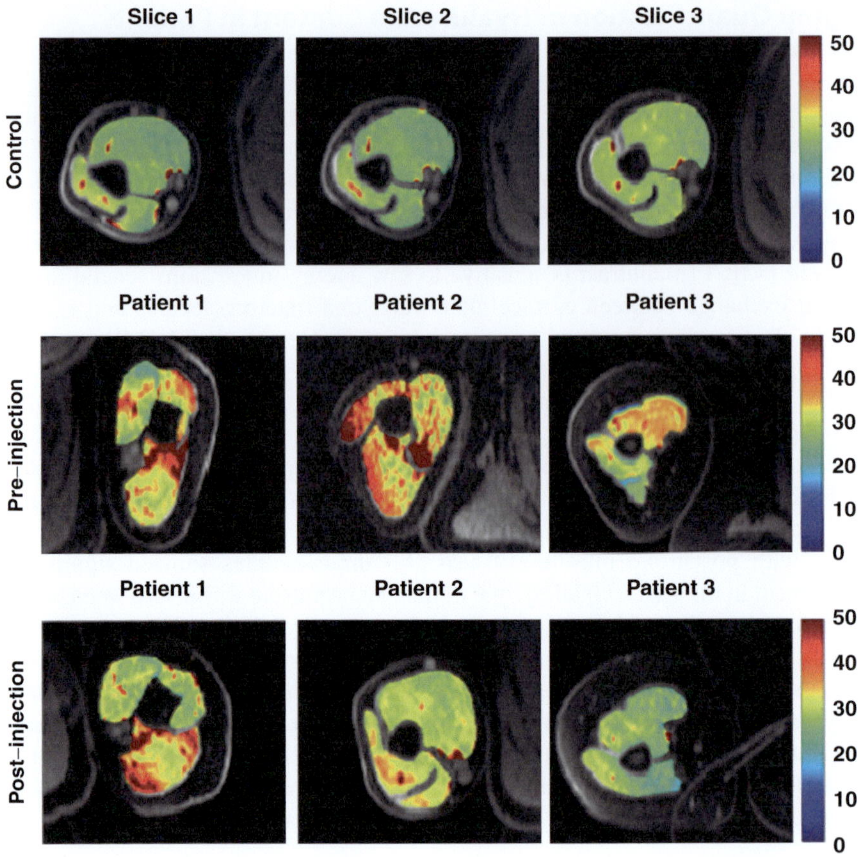

Fig. 13.8 Representative T1ρ maps of the upper arm in controls (top row) and patients with post-stroke muscle stiffness before (middle row) and after (bottom row) hyaluronidase injection treatment. Note the difference in relaxation times and the shape of the muscle before and after the injections. (From Menon R (2019), with permission)

the short component increased in the biceps and triceps muscles due to increased GAG accumulation (As (%)) (Table 13.2). In contrast, the relaxation time of the long component increased due to excessive free water in the ECM. Following treatment with hyaluronidase, note the shift of the mono-exponential and the bi-exponential short and long components with their corresponding fractions to values approaching those in controls. The changes in the fraction of the short component and the relaxation times of the long component provide an understanding of the role of intramuscular fluid accumulation in producing muscle stiffness. The results suggest that muscle stiffness is characterized by increased muscle GAG content and free water, both of which can be reduced with hyaluronidase injections. This pilot study demonstrates the application of bi-exponential T1rho mapping as a marker for GAG content in the muscle and as a potential treatment monitoring tool for patients with muscle stiffness [75].

Table 13.2 Summary of $T_{1\rho}$ mapping results

						P-values		
ROI	Fitting method	Parameter	Controls (n = 5)	Patients – pre (n = 5)	Patients – post (n = 3)	Patients vs. controls	Pre- vs. postinjection	Postinjection vs. controls
Biceps	Mono-exponential	Tlρm (ms)	26.7 ± 0.54	35.5 ± 2.93	29.45 ± 1.23	0.006	0.055	0.660
	Bi-exponential	Tlρs (ms)	7.12 ± 1.97	4.16 ± 3.25	7.72 ± 3.28	0.490	0.510	0.890
		Tlρl (ms)	37.32 ± 2.01	46.33 ± 5.57	48.14 ± 7.19	0.010	0.820	0.011
		As (%)	31.68 ± 8.54	52.21 ± 14.43	42.53 ± 9.17	0.031	0.410	0.070
		Al (%)	68.32 ± 8.54	47.79 ± 14.43	57.47 ± 9.17	0.031	0.410	0.070
Triceps	Mono-exponential	Tlρm (ms)	30.29 ± 2.23	34.57 ± 4.48	32.91 ± 4.9	0.138	0.730	0.500
	Bi-exponential	Tlρs (ms)	8.02 ± 3.26	6.06 ± 4.45	6.84 ± 1.40	0.930	0.90	0.460
		Tlρl (ms)	38.99 ± 4.89	50.5 ± 9.25	44.12 ± 6.13	0.004	0.280	0.150
		As (%)	28.06 ± 7.32	52.66 ± 20.29	42.54 ± 23.00	0.040	0.450	0.190
		Al (%)	71.94 ± 7.32	47.34 ± 20.29	57.46 ± 23.00	0.040	0.450	0.190

Mean T1rho values (± SD) for mono-exponential mean signal ($T_{1\rho m}$) and bi-exponential short signal and fraction ($T_{1\rho s}$, A_s) and long signal and fraction ($T_{1\rho l}$, A_l) in the biceps and triceps regions of interest (ROI) for controls and patients pre- and post hyaluronidase injection. (From Menon R (2021), with permission)

Patient and Muscle Selection for Treatment

The Preinjection Consultation

As for the use of any invasive treatment, including hyaluronidase injections, the preinjection evaluation visit should include a discussion with the patient about treatment goals, explanation of the treatment and procedure, and informed consent.

It must be clearly explained that treatment with hyaluronidase injections for muscle stiffness is off-label and is not yet approved by the FDA for this indication. The pros and cons of the injection of hyaluronidase versus other treatments, including the side effects such as the possibility of an allergic reaction and contingencies in case of one, should be explained. Other side effects can include temporary muscle soreness. The package insert may be provided along with literature on its off-label use for muscle stiffness.

A thorough explanation of the treatment must be provided by the clinician to the patient and family, regarding what it will entail, which muscles will be injected, the approximate number of injections, as well as the potential benefits and side effects. The pros include that it does not cause muscle weakness and that its effects can be additive with repeated treatments as shown in Fig. 13.6, although the incidence of tolerance is not known. The cons include the need for repeated treatments and that it cannot reverse fibrosis or contracture once these are established. Treatment goals must be discussed with the patient and family as suggested by the algorithm in Chap. 8.

Selection of Muscles

The selection of muscles for treatment depends on the goals of the treatment, the degree of stiffness, and the presence of fibrosis. Once these are determined, synergistically acting stiff muscles in one or more spatial planes along the myofascial chain may be selected for injection. Agonist and antagonist muscles across a joint must be treated in the same session for optimal effect [1]. The selection of muscles for injection and dosing requires specific training.

Clinical differentiation between muscle stiffness and contracture may be difficult in patients with severe muscle stiffness. This is important as there may be a critical window of opportunity in patients who are not yet contracted, as described in Chap. 6. Ultrasonography is a useful tool to visualize muscle tissue and infer its composition by assessing its echogenicity [76, 77]. Echo-intensity denotes the brightness of an image caused by the reflection of sound waves and is influenced by sound beam characteristics and tissue density [78]. Healthy muscles look dark with sharp bright lines on B-mode ultrasonography. The dark signal is hypoechoic, and the bright lines represent hyperechoic signal from collagen fibers in the endomysium and perimysium. Hyperechoic signal can be produced by fibrosis but also by fatty infiltration [79–81].

A qualitative assessment of muscle echo-intensity may be made using the grading described by the Heckmatt rating scale (Fig. 13.9a) [82]. The use of the Heckmatt rating scale has demonstrated that muscles showing high echo-intensity have a poorer response to treatment of spasticity with botulinum toxin injections [83–86]. On the other hand, trigger points (TrPs) are defined as stiff nodules in a taut band of muscle that present a hypoechoic signal [87, 88]. However, gray-scale ultrasonography cannot assess the mechanical properties of the muscle such as its stiffness, i.e., the ability of the muscle to be compressed, elongated, stretched, or manipulated.

Hence, shear wave elastography (SWE) has emerged as a quantitative measure of passive stiffness in individuals with spasticity and muscle stiffness, where an acoustic radiation force impulse or shear wave is generated by a special transducer and the local tissue deformation is evaluated using ultrasound imaging [89–92]. However, the use of SWE is limited by interobserver and technical variability, an inability to assess deeper muscles due to attenuation of the shear wave as it passes through the tissue, lack of standard protocols, and the need for specialized equipment [93–96].

The myotonometer is a handheld instrument which provides a mechanical impact to the muscle and measures the decaying oscillations that travel through it. The device can provide quantitative measurements of muscle properties such as tone, stiffness, and elasticity [97], which have been found to be reliable in assessing changes in muscle mechanical properties in individuals with spasticity [98–103]. The measurements of muscle properties with the myotonometer are highly correlated with those made using SWE [104], but they also suffer from similar drawbacks such as high interobserver and technical variability, inability to assess deeper muscles due to attenuation of the impulse as it passes through the tissue, lack of standard protocols, and the need for specialized equipment. Therefore, a more practical method in the clinical setting may be to qualitatively assess the compressibility of the underlying muscle by manual palpation to estimate the resistance of the tissue to displacement using the stiffness rating scale (Fig. 13.9b) [105].

The combined use of the qualitative assessment of muscle stiffness using the stiffness rating scale and of muscle echo-intensity using the Heckmatt rating scale is proposed to differentiate between severe muscle stiffness and contracture in the clinical setting. The stiffness-echogenicity matrix (SEM) combines echo-intensity using the Heckmatt rating scale on the x-axis with stiffness rating on the y-axis (Fig. 13.10). The combined echo-intensity and stiffness grades range from 1A (acutely denervated flaccid muscle) to 4D (noncompressible stiff and contracted muscle), representing a wide spectrum of conditions seen in clinical practice. It is proposed that muscles demonstrating high stiffness grades but low muscle echo-intensity on ultrasound, represented in the red box, are more likely to respond to treatment with hyaluronidase. Therefore, when there is a question about fibrosis or contracture, qualitative ultrasound may assist the clinician in decision-making.

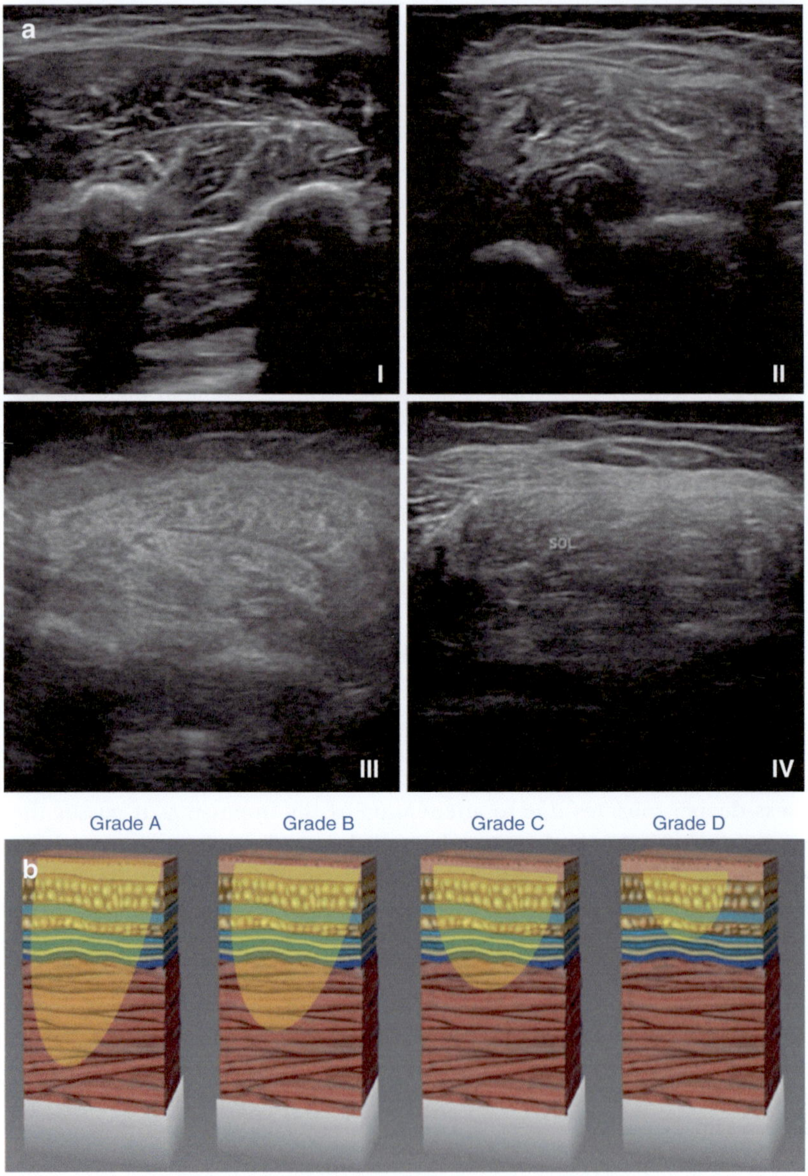

Fig. 13.9 Qualitative assessment of muscle stiffness and echogenicity. (**a**) Muscle echo can be graded by ultrasound using the Heckmatt rating scale, where the grades represent the following: I = Normal, II = Increase in echo intensity while bone echo is still distinct, III = Marked increase in muscle echo intensity with reduced bone echo, IV = Very high muscle echo intensity and complete loss of bone echo. (**b**) The stiffness rating scale assesses the compressibility of the underlying muscle by palpation to estimate the resistance of the tissue to displacement, where the grades represent the following: A = The muscle feels soft to the palpating thumb or index finger. It is possible to compress 75% of the relaxed muscle tissue, B = It is possible to compress only 50% of the relaxed muscle tissue due to mild resistance, C = It is possible to compress only 25% of the relaxed muscle tissue due to moderate resistance, D = It is impossible to compress the relaxed muscle tissue due to high resistance (bone-like). (From Stecco A (2019), with permission)

STIFFNESS–ECHOGENICITY MATRIX		ECHOGENICITY RATING			
		1	2	3	4
STIFFNESS RATING	A	1A Acute denervation	2A Atrophic muscle	3A Sacrcopenia	4A Severe Sacrcopenia
	B	1B Hypertrophic muscle	2B Normal	3B Early peripheral neurogenic	4B Early myogenic
	C	1C Densification	2C Chronic densification	3C Late peripheral neurogenic	4C Late myogenic
	D	1D Trigger points	2D Early central neurogenic	3D Central neurogenic	4D Late central neurogenic

Fig. 13.10 The Stiffness Echogenicity Matrix (SEM) combines qualitative rating of muscle stiffness using the stiffness rating scale on the y-axis with rating of muscle echo-intensity using the Heckmatt rating scale on the x-axis. The cells in the SEM represent a wide spectrum of conditions seen in clinical practice. The color of each cell in the matrix reflects the echo-intensity on grayscale ultrasound. The red box highlights muscles with high stiffness but low echo that may respond to treatment with hyaluronidase. (From Stecco A (2019), with permission)

The Injection

In previous studies, we diluted the commercially available hyaluronidase so as to optimize the volume and pressure of the injection [106]. Dilution also resulted in a lower dosage overall across all the muscles injected as the goal is to inject just enough enzyme to catabolize excessive HA in the stiff muscles. The dilution and dosage for individual muscles may vary based on the degree of muscle stiffness and the underlying disease and requires additional study. As with any invasive procedure, aseptic technique must be used, and precautions must be taken to avoid intravascular injection.

Hyaluronidase injections do not target the motor end plate; hence, the use of electromyography or electrical stimulation guidance is not necessary. However, ultrasound guidance may be helpful to confirm the anatomy in regions where surface anatomy is not clear or where there are critical neurovascular structures.

After Injection

Patients should be advised to use a warm compress for local soreness around the injection sites. Given that immobility can contribute to the accumulation and biophysical alteration of HA, patients should be encouraged to perform passive, active-passive (bimanually assisted), and/or active movements and stretching exercises to restore muscle length. Therapy to retrain functional movements and prevent compensatory muscle use may also be necessary. It is helpful to assess the patient 2–4 weeks after the injections to determine the effect of treatment and dosing and muscle selection for future injections.

Measuring Outcomes

Standardized measures before and after treatment are integral components of the assessment process. The most proximate outcome of the treatment of muscle stiffness with hyaluronidase is a change in passive range of motion at multiple joints in the limb, which may depend on the muscles selected for treatment, the degree of stiffness, and the presence of fibrosis, as well as on baseline movement ability. Functional outcomes are important to patients, and must also be assessed, although these may take time to change. Reduction in discomfort, pain, and the ability to participate in daily life roles are also important to assess.

Conclusions

Although spasticity develops because of injury to the CNS, peripheral non-neural mechanisms contribute to the ensuing muscle stiffness. The hyaluronan hypothesis postulates that the accumulation and biophysical alteration of hyaluronan within the ECM of muscle can lead to muscle stiffness. The use of hyaluronidase has emerged as a potential treatment to catabolize the excessive hyaluronan, which if left untreated may contribute to progression to muscle fibrosis and contracture. Randomized controlled clinical trials are needed to confirm preliminary findings of the efficacy of hyaluronidase in the treatment of muscle stiffness and in the prevention of fibrosis and muscle contracture. A better understanding of the mechanisms underlying muscle stiffness, the basis for treatment with hyaluronidase, and the dosing parameters, can potentially transform clinical practice for the treatment of muscle stiffness in both spastic and non-spastic patient populations.

Disclosures This chapter discusses the off-label use of hyaluronidase for treatment of muscle stiffness. Drs. Preeti Raghavan and Antonio Stecco are co-founders of MovEase, Inc.

References

1. Raghavan P, et al. Human recombinant hyaluronidase injections for upper limb muscle stiffness in individuals with cerebral injury: a case series. EBioMedicine. 2016;9:306–13.
2. Stecco A, Stecco C, Raghavan P. Peripheral mechanisms of spasticity and treatment implications. Curr Phys Med Rehabil Rep. 2014;2(2):121–7.
3. Piehl-Aulin K, et al. Hyaluronan in human skeletal muscle of lower extremity: concentration, distribution, and effect of exercise. J Appl Physiol (1985). 1991;71(6):2493–8.
4. Purslow PP, Trotter JA. The morphology and mechanical properties of endomysium in series-fibred muscles: variations with muscle length. J Muscle Res Cell Motil. 1994;15(3):299–308.
5. Cowman MK, et al. Viscoelastic properties of hyaluronan in physiological conditions. F1000Res. 2015;4:622.
6. Okita M, et al. Effects of reduced joint mobility on sarcomere length, collagen fibril arrangement in the endomysium, and hyaluronan in rat soleus muscle. J Muscle Res Cell Motil. 2004;25(2):159–66.

7. Calve S, et al. Hyaluronic acid, HAS1, and HAS2 are significantly upregulated during muscle hypertrophy. Am J Physiol Cell Physiol. 2012;303(5):C577–88.
8. Menon RG, et al. T1rho-mapping for musculoskeletal pain diagnosis: case series of variation of water bound glycosaminoglycans quantification before and after fascial manipulation((R)) in subjects with elbow pain. Int J Environ Res Public Health. 2020;17(3).
9. Meyer GA, McCulloch AD, Lieber RL. A nonlinear model of passive muscle viscosity. J Biomech Eng. 2011;133(9):091007.
10. Elliott DM, et al. Effect of altered matrix proteins on quasilinear viscoelastic properties in transgenic mouse tail tendons. Ann Biomed Eng. 2003;31(5):599–605.
11. Richter RP, et al. Glycosaminoglycans in extracellular matrix organisation: are concepts from soft matter physics key to understanding the formation of perineuronal nets? Curr Opin Struct Biol. 2018;50:65–74.
12. Gibbs DA, et al. Rheology of hyaluronic acid. Biopolymers. 1968;6(6):777–91.
13. Matteini P, et al. Structural behavior of highly concentrated hyaluronan. Biomacromolecules. 2009;10(6):1516–22.
14. Geiringer SR, deLateur BJ. Physiatric therapeutics. 3. Traction, manipulation, and massage. Arch Phys Med Rehabil. 1990;71(4-S):S264–6.
15. deLateur BJ, Hinderer SR. Physiatric therapeutics. 2. Therapeutic heat and cold, electrotherapy, and therapeutic exercise. Arch Phys Med Rehabil. 1990;71(4-S):S260–3.
16. Li S, et al. Different effects of cold stimulation on reflex and non-reflex components of post-stroke spastic hypertonia. Front Neurol. 2017;8:169.
17. Magnusson SP. Passive properties of human skeletal muscle during stretch maneuvers. A review. Scand J Med Sci Sports. 1998;8(2):65–77.
18. Gao F, et al. Effects of repeated ankle stretching on calf muscle-tendon and ankle biomechanical properties in stroke survivors. Clin Biomech (Bristol, Avon). 2011;26(5):516–22.
19. Stecco C, et al. Hyaluronan within fascia in the etiology of myofascial pain. Surg Radiol Anat. 2011;33(10):891–6.
20. Margalef R, et al. Experimental myofascial trigger point creation in rodents. J Appl Physiol (1985). 2019;126(1):160–9.
21. Fukami Y. Studies of capsule and capsular space of cat muscle spindles. J Physiol. 1986;376:281–97.
22. Kwok JC, Carulli D, Fawcett JW. In vitro modeling of perineuronal nets: hyaluronan synthase and link protein are necessary for their formation and integrity. J Neurochem. 2010;114(5):1447–59.
23. Kwok JC, et al. Extracellular matrix and perineuronal nets in CNS repair. Dev Neurobiol. 2011;71(11):1073–89.
24. Smith PD, et al. "GAG-ing with the neuron": the role of glycosaminoglycan patterning in the central nervous system. Exp Neurol. 2015;274(Pt B):100–14.
25. Carulli D, Kwok JC, Pizzorusso T. Perineuronal nets and CNS plasticity and repair. Neural Plast. 2016;2016:4327082.
26. Duran-Reynals F. Exaltation de l'activité du virus vaccinal par les extraits de certains organs. Comptes Rendus des Séances de la Société de Biologie et de Ses Filiales. 1928;99:6–7.
27. Chain E, Duthie ES. Identity of hyaluronidase and spreading factor. Br J Exp Pathol. 1940;21:324–38.
28. Meyer K. Hyaluronidases. In: Boyer PD, editor. The enzymes. New York: Academic Press; 1971. p. 307–20.
29. Roden L, et al. Enzymic pathways of hyaluronan catabolism. Ciba Found Symp. 1989;143:60–76; discussion 76–86, 281–5.
30. Csoka AB, Frost GI, Stern R. The six hyaluronidase-like genes in the human and mouse genomes. Matrix Biol. 2001;20(8):499–508.
31. Stern R. Devising a pathway for hyaluronan catabolism: are we there yet? Glycobiology. 2003;13(12):105R–15R.
32. Bourguignon V, Flamion B. Respective roles of hyaluronidases 1 and 2 in endogenous hyaluronan turnover. FASEB J. 2016;30(6):2108–14.

33. Kobayashi T, Chanmee T, Itano N. Hyaluronan: metabolism and function. Biomolecules. 2020;10(11).
34. Culty M, Nguyen HA, Underhill CB. The hyaluronan receptor (CD44) participates in the uptake and degradation of hyaluronan. J Cell Biol. 1992;116(4):1055–62.
35. Afify AM, et al. Purification and characterization of human serum hyaluronidase. Arch Biochem Biophys. 1993;305(2):434–41.
36. Yoshida H, et al. KIAA1199, a deafness gene of unknown function, is a new hyaluronan binding protein involved in hyaluronan depolymerization. Proc Natl Acad Sci U S A. 2013;110(14):5612–7.
37. Yamamoto H, et al. A mammalian homolog of the zebrafish transmembrane protein 2 (TMEM2) is the long-sought-after cell-surface hyaluronidase. J Biol Chem. 2017;292(18):7304–13.
38. Yamaguchi Y, et al. TMEM2: a missing link in hyaluronan catabolism identified? Matrix Biol. 2019;78-79:139–46.
39. McGary CT, et al. Degradation and intracellular accumulation of a residualizing hyaluronan derivative by liver endothelial cells. Hepatology. 1993;18(6):1465–76.
40. McGary CT, Raja RH, Weigel PH. Endocytosis of hyaluronic acid by rat liver endothelial cells. Evidence for receptor recycling. Biochem J. 1989;257(3):875–84.
41. Zhou B, et al. Purification and subunit characterization of the rat liver endocytic hyaluronan receptor. J Biol Chem. 1999;274(48):33831–4.
42. Fraser JR, Appelgren LE, Laurent TC. Tissue uptake of circulating hyaluronic acid. A whole body autoradiographic study. Cell Tissue Res. 1983;233(2):285–93.
43. Fraser JR, et al. Plasma clearance, tissue distribution and metabolism of hyaluronic acid injected intravenously in the rabbit. Biochem J. 1981;200(2):415–24.
44. Day TD. The permeability of interstitial connective tissue and the nature of the interfibrillary substance. J Physiol. 1952;117(1):1–8.
45. Craig AS, Eikenberry EF, Parry DA. Ultrastructural organization of skin: classification on the basis of mechanical role. Connect Tissue Res. 1987;16(3):213–23.
46. Verzijl N, et al. Effect of collagen turnover on the accumulation of advanced glycation end products. J Biol Chem. 2000;275(50):39027–31.
47. Laurent UB, Dahl LB, Reed RK. Catabolism of hyaluronan in rabbit skin takes place locally, in lymph nodes and liver. Exp Physiol. 1991;76(5):695–703.
48. Fraser JR, Laurent TC. Turnover and metabolism of hyaluronan. Ciba Found Symp. 1989;143:41–53; discussion 53–9, 281–5.
49. Locke RK. Treatment of spastic flatfoot with procaine-hyaluronidase and stretching. J Natl Assoc Chirop. 1952;42(11):36–8.
50. Frost GI, Csoka T, Stern R. The hyaluronidases: a chemical, biological and clinical overview. Trends Glycosci Glycotechnol. 1996;8:419–34.
51. Farr C, et al. Clinical pharmacology and possible applications of hyaluronidase with reference to Hylase "Dessau". Wien Med Wochenschr. 1997;147(15):347–55.
52. Eberhart AH, Weiler CR, Erie JC. Angioedema related to the use of hyaluronidase in cataract surgery. Am J Ophthalmol. 2004;138(1):142–3.
53. Williams RG. The effects of continuous local injection of hyaluronidase on skin and subcutaneous tissue in rats. Anat Rec. 1955;122(3):349–61.
54. Lin Y, et al. A hyaluronidase activity of the sperm plasma membrane protein PH-20 enables sperm to penetrate the cumulus cell layer surrounding the egg. J Cell Biol. 1994;125(5):1157–63.
55. Bookbinder LH, et al. A recombinant human enzyme for enhanced interstitial transport of therapeutics. J Control Release. 2006;114(2):230–41.
56. Kang DW, et al. Recombinant human hyaluronidase PH20 (rHuPH20) facilitates subcutaneous infusions of large volumes of immunoglobulin in a swine model. Drug Deliv Transl Res. 2012;2(4):254–64.
57. Sharma DSC, Lahiri MA. Use of hyaluronidase in plastic surgery: a review. J Plast Reconstr Aesthet Surg. 2021;74(7):1610–4.

58. Searle T, Ali FR, Al-Niaimi F. Hyaluronidase in dermatology: uses beyond hyaluronic acid fillers. J Drugs Dermatol. 2020;19(10):993–8.
59. Helm Ii S, Racz G. Hyaluronidase in neuroplasty: a review. Pain Physician. 2019;22(6):555–60.
60. Dunn AL, et al. Hyaluronidase: a review of approved formulations, indications and off-label use in chronic pain management. Expert Opin Biol Ther. 2010;10(1):127–31.
61. Bailey SH, Fagien S, Rohrich RJ. Changing role of hyaluronidase in plastic surgery. Plast Reconstr Surg. 2014;133(2):127e–32e.
62. Seifter J. Studies on the pharmacology and toxicology of testicular hyaluronidase. Ann N Y Acad Sci. 1950;52(7):1141–55.
63. Mayer NH. New treatment approaches on the horizon for spastic hemiparesis. PM R. 2018;10(9 Suppl 2):S144–50.
64. Raghavan P. Emerging therapies for spastic movement disorders. Phys Med Rehabil Clin N Am. 2018;29(3):633–44.
65. Keenan KE, et al. Prediction of glycosaminoglycan content in human cartilage by age, T1rho and T2 MRI. Osteoarthr Cartil. 2011;19(2):171–9.
66. Mlynarik V, et al. Transverse relaxation mechanisms in articular cartilage. J Magn Reson. 2004;169(2):300–7.
67. Wang L, Regatte RR. T(1)rho MRI of human musculoskeletal system. J Magn Reson Imaging. 2015;41(3):586–600.
68. Sharafi A, Chang G, Regatte RR. Bi-component T1rho and T2 relaxation mapping of skeletal muscle in-vivo. Sci Rep. 2017;7(1):14115.
69. Peng XG, et al. Noninvasive assessment of age, gender, and exercise effects on skeletal muscle: initial experience with T1 rho MRI of calf muscle. J Magn Reson Imaging. 2017;46(1):61–70.
70. Paul CPL, et al. Quantitative MRI in early intervertebral disc degeneration: T1rho correlates better than T2 and ADC with biomechanics, histology and matrix content. PLoS One. 2018;13(1):e0191442.
71. Samartzis D, et al. Novel diagnostic and prognostic methods for disc degeneration and low back pain. Spine J. 2015;15(9):1919–32.
72. Sepponen RE, et al. A method for T1 rho imaging. J Comput Assist Tomogr. 1985;9(6):1007–11.
73. Gilani IA, Sepponen R. Quantitative rotating frame relaxometry methods in MRI. NMR Biomed. 2016;29(6):841–61.
74. Menon RG, Raghavan P, Regatte RR. Quantifying muscle glycosaminoglycan levels in patients with post-stroke muscle stiffness using T1rho MRI. Sci Rep. 2019;9(1):14513.
75. Menon RG, Raghavan P, Regatte RR. Pilot study quantifying muscle glycosaminoglycan using bi-exponential T1rho mapping in patients with muscle stiffness after stroke. Sci Rep. 2021;11(1):13951.
76. Pillen S, van Alfen N. Skeletal muscle ultrasound. Neurol Res. 2011;33(10):1016–24.
77. Correa-de-Araujo R, et al. The need for standardized assessment of muscle quality in skeletal muscle function deficit and other aging-related muscle dysfunctions: a symposium report. Front Physiol. 2017;8:87.
78. Iftekharuddin KM, Awwal AAS. Field guide to image processing. SPIE field guides. Bellingham, WA: SPIE Press; 2012.
79. Pillen S, et al. Skeletal muscle ultrasound: correlation between fibrous tissue and echo intensity. Ultrasound Med Biol. 2009;35(3):443–6.
80. Nijboer-Oosterveld J, Van Alfen N, Pillen S. New normal values for quantitative muscle ultrasound: obesity increases muscle echo intensity. Muscle Nerve. 2011;43(1):142–3.
81. Reimers K, et al. Skeletal muscle sonography: a correlative study of echogenicity and morphology. J Ultrasound Med. 1993;12(2):73–7.
82. Heckmatt JZ, Leeman S, Dubowitz V. Ultrasound imaging in the diagnosis of muscle disease. J Pediatr. 1982;101(5):656–60.
83. Kenis-Coskun O, et al. Reliability of quantitative ultrasound measurement of flexor digitorum superficialis and profundus muscles in stroke. J Comp Eff Res. 2020;9(18):1293–300.

84. Picelli A, et al. Ultrasonographic evaluation of botulinum toxin injection site for the medial approach to tibialis posterior muscle in chronic stroke patients with spastic equinovarus foot: an observational study. Toxins (Basel). 2017;9(11).
85. Hara T, et al. Effects of botulinum toxin A therapy and multidisciplinary rehabilitation on lower limb spasticity classified by spastic muscle echo intensity in post-stroke patients. Int J Neurosci. 2018;128(5):412–20.
86. Picelli A, et al. Is spastic muscle echo intensity related to the response to botulinum toxin type A in patients with stroke? A cohort study. Arch Phys Med Rehabil. 2012;93(7):1253–8.
87. Sikdar S, et al. Assessment of myofascial trigger points (MTrPs): a new application of ultrasound imaging and vibration sonoelastography. Annu Int Conf IEEE Eng Med Biol Soc. 2008;2008:5585–8.
88. Ozcakar L, et al. Ultrasound imaging for sarcopenia, spasticity and painful muscle syndromes. Curr Opin Support Palliat Care. 2018;12(3):373–81.
89. Brandenburg JE, et al. Quantifying passive muscle stiffness in children with and without cerebral palsy using ultrasound shear wave elastography. Dev Med Child Neurol. 2016;58(12):1288–94.
90. Jakubowski KL, et al. Passive material properties of stroke-impaired plantarflexor and dorsiflexor muscles. Clin Biomech (Bristol, Avon). 2017;49:48–55.
91. Brandenburg JE, et al. Quantifying effect of onabotulinum toxin a on passive muscle stiffness in children with cerebral palsy using ultrasound shear wave elastography. Am J Phys Med Rehabil. 2018;97(7):500–6.
92. Vigotsky AD, Rouse EJ, Lee SSM. Mapping the relationships between joint stiffness, modeled muscle stiffness, and shear wave velocity. J Appl Physiol (1985). 2020;129(3):483–91.
93. Boulard C, Gautheron V, Lapole T. Mechanical properties of ankle joint and gastrocnemius muscle in spastic children with unilateral cerebral palsy measured with shear wave elastography. J Biomech. 2021;124:110502.
94. Zuniga LDO, Lopez CAG, Gonzalez ER. Ultrasound elastography in the assessment of the stiffness of spastic muscles: a systematic review. Ultrasound Med Biol. 2021;47(6):1448–64.
95. Tran A, Gao J. Quantitative ultrasound to assess skeletal muscles in post stroke spasticity. J Cent Nerv Syst Dis. 2021;13:1179573521996141.
96. Lehoux MC, et al. Shear wave elastography potential to characterize spastic muscles in stroke survivors: literature review. Clin Biomech (Bristol, Avon). 2020;72:84–93.
97. Leonard CT, et al. Myotonometer intra- and interrater reliabilities. Arch Phys Med Rehabil. 2003;84(6):928–32.
98. Chuang LL, et al. Quantitative mechanical properties of the relaxed biceps and triceps brachii muscles in patients with subacute stroke: a reliability study of the myoton-3 myometer. Stroke Res Treat. 2012;2012:617694.
99. Li X, et al. Assessing muscle compliance in stroke with the Myotonometer. Clin Biomech (Bristol, Avon). 2017;50:110–3.
100. Chuang LL, Wu CY, Lin KC. Reliability, validity, and responsiveness of myotonometric measurement of muscle tone, elasticity, and stiffness in patients with stroke. Arch Phys Med Rehabil. 2012;93(3):532–40.
101. Chuang LL, et al. Relative and absolute reliabilities of the myotonometric measurements of hemiparetic arms in patients with stroke. Arch Phys Med Rehabil. 2013;94(3):459–66.
102. Aarrestad DD, et al. Intra- and interrater reliabilities of the Myotonometer when assessing the spastic condition of children with cerebral palsy. J Child Neurol. 2004;19(11):894–901.
103. Rydahl SJ, Brouwer BJ. Ankle stiffness and tissue compliance in stroke survivors: a validation of Myotonometer measurements. Arch Phys Med Rehabil. 2004;85(10):1631–7.
104. Lee Y, Kim M, Lee H. The measurement of stiffness for major muscles with shear wave elastography and myoton: a quantitative analysis study. Diagnostics (Basel). 2021;11(3).
105. Stecco A, et al. Stiffness and echogenicity: development of a stiffness-echogenicity matrix for clinical problem solving. Eur J Transl Myol. 2019;29(3):8476.
106. Hechter O. Studies on spreading factors: I. The importance of mechanical factors in hyaluronidase action in skin. J Exp Med. 1947;85(1):77–97.

Emerging Non-Pharmacologic Treatments 14

Manuel F. Mas, Gerard E. Francisco, and Sheng Li

Scientific knowledge is a body of statements of varying degrees of certainty – some most unsure, some nearly sure, none absolutely certain.
—Richard Feynman, The Value of Science, 1955.

- There are many potentially promising emerging non-pharmacologic treatments available for spasticity. These include peripheral electrical stimulation at the level of the skin (transcutaneous electrical nerve stimulation, TENS) and muscle (neuromuscular electrical stimulation, NMES; functional electrical stimulation, FES; breathing-controlled electrical stimulation, BreEStim), spinal cord stimulation (SCS), transcranial direct current stimulation (tDCS), transcranial magnetic stimulation (TMS), acupuncture, whole body vibration, and extracorporeal shock wave therapy.
- These treatments have been studied mostly in patients with stroke, spinal cord injury, multiple sclerosis, and cerebral palsy.

M. F. Mas
University of Puerto Rico, School of Medicine, Department of Physical Medicine, Rehabilitation and Sports Medicine, San Juan, PR, USA

McGovern Medical School, The University of Texas Health Science Center at Houston, Department of Physical Medicine and Rehabilitation, Houston, TX, USA

TIRR Memorial Hermann Hospital, Houston, TX, USA

G. E. Francisco · S. Li (✉)
McGovern Medical School, The University of Texas Health Science Center at Houston, Department of Physical Medicine and Rehabilitation, Houston, TX, USA

TIRR Memorial Hermann Hospital, Houston, TX, USA
e-mail: Sheng.Li@uth.tmc.edu

P. Raghavan (ed.), *Spasticity and Muscle Stiffness*,
https://doi.org/10.1007/978-3-030-96900-4_14

- However, the details regarding their mechanisms of action, treatment parameters such as the intensity, duration, and site of stimulation, and efficacy in combination with other modalities still need to be worked out. Both mechanistic parameter finding studies and larger randomized controlled clinical studies using precise measurements of the components of spastic paresis are needed to better define the role of these emerging treatments.
- At present, none of these treatments can be readily recommended as standard of care to reduce spasticity. However, due to their low side effect profile, they may be reasonable adjuncts to other more established modalities in clinical care.

Introduction

Spasticity is one of the most physically debilitating conditions that interferes with functional improvement [1]. It occurs in up to 43% of individuals with a stroke [2], in 66% of those with multiple sclerosis (MS) [3], in 70% of children with cerebral palsy (CP) [3], and in close to 80% of those with spinal cord injury (SCI) [4]. A wide spectrum of non-pharmacologic treatment options exist for the treatment of spastic paresis [5]. Mainstream therapies include physical and occupational therapy (PT and OT, for range of motion, stretching, strengthening, balance and coordination training, and functional training) and physical modalities (e.g., splinting and casting, Kinesio Taping®). These therapies are used across the various phases of rehabilitation (see also Chap. 8). Conventional spasticity management usually refers to both pharmacologic and rehabilitative treatments [6], although rehabilitation can encompass a broad range of therapy options. However, despite this, the treatment of spasticity remains challenging for both clinicians and patients.

The quest to better serve patients has led to the emergence of many new treatments. Of these, neuromodulation using both peripheral and central electrical stimulation and central magnetic stimulation has robust data available for review. This chapter focuses primarily on electrical and magnetic stimulation in four populations that commonly present with spastic paresis: stroke, SCI, MS and CP. Other less studied therapies are also explored. Evidence for each modality and diagnostic group is synthesized from the published literature. It is important to note that the focus of this review is on spasticity, although some of these treatments may be beneficial for motor performance.

Peripheral Electrical Stimulation

The use of electrical stimulation (ES) to produce movement was recognized in experiments performed as early as 1790 by Luigi Galvani and 1831 by Michael Faraday [7, 8]. ES has been used for a vast range of applications using varying stimulation parameters, number of channels, sites of stimulation, and types of stimulation [9]. Although the intricacies of ES are beyond the scope of this chapter, we review the key parameters. Frequency of ES refers to the number of pulses produced per second during stimulation and is stated in hertz (Hz). The frequency used in most clinical regimens is 20–50 Hz [10, 11]. The ramp time is the time duration from turning on the stimulation to reaching the desired frequency and can be adjusted to the patient's comfort level. Pulse width or duration refers to the time span of a single pulse of ES and is commonly expressed in microseconds. The intensity or amplitude of the current is usually reported in milliamperes (mA), with higher intensities eliciting stronger depolarizing effects on structures underlying the electrodes [7]. The ES current is delivered using electrodes placed on the patient's skin. The larger the surface of the electrode, the greater the volume of the underlying tissue that will be activated, whereas smaller electrodes deliver a more focused current. Optimal electrode placement is still an area of debate – some clinicians prefer placing them over the muscle belly, whereas others prefer placing them over the motor point. Rehabilitation therapists usually place the electrodes over the muscle belly [7].

The most common types of ES include neuromuscular electrical stimulation (NEMS), transcutaneous electrical nerve stimulation (TENS), and functional electrical stimulation (FES). NMES employs an electrical current of sufficient intensity to elicit muscle contraction. It is typically provided at higher frequencies such as 20–50 Hz and is often simply referred to as ES. FES applies stimulation to a set of muscles involved in a task to facilitate a functional activity; here the timing of stimulation of the various muscles is important [12]. TENS consists of the application of low-intensity continuous electrical current to the cutaneous nerve fibers with no apparent muscular stimulation [13]. Each of these types of ES has been studied for the treatment of spasticity in various patient populations. However, the mechanisms underlying the use of ES in spasticity management remain unclear.

Stroke

Table 14.1 summarizes the evidence on the use of ES for spasticity after a stroke. Hesse et al. performed a randomized, placebo-controlled study to evaluate the effects of ES in combination with botulinum toxin (BoNT) on chronic upper limb spasticity. Patients who were treated with a combination of BoNT and ES showed greater facilitation of hand hygiene (cleaning the palm) when compared to the groups receiving the toxin or placebo without ES [14]. The authors propose that ES of the neuromuscular unit may enhance the rate of uptake and the latency of onset of BoNT. In a study comparing PT using inhibitory Bobath techniques for ankle plantar flexor spasticity, with and without ES to the ankle dorsiflexors in 40 patients, the combined treatment significantly increased passive ankle joint dorsiflexion and muscle strength while significantly decreasing ankle plantar flexor spasticity [15]. In an innovative application of FES with a leg-cycling wheelchair, hemiplegic subjects with higher muscle tone showed significantly reduced leg spasticity with FES when compared to those who performed leg-cycling without FES or used a manual wheelchair [16]. Similarly, treatment for 12 weeks with a combination of conventional therapy and FES to the peroneal nerve and anterior tibial muscle in stroke survivors with foot drop led to a significant reduction in plantar flexor spasticity when compared with conventional therapy alone [17]. However, ES to tibialis anterior and soleus muscles in combination with a passive locomotion-like stretching regimen did not lead to a difference in the Modified Ashworth Scale (MAS) score compared to those treated without ES [18]. In a large randomized controlled trial of 90 acute stroke patients treated with 30-minute sessions of NMES to the wrist and

Table 14.1 Summary of evidence for electrical stimulation modalities for spasticity management in patients with stroke

Author, year	Design	Patients	Intervention	Outcome	Results
Hesse et al. 1998 [14]	Randomized, controlled, double-blind	$N = 24$ (6/grp) Chronic stroke with upper extremity spasticity	Grp A: BoNT + ES Grp B: BoNT only to 6 muscles Grp C: Placebo + ES Grp D: Placebo BoNT = 1000 units ES parameters: 30 min for 3 sessions/day × 3 days	MAS, ADLs at 2, 6, and 12 weeks	BoNT + ES resulted in most tone reduction, particularly at the elbow and wrist joints No difference in tone across elbow, wrist, and finger joints Better hand hygiene in group with BoNT + ES
Bakhtiary & Fatemy 2008 [15]	Randomized, controlled	$N = 40$ Chronic stroke with plantar flexor spasticity	Grp A: ES + PT: 20 min ES to DF + PT daily × 20 sessions Grp B: PT only	MAS, ROM	Greater reduction in PF spasticity in the combined group Greater increase in ROM of ankle joint No difference in H-reflex
Lo et al. 2009 [16]	Pre-Post	$N = 17$ Stroke with lower extremity spasticity	Grp A: FES-assisted leg cycling wheelchair Grp B: Leg cycling wheelchair Grp C: Manual wheelchair	MAS, H/M ratio and relaxation index	MAS and H/M ratio significantly decreased in both leg cycling groups, but decreased more in the FES-assisted leg cycling group in those with higher muscle tone
Sabut et al. 2011 [17]	Randomized, controlled	$N = 51$ Chronic stroke with foot drop	Grp A: FES + PT: 20–30 min FES to peroneal nerve Grp B: PT only 1 hour/day, 5 days/week, × 12weeks	MAS for PF spasticity ROM	Significant decrease in spasticity, 38.3% in FES + PT and 21.2% in PT only groups DF strength increased by 56.6% in FES + PT and 27.7% in PT only groups
Yamaguchi et al. 2012 [18]	Randomized, controlled	$N = 27$ Subacute stroke	Grp A: ES + passive stretching Grp B: ES only Grp C: Stretching only	Gait speed, MAS NOTE: Only immediate effects of ES tested	No significant difference in MAS or change in MAS among three groups Gait velocity increased in all 3 groups

Malhotra et al. 2013 [19]	Randomized, controlled	$N = 90$ 1–6 weeks post stroke	Grp A: NMES (30 min) to wrist/ finger extensors + OT Grp B: OT only	MAS, pain, contractures	No significant effect on spasticity and some effect on stiffness Reduced pain
Cho et al. 2013 [20]	Randomized, controlled	$N = 42$ Chronic stroke	Grp A: TENS to gastrocnemius for 60 min + PT Grp B: Placebo + PT	MAS, balance	Significant reduction in gastrocnemius spasticity after TENS Improved balance with TENS Returned to baseline in 1 day
Karakoyun et al. 2015 [21]	Controlled	$N = 27$ chronic stroke $N = 24$ healthy	30 min single session TENS to lower extremity	MAS Walking speed H/M ratio	Significant decrease in spasticity Increase in walking speed Lower M wave amplitude Higher H/M ratio
Laddha et al. 2016 [22]	Randomized, controlled	$N = 30$ Stroke with PF spasticity	Grp A: Exercise Grp B: TENS 30 min + Exercise Grp C: TENS 60 min + Exercise 5 sessions/week × 6 weeks	MAS PF Ankle ROM Clonus at baseline, 3 weeks, and 6 weeks Timed Up and Go test	Decrease in PF spasticity and clonus greater in the TENS groups No significant difference between the two TENS groups Increase in walking speed in all groups

Grp group, *BoNT* botulinum toxin, *ES* electrical stimulation, *min* minute, *MAS* Modified Ashworth Scale, *ADL* activities of daily living, *PT* physical therapy, *DF* dorsiflexor, *ROM* range of motion, *PF* plantar flexor, *H/M ratio* H-reflex/M-wave ratio, *FES* functional electrical stimulation, *NMES* neuromuscular electrical stimulation, *OT* occupational therapy, *TENS* transcutaneous electrical nerve stimulation finger extensors followed by physiotherapy, there was no significant change in objective measurement of spasticity when compared to those who were treated with physiotherapy alone, although pain was better controlled [19]. The rate of recovery in passive range of motion was however significantly better in the treatment arm in both the nonfunctional and functional groups over 36 weeks. Taken together, these studies suggest that ES of the muscle with NMES and FES can reduce spasticity in combination with active therapy, but not with a passive stretching regimen in patients with chronic stroke, and it can enhance the recovery of passive range of motion in acute stroke patients. These effects may be due to the enhancement of muscle function in combination with movement therapy rather than due to a direct effect on spasticity.

On the other hand, TENS appears to have a transient effect on spasticity. In a placebo-controlled study, chronic stroke patients had significant reduction of ankle plantar flexor spasticity and improved balance after one trial of TENS to the gastrocnemius muscle [20]. Similar findings were observed after a 30-minute trial of TENS to the tibialis anterior muscle with significant decrease in lower extremity spasticity and improved walking speed [21]. These benefits returned to baseline within one day of treatment, however. In another study, TENS was applied over the common peroneal nerve of stroke patients to evaluate its effects on ankle plantar flexor spasticity. TENS treatment produced significant reduction of ankle plantar flexor spasticity when compared to the therapy group. However, in another study there was no difference in spasticity when comparing 30- and 60-minute sessions of TENS over a period of 6 weeks [22]. Recent systematic reviews on TENS for spasticity following stroke support its repeated use as an adjunct therapy to reduce spasticity in spastic paretic plantar flexors [23, 24]. In contrast to the transient effect of TENS, a novel ES modality, breathing-controlled electrical stimulation (BreEStim), appears to have a longer-term effect on poststroke spasticity. BreEStim applies ES to finger extensors in a coupled manner during the voluntary inspiratory phase of breathing. After a single 30-minute treatment session, spasticity in the finger flexors reduced significantly, and the reduction lasted for at least 4 weeks [25].

The studies reviewed above suggest that ES is a promising tool to decrease upper and lower extremity spasticity in stroke survivors, although there has been a greater focus on lower extremity spasticity. There is, however, no consensus on the specific type of ES technique to be used, whether muscles or nerves are to be stimulated, or the length of treatment. There is also a reliance on the use of the MAS in most studies, which may not be the most objective assessment tool for spasticity [26, 27] (also see Chap. 3). Questions also remain about the duration of improvement after the treatment period has ended. Yet, ES can be considered a safe adjunct to enhance the effect of PT and OT in the treatment of spastic movement disorder.

Spinal Cord Injury

In contrast to the stroke population, ES has been more commonly utilized in conjunction with functional training in SCI (Table 14.2). Bajd et al. performed one of the first studies evaluating the effects of ES on spasticity following SCI. TENS was applied to dermatomes belonging to the same spinal cord level as the spastic muscles in six patients. There was a noticeable decrease in spasticity in three of the six patients on the pendulum test to assess spasticity in the knee extensors [28]. In subsequent studies,

Table 14.2 Summary of evidence for electrical stimulation modalities for spasticity management in patients with spinal cord injury

Author, year	Design	Patients	Intervention	Outcome	Results
Bajd et al. 1985 [28]	Pre-Post pilot	$N = 6$	TENS to the dermatome of spastic muscles	Pendulum test for knee extensors	Noticeable decrease in spasticity in 3 subjects No change in other 3 subjects
Robinson et al. 1988 [29]	Pre-Post (short-term use)	$N = 12$	ES induced quadriceps exercise re-conditioning protocol 20 min ×2/day	Normalized relaxation index from pendulum test	Significant decrease in spasticity after ES No carryover 24 hours later
Robinson et al. 1988 [30]	Pre-Post (long-term use)	$N = 31$	ES induced quadriceps exercise re-conditioning protocol 20 min ×2/day, 6 day/week, ×8 weeks	Normalized relaxation index from pendulum test	For most, spasticity increased after 4 weeks, but decreased after 8 weeks Benefit evident in incomplete quadriplegics
Skold et al. 2002 [31]	Controlled	$N = 15$ Motor complete SCI	Grp A: FES cycling ×3/week, ×6 months Grp B: Control	MAS EMG Resistive torque Self-rating	No change in leg muscle spasticity Leg muscle volume increased by 10% at end of 6 months of FES cycling
Ralston et al. 2013 [32]	Randomized, crossover	$N = 14$ Motor complete SCI	Treatment: FES cycling ×4/week, ×2 weeks One week washout period Control/sham	Urine output MAS	No significant effect of FES cycling on LE spasticity, urine output, or LE swelling, though results were favorable
Reichenfelser et al. 2012 [33]	Pre-Post	$N = 23$ Incomplete SCI	Treatment: FES cycling 20 min/session, ×18 sessions	Passive resistance Power output	Increase in power output Significant decrease in spasticity

(continued)

Table 14.2 (continued)

Author, year	Design	Patients	Intervention	Outcome	Results
Carty et al. 2013 [34]	Pre-Post	*N* = 14 T4-T11 SCI, average 10 years postinjury	Treatment: NMES to quadriceps/hamstring muscles, ×8 weeks	Spinal cord assessment tool for spastic reflexes	Significant increase in LE lean mass Reduction in spasticity
Kuhn et al. 2014 [35]	Pre-Post	*N* = 30 Chronic SCI	Treatment: 20 min FES cycling program 2 days/week 4 weeks	Muscle cross-section Muscle/Leg circumference Spasticity Walking ability	Spasticity decreased in multiple muscle groups Increase in muscle cross-section and circumference
Ping Ho Chung & Kam Kwan Cheng 2010 [36]	Randomized, controlled	*N* = 18 SCI with LE spasticity	Grp A: 60 min TENS to common peroneal nerve. Grp B: Sham Single session study	Composite spasticity score	Significant reduction in spasticity by 29.5% in TENS group Reduction in ankle clonus by 29.6% in TENS group
Oo 2014 [37]	Randomized, controlled	*N* = 16 Subacute SCI with spasticity	Treatment group: 60 min TENS over bilateral common peroneal nerves + 30 min PT Control group: 30 min PT 15 sessions	Composite spasticity score	Significant decrease in spasticity in treatment group
Sivaramakrishnan et al. 2017 [38]	Double-blind, randomized, crossover	*N* = 10 SCI with LE spasticity	TENS or FES (30 min) in a crossover manner separated by 24 hours	MAS Spinal cord assessment tool for spastic reflexes	No difference between TENS/FES. Significant reduction in spasticity for 1–4 hours with both modalities

TENS transcutaneous electrical nerve stimulation, *ES* electrical stimulation, *min* minute, *Grp* group, *FES* functional electrical stimulation, *MAS* Modified Ashworth Scale, *EMG* electromyography, *LE* lower extremity, *SCI* spinal cord injury, *NMES* neuromuscular electrical stimulation, *PT* physical therapy which also measured spasticity using the pendulum test, 20 minutes of cyclic ES significantly decreased spasticity in 12 SCI patients [29]. The same group also studied the long-term effects of ES using an extension of the same protocol for 8 weeks – they noted an increase in spasticity in the paralyzed quadriceps muscles after 4 weeks of ES, but a reduction in spasticity after 8 weeks especially in the incomplete quadriplegics [30].

Interestingly, spasticity was found to be unchanged in motor complete quadriplegic SCI patients after 6 months of FES combined with cycling, although lower extremity muscle mass increased by 10% [31]. These results were corroborated by a more recent study of FES cycling in a 4-week randomized crossover trial in patients with recent motor complete SCI patients. There was no significant change in spasticity [32]. On the other hand, incomplete SCI patients who performed FES cycling for 18 sessions had increased power output and a significant decrease in spasticity [33]. In a mixed group of SCI patients, 8 weeks of NMES to the quadriceps and hamstring muscles showed a significant reduction in spasticity using the spinal cord assessment tool for spastic reflexes, but results on other measures were mixed. There was however a significant increase in lean body mass [34]. The effect of FES cycling was again studied in a mixed group of SCI patients during a four-week period, two days each week, and showed improvement in spasticity as well as increase in muscle mass [35]. Taken together, these studies suggest that muscle ES in SCI can reduce spasticity by augmenting active use of the muscle in those individuals who can still activate their muscles (incomplete quadriplegics), but not in those who cannot activate their muscles (complete quadriplegics). However, it can increase muscle mass even in those who have complete injury.

The use of TENS in a placebo-controlled, randomized controlled trial in SCI patients over the common peroneal nerve for 60 minutes led to an immediate significant increase in passive range of motion of ankle dorsiflexion and decrease in ankle clonus and spasticity [36]. A more recent study of TENS applied to bilateral common peroneal nerves for 30 minutes during a three-week course in combination with PT showed both immediate (within session) and long-term (across session) decreases in spasticity as measured by a composite spasticity score [37]. In a study comparing the effects of TENS and FES on hip adductors and knee extensors in a group of mostly incomplete SCI patients, both muscle and cutaneous ES modalities had similar effects on immediate spasticity that lasted for at least 4 hours post treatment [38].

The studies above show that individuals with SCI can benefit from ES for the reduction of spasticity, especially when it is combined with functional activities and especially in patients with incomplete SCI. In addition, muscle ES leads to the increase in muscle strength and volume in treated muscles. Yet, spasticity was not equally assessed in all studies, and different ES techniques were utilized. The only study comparing muscle and cutaneous ES modalities (FES vs. TENS) showed that both lead to an immediate reduction in spasticity. These results suggest that the use of FES and TENS can both be used as adjuncts to PT.

Multiple Sclerosis

When compared to stroke and SCI populations, ES has been studied much less in patients with MS, and the studies have used cutaneous rather than muscle stimulation (Table 14.3). TENS applied to the spastic plantar flexor muscles for 20 minutes per day for 4 weeks led to a statistically significant reduction in spasticity as assessed by myoelectric activity on electromyography and the MAS. This did not translate into improved ambulation however [39]. In another study, patients with MS used TENS over spastic muscles for either 60 minutes or 8 hours a day for 2 weeks. Spasticity, as measured by the global spasticity score, did not differ between the two groups. However, there was a greater reduction in spasms with 8 hours of TENS a day [40]. More recently, lower extremity spasticity was assessed after self-applied TENS versus oral baclofen. After 4 weeks, spasticity decreased in both groups, but the TENS group showed a statistically significant decrease in the MAS score [41]. These studies demonstrate that TENS is helpful in the reduction of spasticity and spasms in patients with MS and may potentially be used instead of oral medications which may exacerbate fatigue in this population.

Cerebral Palsy

As in MS, ES has not been studied extensively in the CP population, and it has primarily been used for wrist and finger spasticity in this population. Scheker et al. designed a therapeutic regimen using NMES and dynamic bracing to reduce upper extremity spasticity in children with CP. The regimen consisted of two 30-minute sessions of NMES

Table 14.3 Summary of evidence for electrical stimulation modalities for spasticity management in patients with multiple sclerosis

Author, year	Design	Patients	Intervention	Outcome	Results
Armutlu et al. 2003 [39]	Pre-Post	$N = 10$	TENS ×20 min/day, ×4 weeks	MAS of ankle plantar flexors Ambulation index	Significant reduction in spasticity No change in ambulation index
Miller et al. 2007 [40]	Randomized, single-blind, crossover	$N = 32$	TENS: 60 min/day vs. 8 hours/day ×2 weeks	Global spasticity score (GSS) Penn spasm score (PSS) VAS for pain	No difference in GSS between the two groups Significant reduction in spasms and pain in the 8 hour group
Shaygannejad et al. 2013 [41]	Randomized, controlled	$N = 52$	TENS ×20 min/day ×4 weeks	MAS of LE muscles pre-post	Significant reduction in spasticity of both extremities

TENS transcutaneous electrical nerve stimulation, *min* minute, *MAS* Modified Ashworth Scale, *VAS* Visual Analog Scale, *LE* lower extremity of the antagonist wrist and finger extensors combined with dynamic orthotic traction during the day and a static brace at night. Treatment ranged from 3 to 43 months and showed reduction in spasticity of the wrist and fingers on the Zancolli classification and a marked improvement in upper extremity function [42]. A subsequent randomized controlled trial using the same regimen showed that the combination of NMES and dynamic bracing significantly improved spasticity and upper extremity function after 6 months of treatment, compared to either intervention alone, and the effects lasted for two months following the end of the treatment [43]. A more recent randomized controlled trial showed that NMES in combination with conventional therapy and orthoses was more effective in reducing wrist and finger flexor spasticity and improving hand function in unilateral spastic CP than conventional therapy alone [44] (Table 14.4). These studies suggest that NMES in conjunction with bracing and conventional therapy can reduce upper extremity spasticity and improve hand function in patients with CP.

In summary, the effects of ES on spasticity have been studied in several patient populations. Patients with chronic poststroke spasticity may benefit from TENS for immediate relief of spasticity as an adjunct to PT or OT, or from FES for plantar flexor spasticity. FES seems to be beneficial for lower extremity spasticity specifically for patients with incomplete SCI. TENS can be particularly useful to reduce spasticity in patients with MS and may be preferable to drug therapy in patients with fatigue. NMES in combination with bracing and conventional therapy decreases upper extremity spasticity and improves function in patients with CP. ES appears to work best in combination with conventional therapy and functional activities. There is still much to be understood about the therapeutic parameters of ES including type of stimulation, stimulation intensity, treatment length, and how it may best be combined with other treatments.

Spinal Cord Stimulation

Spinal cord stimulation (SCS) consists of inserting a percutaneous or surgical paddle lead containing multiple stimulating electrodes typically into the epidural space [45]. These leads are connected to a pulse generator containing a battery and programmable components. Implantation requires a surgical procedure. Stimulation parameters and location of the electrodes vary. SCS has emerged as a standard of care treatment for chronic neuropathic pain [46]. In the United States, it is routinely used for failed back surgery syndrome and complex regional pain syndrome [47]. Yet, it remains a controversial treatment for severe spasticity [45]. A retrospective study of the possible long-term efficacy of epidural SCS for spasticity was conducted on 17 patients. Only 1 out of the 17 SCI patients with an epidural spinal cord stimulator reported symptomatic spasticity relief. The authors concluded that the epidural spinal cord stimulator lacks long-term efficacy for the relief of spasticity and pain and is not cost-effective [48]. In a subsequent retrospective study of 71 patients with CP or SCI who received SCS, a decrease in muscle tone was observed in all patients with spinal spasticity, but only in patients with spastic lower limb paraparesis of cerebral origin. There was no change in patients with tetraplegia. However, in 11% of patients, the therapy could be

Table 14.4 Summary of evidence for electrical stimulation modalities for spasticity management in patients with cerebral palsy

Author, year	Design	Patients	Intervention	Outcome	Results
Scheker et al. 1999 [42]	Pre-Post	*N* = 19 Spastic CP	30 min NMES to finger extensors ×2/day, for 3–43 months	Zancolli classification	Moved up 1–3 levels on the Zancolli Improvement in UE function
Ozer et al. 2006 [43]	Randomized, controlled, blinded assessment	*N* = 24 Spastic hemiplegic CP	Grp 1: NMES alone, 30 min ×2/day Grp 2: 30 min bracing, ×2/day Grp 3: Combined NMES and bracing ×6 months Monthly follow-up for 3 months	Zancolli classification Melbourne assessment Grip strength	Only the combined group showed significant improvement in all 3 measures Improvement lasted for 2 months following end of treatment
Yildizgoren et al. 2014 [44]	Randomized, controlled	*N* = 24 Spastic hemiplegic CP	Treatment: 30 min/day ES to wrist extensors ×5days/week, ×6weeks + Conventional exercises Control: Conventional exercises	Zancolli classification Manual Ability classification Abilhand-Kids test	Significant increase in active wrist extension and decrease in spasticity in wrist flexors at fourth and sixth week in treatment group Significant decrease in spasticity in wrist flexors at sixth week in control group

CP cerebral palsy, *min* minute, *NMES* neuromuscular electrical stimulation, *UE* upper extremity, *Grp* group, *ES* electrical stimulation discontinued after several years of treatment, suggesting that chronic stimulation could perhaps permanently mitigate spasticity in a select group of patients [49]. Epidural SCS led to a significant reduction in spasms in SCI patients followed for 24 months postimplantation, who were refractory to other treatments [50]. No studies are available for analysis of the effects of SCS in patients with stroke or MS.

Taken together, there is limited evidence documenting the efficacy of SCS to decrease spasticity in patients with spastic paraparesis from SCI and CP, although some accounts appear promising. Clinicians and patients must take into account the high cost of this treatment [48]. However, improvements in stimulator technology and details on the ideal location of the electrodes and stimulation parameters warrant revisiting this treatment modality in future studies.

Transcranial Direct Current Stimulation

Transcranial direct current stimulation (tDCS) is a noninvasive technique that can induce sustained changes in excitability in the brain [51]. It can modulate spontaneous neuronal firing rates, as well as synaptic and non-synaptic plasticity [52]. The components of tDCS are a constant current stimulator and surface electrodes. Current stimulators generally have a voltage setting from 0 to 4 mA and can supply up to 80 mA per minute per session. For motor cortical stimulation, the stimulating electrode is usually placed over the motor cortex, and the reference electrode is placed over the contralateral supraorbital ridge (Fig. 14.1). Current intensities vary between 1 and 2 mA and are commonly applied for 10–20 minutes. Stimulation can be either anodal or cathodal. Anodal stimulation increases cortical excitability while cathodal stimulation decreases it [51].

Stroke

Most of the studies on tDCS have been conducted in the stroke population (Table 14.5). In a study by Qu et al., patients with upper limb spasticity after a stroke were randomized to a treatment group that received tDCS and PT or a control group that received PT only. Cathodal tDCS was applied to the primary sensorimotor cortex of the affected side. After one month, the treatment group that received tDCS showed a significant reduction in spasticity, which was not noted in the control group [53]. In another study, dual tDCS (anode over the affected motor cortex (M1) and cathode over contralateral M1) was compared with cathodal tDCS (cathode over contralateral M1) in patients with chronic poststroke upper extremity spasticity in a crossover, double-blind study. Although both tDCS paradigms decreased spasticity, cathodal tDCS had a larger effect on spasticity supported by changes in H-reflex modulation (decreased amplitude and increased latency) [54]. tDCS has also been studied in combination with motor and sensory training. When combined with virtual reality therapy, it significantly reduced wrist spasticity compared with virtual reality and sham tDCS alone [55]. Combined therapy using tDCS and robot-assisted arm training (AT) in patients with upper limb

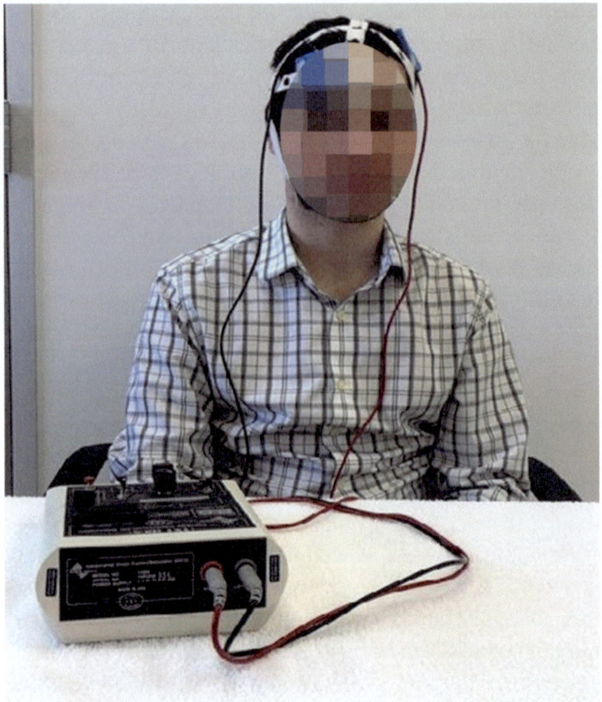

Fig. 14.1 Common setup for transcranial direct current stimulation

impairment due to chronic stroke was tested in a randomized, double-blind, crossover study of anodal tDCS on the affected hemisphere (tDCS(a) + AT) and cathodal tDCS on the unaffected hemisphere (tDCS(c) + AT). Interestingly, cathodal tDCS was more effective than anodal tDCS in reducing distal upper limb spasticity for right, but not left, hemispheric lesions when combined with robotic therapy [56]. In contrast, in a sham-controlled trial, chronic stroke patients exposed to tDCS with sensory modulation and passive movements on the paretic hand had limited immediate improvement of spasticity and no long-term effects [57].

Taken together, these studies suggest that tDCS may be a useful adjunct to active therapies in reducing spasticity. A systematic review performed in 2016 concluded that there is moderate-to-low quality evidence for no effect of tDCS in improving spasticity immediately after the intervention in poststroke patients [58]. As with other modalities, there are still many variables to study including timing and length of treatment, anodal versus cathodal stimulation, and area and side of stimulation.

Cerebral Palsy

The literature is sparse on the use of tDCS for CP. In 2014, Aree-uea et al. performed a sham-controlled trial to investigate the anti-spasticity effects of anodal tDCS in individuals with spastic CP. The left primary motor cortex was targeted for five consecutive

Table 14.5 Transcranial direct current stimulation for spasticity management in patients with stroke

Author, year	Design	Patients	Intervention	Outcome	Results
Qu et al. 2009 [53]	Randomized, controlled	$N = 50$ Stroke with UE spasticity	Treatment: Ipsilesional tDCS + PT Control: PT only	MAS UE FMA Barthel Index	Significant improvement in all measures for treatment group Only significant improvement on FMA in control group
Del Felice et al. 2016 [54]	Crossover, double-blind	$N = 10$ Stroke with UE spasticity	Dual tDCS vs. cathodal tDCS One tDCS treatment followed by the other tDCS treatment after 3 months 20 min for 5 days	MAS Postural Assessment Scale Bhakta finger flexion scale	Cathodal tDCS was superior in reducing spasticity
Viana et al. 2014 [55]	Double-blind, randomized, controlled	$N = 20$ Stroke with UE impairment	Treatment: tDCS + Virtual reality therapy Control: Sham tDCS + Virtual reality therapy	MAS UE FMA Wolf Motor Function Test	Significant difference in improvement in wrist spasticity in tDCS group
Ochi et al. 2013 [56]	Double-blind, randomized crossover	$N = 18$ Chronic stroke with moderate-to-severe arm paresis	Treatments: Anotal tDCS + Robotic AT Cathodal tDCS + Robotic AT 1 mA of tDCS during the first 10 min of AT for 5 days	MAS UE FMA Motor Activity Log	Distal spasticity was significantly improved with cathodal tDCS + Robotic AT for right hemispheric lesions, but not for left hemispheric lesions
Koh et al. 2017 [57]	Double-blind, randomized, controlled	$N = 25$ Chronic stroke	Grp1: Bilateral tDCS + sensory modulation + passive movements Grp2: Sham tDCS + passive movements	UE FMA MAS Action Research Arm Test Barthel Index	No significant difference between groups Trend for improvement in spasticity and function in tDCS group

UE upper extremity, *tDCS* transcranial direct current stimulation, *PT* physical therapy, *MAS* Modified Ashworth Scale, *FMA* Fugl-Meyer Assessment, *AT* arm training, *min* minute, *Grp* group days. Children who were exposed to tDCS had significantly greater reduction in spasticity on the MAS after treatment that persisted in some joints for 48 hours, but not in passive range of motion [59]. Studies are currently being performed to better understand the benefits of tDCS for spasticity in individuals with CP [60].

Multiple Sclerosis

The literature on the use of tDCS for spasticity due to MS is also sparse. One randomized, sham-controlled study of anodal tDCS to the primary motor cortex of the more affected side for 5 days did not show a significant improvement in spasticity, and the findings were no different in patients with MS who received the sham treatment [61]. Thus, the only available study exploring the use of tDCS for MS did not support its efficacy.

In summary, although there is a larger body of evidence evaluating the use of tDCS to decrease spasticity in the stroke population, its application and benefits are uncertain. Other conditions have scant research. However, cathodal tDCS appears to enhance the effect of active therapy and may have a secondary effect on spasticity.

Repetitive Transcranial Magnetic Stimulation

Repetitive transcranial magnetic stimulation (rTMS) is a noninvasive, transcranial intervention that generates a strong magnetic field to a specific area of the cerebral cortex by way of an electrical coil [62]. The coil is usually shaped like the number eight and is placed over the scalp of the patient (Fig. 14.2). This coil is connected to a pulse generator or stimulator, that delivers a changing electric current to the coil. A magnetic field is produced via electromagnetic induction which penetrates the skull noninvasively and subsequently causes electrical current to stimulate the cortex under the coil. Pulses are delivered at a set frequency and intensity to change cortical excitability, thus modulating brain function [63]. Different frequencies can either inhibit or excite the stimulated area [64]. Generally, 5–10 Hz is considered an excitatory frequency while less than 1 Hz is an inhibitory frequency for rTMS. The goal of interventions with rTMS is to re-establish interhemispheric balance by exciting the injured hemisphere and inhibiting the contralesional one [65].

Stroke

Several studies have evaluated the use of rTMS for poststroke spasticity (Table 14.6). In a study of chronic, hemiparetic patients with unchanged paresis for more than 5 years, movement was evoked in the paretic arm using a single pulse of TMS, and rTMS at 1 Hz was applied to either one or both hemispheres. Interestingly, spasticity could be modified by stimulation of either the ipsilesional or the contralesional hemisphere [66]. However, stimulation of the contralesional hemisphere using 1 Hz rTMS

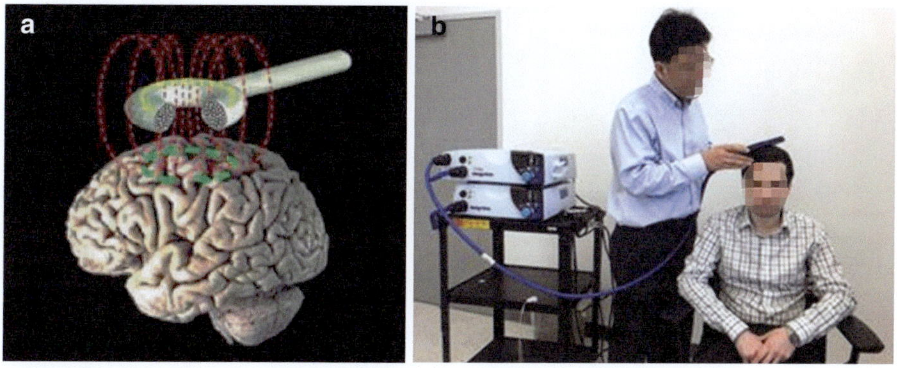

Fig. 14.2 Illustration of transcranial magnetic stimulation (TMS) mechanisms and setup. (**a**) Repetitive transcranial magnetic stimulation (rTMS) coil and stimulation area underneath. (**b**) Common setup for TMS

has been used more commonly. Kakuda et al. performed a series of uncontrolled studies that applied 1 Hz rTMS to the contralesional hemisphere followed by OT. Initial results showed improvement in hand function and decrease in spasticity on the MAS in some upper limb flexors after a 15-day treatment protocol [67]. A follow-up study in a separate cohort showed that MAS scores were significantly decreased in the finger and wrist flexors both immediately after the 15-day protocol and 4 weeks later. Hand function was improved as well [68]. This protocol combined with daily administration of 100 mg of levodopa was also found to be effective in improving paretic arm motor function right after treatment in five patients. However, spasticity barely changed [69]. The same group also explored the changes in motor neuron excitability as measured by F-wave parameters and found that the 15-day rTMS/OT protocol produced significant reduction in motor neuron excitability [70]. Although all these studies stimulated the contralesional hemisphere at 1 Hz, they did not have a control group, and the sample sizes were low, making it difficult to know if it was the rTMS or the OT that led to reduction in spasticity.

In a randomized double-blind crossover study, rTMS at 1 Hz was applied to the contralesional motor cortex of patients with chronic hemiplegic stroke combined with repetitive facilitation exercises for two weeks versus two weeks of sham rTMS only. Although motor function improved significantly during the rTMS motor facilitation protocol compared to the sham sessions, spasticity did not significantly change during either of them [71]. However, another randomized controlled study tested the effect of rTMS at 1 Hz to the contralesional primary motor cortex combined with PT for ten sessions compared to sham rTMS and PT and found a significant decrease in upper limb spasticity in chronic stroke patients with rTMS which was not observed in the control group [72]. However, these two studies had a low sample size, and the results are still inconclusive on the effect of rTMS versus therapy on spasticity. Nevertheless, rTMS can potentially be used as an adjunct to therapy.

In another study, rTMS and OT were combined with botulinum toxin injections (BoNT) to the paretic arm to evaluate spasticity and motor function; BoNT was injected

Table 14.6 Repetitive transcranial magnetic stimulation for spasticity management in patients with stroke

Author, year	Design	Patients	Intervention	Outcome	Results
Mally & Dinya 2008 [66]	Pre-Post	$N = 64$ Chronic stroke with unchanged paresis for more than 5 years	1 Hz rTMS directed to area that evoked movement in paretic arm 4 Groups based on rTMS stimulation areas Twice a day/1 week	MAS	Reduction in spasticity by stimulation of either hemisphere Movement induction only by stimulation of intact motor pathway
Kakuda et al. 2010 [67]	Pre-Post	$N = 15$ Chronic stroke with UE spasticity	1 Hz rTMS to contralesional hemisphere + OT 22 sessions in 15 days	MAS UE FMA Wolf Motor Function Test	Some decrease in spasticity in 12 patients Function increased in all patients
Kakuda et al. 2011 (a) [68]	Pre-Post	$N = 39$ Chronic stroke with UE spasticity	1 Hz rTMS to contralesional hemisphere + OT 22 sessions in 15 days	MAS UE FMA Wolf Motor Function Test	Significant decrease in finger/wrist flexor spasticity at discharge and 4 weeks after treatment
Kakuda et al. 2011 (b) [69]	Pre-Post	$N = 5$ Chronic stroke with UE spasticity	1 Hz rTMS to contralesional hemisphere + OT + daily levodopa rTMS for 40 min daily	MAS UE FMA Wolf Motor Function Test	No significant difference in spasticity
Kondo et al. 2015 [70]	Pre-Post	$N = 10$ Poststroke with UE spastic hemiparesis	Low frequency rTMS (1 session, 40 min) + OT per day for 15 days	F-wave parameters MAS UE FMA	Significant decrease in spasticity No change in F-wave frequency
Etoh et al. 2013 [71]	Randomized, double-blind, crossover	$N = 18$ Stroke with UE hemiplegia	Grp1: 1 Hz rTMS + OT Grp2: Sham rTMS 2 weeks for each rTMS treatment	MAS UE FMA Action Research Arm Test Simple hand function testing	No significant change in spasticity Improvement in motor function only during motor rTMS sessions
Barros Galvao et al. 2014 [72]	Randomized, sham-controlled	$N = 20$ Poststroke UE spasticity	Treatment: 1 Hz rTMS to contralesional hemisphere (10 sessions, 3 days/week) + PT Control: Sham rTMS + PT 4 week follow-up	MAS FIM Range of Motion UE FMA	Significant reduction in spasticity in the treatment group

Kakuda et al. 2012 [73]	Pre-Post	$N = 14$ Chronic stroke with UE spasticity	1 Hz rTMS to contralesional hemisphere + OT + BoNT 22 rTMS sessions in 15 days, 60 min per session	MAS UE FMA Wolf Motor Function Test Motor Activity Log	Improvement in spasticity in all muscles tested Improvement in function
Yamada et al. 2014 [74]	Retrospective, controlled	$N = 80$ Poststroke with spastic hemiparesis	Grp1: BoNT followed by 1 Hz rTMS to contralesional hemisphere (12 sessions/40 min each) + OT Grp2: 1 Hz rTMS to contralesional hemisphere (12 sessions/40 min each) + OT 15 day course	MAS UE FMA Wolf Motor Function Test	Significant improvement in spasticity and function in both groups BoNT group had significant decrease in finger flexor spasticity compared to the no BoNT group
Rastgoo et al. 2016 [75]	Randomized, sham-controlled	$N = 20$ Poststroke with LE spasticity	Treatment: rTMS to contralesional hemisphere, 5 daily sessions Control: Sham rTMS	MAS H-reflex LE FMA Timed Up and Go Test	Improvement in spasticity with active rTMS
Naghdi et al. [76]	Pre-Post	$N = 7$ Poststroke with LE spasticity	1 Hz TMS, 20 min to contralesional hemisphere 5 sessions	MAS	Improvement in ankle plantar flexor spasticity
Terreaux et al. [77]	Prospective, randomized, double-blind, crossover	$N = 5$ Spastic hemiparesis	1 Hz rTMS 10 Hz rTMS Placebo	MAS	No change in placebo or 10 Hz treatment Spasticity reduction did not reach statistical significance in 1 Hz rTMS group
Yamada et al. 2013 [78]	Pre-Post	$N = 8$ Poststroke with UE hemiparesis	Bihemispheric rTMS (10 sessions/40 min per session) + OT 15-day course	MAS UE Fugl-Meyer Wolf Motor Function Test Motor	Decrease in wrist, elbow, and finger spasticity Improvement in function

rTMS repetitive transcranial magnetic stimulation, *MAS* Modified Ashworth Scale, *UE* upper extremity, *OT* occupational therapy, *FMA* Fugl-Meyer Assessment, *min* minute, *Grp* group, *PT* physical therapy, *FIM* functional independence measure, *BoNT* botulinum toxin, *LE* lower extremity

4 weeks prior to the rTMS/OT protocol. After treatment, patients showed improved MAS scores across all examined muscle groups at discharge and 4 weeks following rTMS/OT. However these results were obtained within the therapeutic window of BoNT injections [73]. The same group of investigators also performed a retrospective controlled study on 80 patients, of whom 42 received rTMS/OT following BoNT injections, whereas 38 received rTMS/OT alone. Both groups showed significant improvement in spasticity, but the addition of BoNT resulted in better improvement of spasticity in the injected muscles [74]. Here again, it is difficult to tease out the effect of rTMS versus therapy and toxin injections.

Lower extremity spasticity in chronic stroke patients has also been assessed after treatment with 1 Hz rTMS directed at the contralesional lower extremity motor area in a randomized sham-controlled crossover trial with one-week follow-up. After five consecutive daily sessions, spasticity reduced by 1 point on the MAS in the rTMS group and was not observed in the sham rTMS group. There was no change in the H/M ratio or function however [75]. Lower extremity spasticity also improved after five consecutive 1 Hz rTMS sessions of 20 minutes as measured by the MAS in a separate small uncontrolled study [76]. As in the upper limb studies, there is little evidence of significant efficacy of rTMS on spasticity in the lower limb, although its use as an adjunct may be acceptable.

Two studies explored the use of high- and low-frequency rTMS treatments. A randomized, double-blind, crossover study tested the effect of rTMS at 1 Hz and 10 Hz frequencies on the premotor cortex against placebo for improvement of lower extremity spasticity in five patients with spastic hemiparesis. There was no significant improvement in the MAS scores at either frequency. However, 1 Hz rTMS did reduce reflex excitability and stiffness in ankle plantar flexors and led to changes in quantitative gait analysis [77]. In another study, bihemispheric rTMS using both 1 Hz and 10 Hz stimulations were combined with intensive OT and significantly decreased spasticity on the MAS at the elbow, wrist, and finger flexors of the upper limb in eight patients with poststroke hemiparesis. However, there was no control group [78]. Thus although there have been a number of studies performed with low-frequency rTMS to the contralesional cortex, a recent systematic review on the use of rTMS for poststroke spasticity concluded that there is limited evidence available to support its use in improving spasticity due to low sample sizes, inadequate duration of treatment, and lack of control arms [79].

Spinal Cord Injury

Compared to stroke, rTMS has not been studied as much in patients with SCI (Table 14.7). In a randomized, double-blind, sham-controlled study, subjects with incomplete cervical or thoracic SCI received 10 daily sessions of real or sham intermittent theta-burst stimulation (iTBS), which is a safe, noninvasive excitatory rTMS protocol that applies short bursts of stimulation at high frequencies. Patients who received real iTBS had significant reduction of the H/M ratio and reduction in spasticity as

Table 14.7 Repetitive transcranial magnetic stimulation for spasticity management in patients with spinal cord injury

Author, year	Design	Patients	Intervention	Outcome	Results
Nardone et al. 2017 [80]	Randomized, double-blind, crossover, sham-controlled	$N = 10$ Incomplete cervical or thoracic SCI	Active vs. Sham intermittent theta burst stimulation	MEP amplitude MAS SCI Assessment Tool for spasticity Neurophysiological parameters	Reduction in spasticity with active stimulation Changes persisted for 1 week
Nardone et al. 2014 [81]	Randomized, double-blind, crossover, sham-controlled	$N = 9$ Incomplete cervical or thoracic SCI	Active vs. Sham rTMS to contralesional hemisphere 5 daily sessions	Reciprocal inhibition MAS SCI Assessment Tool for spasticity	Active rTMS reduced LE spasticity
Kumru et al. 2010 [82]	Sham-controlled	$N = 15$ Incomplete SCI	Active vs. Sham high-frequency rTMS 5 daily sessions	MAS VAS SCI Spasticity Evaluation Tool	Improvement in spasticity with active rTMS only Improvement lasted for at least 1 week

SCI spinal cord injury, *MEP* motor evoked potential, *MAS* Modified Ashworth Scale, *rTMS* Repetitive transcranial magnetic stimulation, *LE* lower extremity, *VAS* Visual Analog Scale measured by the MAS which persisted for one week. This was not observed in the sham group [80]. The same group of investigators found that rTMS to the contralesional motor area also significantly reduced lower extremity spasticity in SCI patients after five daily sessions, which again was not noted in the sham rTMS group [81]. In yet another study, high-frequency rTMS directed to the leg motor area for five daily sessions significantly reduced lower limb spasticity in incomplete SCI patients. These improvements lasted for one week and were not seen in the sham rTMS group [82]. Compared to the stroke population, rTMS studies in SCI use high-frequency stimulation, which was shown to decrease lower extremity spasticity. As with other modalities, details regarding frequency and location to direct rTMS need to be better studied.

Multiple Sclerosis

There are very few studies evaluating rTMS for spasticity due to MS. In 2016, high-frequency (10 Hz) rTMS was compared with iTBS in reducing spasticity in 22 patients with secondary progressive MS who were pseudorandomized into the two groups. Stimulation was directed at the primary motor area of both legs. After ten sessions, both groups showed significant improvement in spasticity as measured by the MAS, and there were no differences between the groups [83]. In another study in patients with relapsing-remitting MS, a single session of 1 Hz rTMS over the primary motor cortex of the leg increased the H/M ratio in the soleus muscle, whereas 5 Hz rTMS decreased the H/M ratio in the soleus muscle and increased corticospinal excitability. However, the results lasted less than 10 minutes. Clinical improvement in lower limb spasticity was achieved with 5 Hz rTMS over a two-week protocol which was not seen with sham rTMS [84]. There is thus currently little evidence to conclusively support the use of rTMS for spasticity in patients with MS [85]. As in the SCI population, the studies focus more on high-frequency rTMS in MS.

Cerebral Palsy

Only one study has used rTMS for spasticity in patients with CP. In 2016, excitatory rTMS of 5 Hz and 10 Hz was applied over the primary motor cortex in 20 patients with spastic CP. The treatment lasted for 15 minutes daily followed by standard therapy for 1 hour for 20 days. Patients experienced a significant decrease in spasticity as measured by the MAS following rTMS compared with the control group which received only standard therapy [86].

In summary, the evidence to support the use of rTMS to reduce spasticity is limited. Studies in the stroke population used mostly low-frequency rTMS, whereas the SCI, MS, and CP patient populations responded better to high-frequency stimulation. Few studies used physiological measurements to determine the stimulation parameters, and most of the studies combined the intervention with therapy making it difficult to tease out the effects of rTMS alone. More mechanistic research is warranted if rTMS is to be used in the treatment of spasticity, especially because the treatment is more involved and expensive than ES and tDCS protocols.

Other Emerging Treatments

Several additional treatments have emerged for spasticity. Whole body vibration may be beneficial in reducing spasticity in patients with CP [87], stroke [88], and SCI [89–91]. However, the evidence is limited. Acupuncture has been shown to significantly reduce spasticity poststroke [92–95]. Most studies focus on either needle or electroacupuncture. A recent systematic review of 22 studies concluded that electroacupuncture combined with routine care has the potential to reduce poststroke spasticity [96]. Laser acupuncture has shown a beneficial effect in reducing spasticity in CP when combined with physiotherapy [97]. Acupuncture can be beneficial in reducing spasticity in patients with MS, although more rigorous studies are needed [98]. Since various acupuncture protocols have been studied, there is not a clear consensus as to the most effective protocol for spasticity reduction for the various diagnoses. Extracorporeal shock wave therapy (ESWT) may be effective in reducing spasticity following stroke [99] and CP [100–102]. As for other electrical and magnetic stimulation modalities, the details of the underlying mechanisms and the most effective parameters are yet to be worked out.

Conclusion

Although many potentially promising treatments for spasticity have been studied, the details need further study. These include the underlying mechanisms, ideal intensity and sites of stimulation, most effective length of treatment, best time to use them, and the benefits of combining them with other treatments. However, the same can be said of several of the more conventional treatments. Spasticity has been frequently used as a catch-all term for positive symptoms in patients with central nervous system injury, but it is almost always accompanied by the negative symptoms of weakness. Indeed, many of the modalities discussed in this chapter such as electrical and magnetic stimulation may stimulate rather than inhibit the spastic muscle, having a greater effect on the negative symptoms. In addition, the measures used to assess spasticity have been imprecise in most of the studies. More rigorous studies can pave the way to fine-tune the treatments and augment the clinician's toolset. Other factors that should be considered when choosing from these treatments include cost, coverage by insurance, and expertise in their use. Although none of the discussed modalities can be recommended as the gold standard at this time, their low side effect profile and available evidence make them reasonable adjuncts to conventional treatment modalities and warrant further study to gain a place among standard treatments.

References

1. Wissel J, Manack A, Brainin M. Toward an epidemiology of poststroke spasticity. Neurology. 2013;80(3 Suppl 2):S13–9.
2. Kong KH, Lee J, Chua KS. Occurrence and temporal evolution of upper limb spasticity in stroke patients admitted to a rehabilitation unit. Arch Phys Med Rehabil. 2012;93(1):143–8.
3. Martin A, Abogunrin S, Kurth H, Dinet J. Epidemiological, humanistic, and economic burden of illness of lower limb spasticity in adults: a systematic review. Neuropsychiatr Dis Treat. 2014;10:111–22.
4. Haisma JA, van der Woude LH, Stam HJ, Bergen MP, Sluis TA, Post MW, et al. Complications following spinal cord injury: occurrence and risk factors in a longitudinal study during and after inpatient rehabilitation. J Rehabil Med. 2007;39(5):393–8.
5. Mayer NH, Esquenazi A. Muscle overactivity and movement dysfunction in the upper motoneuron syndrome. Phys Med Rehabil Clin N Am. 2003;14(4):855–83, vii–viii.
6. Khan F, Amatya B, Bensmail D, Yelnik A. Non-pharmacological interventions for spasticity in adults: an overview of systematic reviews. Ann Phys Rehabil Med. 2017;16.
7. Doucet BM, Lam A, Griffin L. Neuromuscular electrical stimulation for skeletal muscle function. Yale J Biol Med. 2012;85(2):201–15.
8. Cambridge NA. Electrical apparatus used in medicine before 1900. Proc R Soc Med. 1977;70(9):635–41.
9. Intiso D, Santamato A, Di Rienzo F. Effect of electrical stimulation as an adjunct to botulinum toxin type A in the treatment of adult spasticity: a systematic review. Disabil Rehabil. 2017;39(21):2123–33.
10. Baker LL, Bowman BR, McNeal DR. Effects of waveform on comfort during neuromuscular electrical stimulation. Clin Orthop Relat Res. 1988;233:75–85.
11. de Kroon J, IJzerman M, Chae J, Lankhorst G, Zilvold G. Relation between stimulation characteristics and clinical outcome in studies using electrical stimulation to improve motor control of the upper extremity in stroke. J Rehabil Med. 2005;37(2):65–74.
12. Maffiuletti NA, Gondin J, Place N, Stevens-Lapsley J, Vivodtzev I, Minetto MA. Clinical use of neuromuscular electrical stimulation for neuromuscular rehabilitation: what are we overlooking? Arch Phys Med Rehabil. 2018;99(4):806–12.
13. Kerr C, McDowell B, McDonough S. Electrical stimulation in cerebral palsy: a review of effects on strength and motor function. Dev Med Child Neurol. 2004;46(3):205–13.
14. Hesse S, Reiter F, Konrad M, Jahnke MT. Botulinum toxin type A and short-term electrical stimulation in the treatment of upper limb flexor spasticity after stroke: a randomized, double-blind, placebo-controlled trial. Clin Rehabil. 1998;12(5):381–8.
15. Bakhtiary AH, Fatemy E. Does electrical stimulation reduce spasticity after stroke? A randomized controlled study. Clin Rehabil. 2008;22(5):418–25.
16. Lo H, Tsai K, Su F, Chang G, Yeh C. Effects of a functional electrical stimulation-assisted leg-cycling wheelchair on reducing spasticity of patients after stroke. J Rehabil Med. 2009;41(4):242–6.
17. Sabut SK, Sikdar C, Kumar R, Mahadevappa M. Functional electrical stimulation of dorsiflexor muscle: effects on dorsiflexor strength, plantarflexor spasticity, and motor recovery in stroke patients. NeuroRehabilitation. 2011;29(4):393–400.
18. Yamaguchi T, Tanabe S, Muraoka Y, Masakado Y, Kimura A, Tsuji T, et al. Immediate effects of electrical stimulation combined with passive locomotion-like movement on gait velocity and spasticity in persons with hemiparetic stroke: a randomized controlled study. Clin Rehabil. 2012;26(7):619–28.
19. Malhotra S, Rosewilliam S, Hermens H, Roffe C, Jones P, Pandyan AD. A randomized controlled trial of surface neuromuscular electrical stimulation applied early after acute stroke: effects on wrist pain, spasticity and contractures. Clin Rehabil. 2013;27(7):579–90.
20. Cho H, In TS, Cho KH, Song CH. A single trial of transcutaneous electrical nerve stimulation (TENS) improves spasticity and balance in patients with chronic stroke. Tohoku J Exp Med. 2013;229(3):187–93.

21. Karakoyun A, Boyraz İ, Gunduz R, Karamercan A, Ozgirgin N. Electrophysiological and clinical evaluation of the effects of transcutaneous electrical nerve stimulation on the spasticity in the hemiplegic stroke patients. J Phys Ther Sci. 2015;27(11):3407–11.
22. Laddha D, Ganesh GS, Pattnaik M, Mohanty P, Mishra C. Effect of transcutaneous electrical nerve stimulation on plantar flexor muscle spasticity and walking speed in stroke patients. Physiother Res Int. 2016;21(4):247–56.
23. Kwong PW, Ng GY, Chung RC, Ng SS. Transcutaneous electrical nerve stimulation improves walking capacity and reduces spasticity in stroke survivors: a systematic review and meta-analysis. Clin Rehabil. 2017;13:26921551774534.
24. Lin S, Sun Q, Wang H, Xie G. Influence of transcutaneous electrical nerve stimulation on spasticity, balance, and walking speed in stroke patients: a systematic review and meta-analysis. J Rehabil Med. 2018;50(1):3–7.
25. Li S, Rymer WZ. Voluntary breathing influences corticospinal excitability of nonrespiratory finger muscles. J Neurophysiol. 2011;105(2):512–21.
26. Gómez-Soriano J, Cano-de-la-Cuerda R, Muñoz-Hellin E, Ortiz-Gutiérrez R, Taylor JS. [Evaluation and quantification of spasticity: a review of the clinical, biomechanical and neurophysiological methods]. Rev Neurol. 2012;55(4):217–26.
27. Banky M, Ryan HK, Clark R, Olver J, Williams G. Do clinical tests of spasticity accurately reflect muscle function during walking: a systematic review. Brain Inj. 2017;31(4):440–55.
28. Bajd T, Gregoric M, Vodovnik L, Benko H. Electrical stimulation in treating spasticity resulting from spinal cord injury. Arch Phys Med Rehabil. 1985;66(8):515–7.
29. Robinson CJ, Kett NA, Bolam JM. Spasticity in spinal cord injured patients: 1. Short-term effects of surface electrical stimulation. Arch Phys Med Rehabil. 1988;69(8):598–604.
30. Robinson CJ, Kett NA, Bolam JM. Spasticity in spinal cord injured patients: 2. Initial measures and long-term effects of surface electrical stimulation. Arch Phys Med Rehabil. 1988;69(10):862–8.
31. Sköld C, Lönn L, Harms-Ringdahl K, Hultling C, Levi R, Nash M, et al. Effects of functional electrical stimulation training for six months on body composition and spasticity in motor complete tetraplegic spinal cord-injured individuals. J Rehabil Med. 2002;34(1):25–32.
32. Ralston KE, Harvey L, Batty J, Bonsan LB, Ben M, Cusmiani R, et al. Functional electrical stimulation cycling has no clear effect on urine output, lower limb swelling, and spasticity in people with spinal cord injury: a randomised cross-over trial. J Physiother. 2013;59(4):237–43.
33. Reichenfelser W, Hackl H, Hufgard J, Kastner J, Gstaltner K, Gföhler M. Monitoring of spasticity and functional ability in individuals with incomplete spinal cord injury with a functional electrical stimulation cycling system. J Rehabil Med. 2012;44(5):444–9.
34. Carty A, McCormack K, Coughlan GF, Crowe L, Caulfield B. Alterations in body composition and spasticity following subtetanic neuromuscular electrical stimulation training in spinal cord injury. J Rehabil Res Dev. 2013;50(2):193–202.
35. Kuhn D, Leichtfried V, Schobersberger W. Four weeks of functional electrical stimulated cycling after spinal cord injury: a clinical cohort study. Int J Rehabil Res. 2014;37(3):243–50.
36. Ping Ho Chung B, Kam Kwan Cheng B. Immediate effect of transcutaneous electrical nerve stimulation on spasticity in patients with spinal cord injury. Clin Rehabil. 2010;24(3):202–10.
37. Oo WM. Efficacy of addition of transcutaneous electrical nerve stimulation to standardized physical therapy in subacute spinal spasticity: a randomized controlled trial. Arch Phys Med Rehabil. 2014;95(11):2013–20.
38. Sivaramakrishnan A, Solomon JM, Manikandan N. Comparison of transcutaneous electrical nerve stimulation (TENS) and functional electrical stimulation (FES) for spasticity in spinal cord injury – A pilot randomized cross-over trial. J Spinal Cord Med. 2017;25:1–15.
39. Armutlu K, Meriç A, Kirdi N, Yakut E, Karabudak R. The effect of transcutaneous electrical nerve stimulation on spasticity in multiple sclerosis patients: a pilot study. Neurorehabil Neural Repair. 2003;17(2):79–82.
40. Miller L, Mattison P, Paul L, Wood L. The effects of transcutaneous electrical nerve stimulation (TENS) on spasticity in multiple sclerosis. Mult Scler. 2007;13(4):527–33.

41. Shaygannejad V, Janghorbani M, Vaezi A, Haghighi S, Golabchi K, Heshmatipour M. Comparison of the effect of baclofen and transcutaneous electrical nerve stimulation for the treatment of spasticity in multiple sclerosis. Neurol Res. 2013;35(6):636–41.
42. Scheker LR, Chesher SP, Ramirez S. Neuromuscular electrical stimulation and dynamic bracing as a treatment for upper-extremity spasticity in children with cerebral palsy. J Hand Surg Am. 1999;24(2):226–32.
43. Ozer K, Chesher SP, Scheker LR. Neuromuscular electrical stimulation and dynamic bracing for the management of upper-extremity spasticity in children with cerebral palsy. Dev Med Child Neurol. 2006;48(7):559–63.
44. Yıldızgören MT, Nakipoğlu Yüzer GF, Ekiz T, Özgirgin N. Effects of neuromuscular electrical stimulation on the wrist and finger flexor spasticity and hand functions in cerebral palsy. Pediatr Neurol. 2014;51(3):360–4.
45. Thiriez C, Gurruchaga J-M, Goujon C, Fénelon G, Palfi S. Spinal stimulation for movement disorders. Neurotherapeutics. 2014;11(3):543–52.
46. Shealy CN, Mortimer JT, Reswick JB. Electrical inhibition of pain by stimulation of the dorsal columns: preliminary clinical report. Anesth Anal. 1967;46(4):489–91.
47. Nagel SJ, Wilson S, Johnson MD, Machado A, Frizon L, Chardon MK, et al. Spinal cord stimulation for spasticity: historical approaches, current status, and future directions. Neuromodulation. 2017;20(4):307–21. https://doi.org/10.1111/ner.12591. Epub 2017 Apr 2. PMID: 28370802.
48. Midha M, Schmitt JK. Epidural spinal cord stimulation for the control of spasticity in spinal cord injury patients lacks long-term efficacy and is not cost-effective. Spinal Cord. 1998;36(3): 190–2.
49. Dekopov AV, Shabalov VA, Tomsky AA, Hit MV, Salova EM. Chronic spinal cord stimulation in the treatment of cerebral and spinal spasticity. Stereotact Funct Neurosurg. 2015;93(2):133–9.
50. Barolat G, Singh-Sahni K, Staas WE, Shatin D, Ketcik B, Allen K. Epidural spinal cord stimulation in the management of spasms in spinal cord injury: a prospective study. Stereotact Funct Neurosurg. 1995;64(3):153–64.
51. Stagg CJ, Nitsche MA. Physiological basis of transcranial direct current stimulation. Neurosci. 2011;17(1):37–53.
52. Nitsche MA, Fricke K, Henschke U, Schlitterlau A, Liebetanz D, Lang N, et al. Pharmacological modulation of cortical excitability shifts induced by transcranial direct current stimulation in humans. J Physiol. 2003;553(Pt 1):293–301.
53. Qu YP, Wu DY, Tu XQ, Qian L, Bin YY, Geng H. Effect of transcranial direct current stimulation on relieving upper-limb spasticity after stroke. Chinese J Cerebrovasc Dis. 2009;6(11):586–9.
54. Del Felice A, Daloli V, Masiero S, Manganotti P. Contralesional cathodal versus dual transcranial direct current stimulation for decreasing upper limb spasticity in chronic stroke individuals: a clinical and neurophysiological study. J Stroke Cerebrovasc Dis. 2016;25(12):2932–41.
55. Viana RT, Laurentino GEC, Souza RJP, Fonseca JB, Silva Filho EM, Dias SN, et al. Effects of the addition of transcranial direct current stimulation to virtual reality therapy after stroke: a pilot randomized controlled trial. NeuroRehabilitation. 2014;34(3):437–46.
56. Ochi M, Saeki S, Oda T, Matsushima Y, Hachisuka K. Effects of anodal and cathodal transcranial direct current stimulation combined with robotic therapy on severely affected arms in chronic stroke patients. J Rehabil Med. 2013;45(2):137–40.
57. Koh C-L, Lin J-H, Jeng J-S, Huang S-L, Hsieh C-L. Effects of transcranial direct current stimulation with sensory modulation on stroke motor rehabilitation: a randomized controlled trial. Arch Phys Med Rehabil. 2017;98(12):2477–84.
58. Elsner B, Kugler J, Pohl M, Mehrholz J. Transcranial direct current stimulation for improving spasticity after stroke: a systematic review with meta-analysis. J Rehabil Med. 2016;48(7):565–70.
59. Aree-uea B, Auvichayapat N, Janyacharoen T, Siritaratiwat W, Amatachaya A, Prasertnoo J, et al. Reduction of spasticity in cerebral palsy by anodal transcranial direct current stimulation. J Med Assoc Thail. 2014;97(9):954–62.

60. Moura RCF, Santos CA, Grecco LAC, Lazzari RD, Dumont AJL, Duarte NC de A, et al. Transcranial direct current stimulation combined with upper limb functional training in children with spastic, hemiparetic cerebral palsy: study protocol for a randomized controlled trial. Trials. 2016;17(1):405.
61. Iodice R, Dubbioso R, Ruggiero L, Santoro L, Manganelli F. Anodal transcranial direct current stimulation of motor cortex does not ameliorate spasticity in multiple sclerosis. Restor Neurol Neurosci. 2015;33(4):487–92.
62. Talelli P, Rothwell J. Does brain stimulation after stroke have a future? Curr Opin Neurol. 2006;19(6):543–50.
63. Corti M, Patten C, Triggs W. Repetitive transcranial magnetic stimulation of motor cortex after stroke: a focused review. Am J Phys Med Rehabil. 2012;91(3):254–70.
64. Kobayashi M, Pascual-Leone A. Transcranial magnetic stimulation in neurology. Lancet Neurol. 2003;2(3):145–56.
65. Hoyer EH, Celnik PA. Understanding and enhancing motor recovery after stroke using transcranial magnetic stimulation. Restor Neurol Neurosci. 2011;29(6):395–409.
66. Mályy J, Dinya E. Recovery of motor disability and spasticity in post-stroke after repetitive transcranial magnetic stimulation (rTMS). Brain Res Bull. 2008;76(4):388–95.
67. Kakuda W, Abo M, Kobayashi K, Momosaki R, Yokoi A, Fukuda A, et al. Low-frequency repetitive transcranial magnetic stimulation and intensive occupational therapy for poststroke patients with upper limb hemiparesis: preliminary study of a 15-day protocol. Int J Rehabil Res. 2010;33(4):339–45.
68. Kakuda W, Abo M, Kobayashi K, Momosaki R, Yokoi A, Fukuda A, et al. Anti-spastic effect of low-frequency rTMS applied with occupational therapy in post-stroke patients with upper limb hemiparesis. Brain Inj. 2011;25(5):496–502.
69. Kakuda W, Abo M, Kobayashi K, Momosaki R, Yokoi A, Fukuda A, et al. Combination treatment of low-frequency rTMS and occupational therapy with levodopa administration: an intensive neurorehabilitative approach for upper limb hemiparesis after stroke. Int J Neurosci. 2011;121(7):373–8.
70. Kondo T, Kakuda W, Yamada N, Shimizu M, Abo M. Effects of repetitive transcranial magnetic stimulation and intensive occupational therapy on motor neuron excitability in poststroke hemiparetic patients: a neurophysiological investigation using F-wave parameters. Int J Neurosci. 2015;125(1):25–31.
71. Etoh S, Noma T, Ikeda K, Jonoshita Y, Ogata A, Matsumoto S, et al. Effects of repetitive trascranial magnetic stimulation on repetitive facilitation exercises of the hemiplegic hand in chronic stroke patients. J Rehabil Med. 2013;45(9):843–7.
72. Barros Galvão SC, Borba Costa dos Santos R, Borba dos Santos P, Cabral ME, Monte-Silva K. Efficacy of coupling repetitive transcranial magnetic stimulation and physical therapy to reduce upper-limb spasticity in patients with stroke: a randomized controlled trial. Arch Phys Med Rehabil. 2014;95(2):222–9.
73. Kakuda W, Abo M, Momosaki R, Yokoi A, Fukuda A, Ito H, et al. Combined therapeutic application of botulinum toxin type A, low-frequency rTMS, and intensive occupational therapy for post-stroke spastic upper limb hemiparesis. Eur J Phys Rehabil Med. 2012;48(1):47–55.
74. Yamada N, Kakuda W, Kondo T, Mitani S, Shimizu M, Abo M. Local muscle injection of botulinum toxin type A synergistically improves the beneficial effects of repetitive transcranial magnetic stimulation and intensive occupational therapy in Post-stroke patients with spastic upper limb hemiparesis. Eur Neurol. 2014;72(5–6):290–8.
75. Rastgoo M, Naghdi S, Nakhostin Ansari N, Olyaei G, Jalaei S, Forogh B, et al. Effects of repetitive transcranial magnetic stimulation on lower extremity spasticity and motor function in stroke patients. Disabil Rehabil. 2016;38(19):1918–26.
76. Naghdi S, Ansari NN, Rastgoo M, Forogh B, Jalaie S, Olyaei G. A pilot study on the effects of low frequency repetitive transcranial magnetic stimulation on lower extremity spasticity and motor neuron excitability in patients after stroke. J Bodyw Mov Ther. 2015;19(4):616–23.

77. Terreaux L, Gross R, Leboeuf F, Desal H, Hamel O, Nguyen JP, et al. Benefits of repetitive transcranial magnetic stimulation (rTMS) for spastic subjects: clinical, functional, and biomechanical parameters for lower limb and walking in five hemiparetic patients. ScientificWorldJournal. 2014;2014:389350.
78. Yamada N, Kakuda W, Kondo T, Shimizu M, Mitani S, Abo M. Bihemispheric repetitive transcranial magnetic stimulation combined with intensive occupational therapy for upper limb hemiparesis after stroke. Int J Rehabil Res. 2013;36(4):323–9.
79. McIntyre A, Mirkowski M, Thompson S, Burhan AM, Miller T, Teasell R. A systematic review and meta-analysis on the use of repetitive transcranial magnetic stimulation for spasticity post-stroke. PM R. 2017;10(3):293–302.
80. Nardone R, Langthaler PB, Orioli A, Höller P, Höller Y, Frey VN, et al. Effects of intermittent theta burst stimulation on spasticity after spinal cord injury. Restor Neurol Neurosci. 2017;35(3):287–94.
81. Nardone R, Höller Y, Thomschewski A, Brigo F, Orioli A, Höller P, et al. rTMS modulates reciprocal inhibition in patients with traumatic spinal cord injury. Spinal Cord. 2014;52(11):831–5.
82. Kumru H, Murillo N, Vidal Samso J, Valls-Sole J, Edwards D, Pelayo R, et al. Reduction of spasticity with repetitive transcranial magnetic stimulation in patients with spinal cord injury. Neurorehabil Neural Repair. 2010;24(5):435–41.
83. Korzhova JE, Chervyakov AV, Poydasheva AG, Kochergin IA, Peresedova AV, Zakharova MN, et al. The application of high-frequency and iTBS transcranial magnetic stimulation for the treatment of spasticity in the patients presenting with secondary progressive multiple sclerosis. Vopr Kurortol Fizioter i Lech Fiz kul'tury. 2016;93(5):8.
84. Centonze D, Koch G, Versace V, Mori F, Rossi S, Brusa L, et al. Repetitive transcranial magnetic stimulation of the motor cortex ameliorates spasticity in multiple sclerosis. Neurology. 2007;68(13):1045–50.
85. Amatya B, Khan F, La Mantia L, Demetrios M, Wade DT. Non pharmacological interventions for spasticity in multiple sclerosis. Cochrane Database Syst Rev. 2013;2:CD009974.
86. Gupta M, Lal Rajak B, Bhatia D, Mukherjee A. Effect of r-TMS over standard therapy in decreasing muscle tone of spastic cerebral palsy patients. J Med Eng Technol. 2016;40(4):210–6.
87. Cheng H-YK JY-Y, Chen C-L, Chuang L-L, Cheng C-H. Effects of whole body vibration on spasticity and lower extremity function in children with cerebral palsy. Hum Mov Sci. 2015;39:65–72.
88. Miyara K, Matsumoto S, Uema T, Hirokawa T, Noma T, Shimodozono M, et al. Feasibility of using whole body vibration as a means for controlling spasticity in post-stroke patients: a pilot study. Complement Ther Clin Pract. 2014;20(1):70–3.
89. Sadeghi M, Sawatzky B. Effects of vibration on spasticity in individuals with spinal cord injury. Am J Phys Med Rehabil. 2014;93(11):995–1007.
90. Ji Q, He H, Zhang C, Lu C, Zheng Y, Tian LX, et al. Effects of whole-body vibration on neuromuscular performance in individuals with spinal cord injury: a systematic review. Clin Rehabil. 2017;31(10):1279–91.
91. Ness LL, Field-Fote EC. Effect of whole-body vibration on quadriceps spasticity in individuals with spastic hypertonia due to spinal cord injury. Restor Neurol Neurosci. 2009;27(6):621–31.
92. Zhao J-G, Cao C-H, Liu C-Z, Han B-J, Zhang J, Li Z-G, et al. Effect of acupuncture treatment on spastic states of stroke patients. J Neurol Sci. 2009;276(1–2):143–7.
93. Hou L, Han S, Gao W, Xu Y, Yang X, Yang W. Aligned acupuncture at muscle regions plus cutaneous needle for upper limb spasticity after stroke: a multicenter randomized controlled trial. J Acupunct Tuina Sci. 20140;12(3):141–5.
94. Zhao W, Wang C, Li Z, Chen L, Li J, Cui W, et al. Efficacy and safety of transcutaneous electrical acupoint stimulation to treat muscle spasticity following brain injury: a double-blinded, multicenter, randomized controlled trial. Sterling M, editor. PLoS One. 2015;10(2):e0116976.
95. Yan T, Hui-Chan CWY. Transcutaneous electrical stimulation on acupuncture points improves muscle function in subjects after acute stroke: a randomized controlled trial. J Rehabil Med. 2009;41(5):312–6.

96. Cai Y, Zhang CS, Liu S, Wen Z, Zhang AL, Guo X, et al. Electroacupuncture for poststroke spasticity: a systematic review and meta-analysis. Arch Phys Med Rehabil. 2017;98(12):2578–2589.e4.
97. Dabbous OA, Mostafa YM, El Noamany HA, El Shennawy SA, El Bagoury MA. Laser acupuncture as an adjunctive therapy for spastic cerebral palsy in children. Lasers Med Sci. 2016;31(6):1061–7.
98. Karpatkin HI, Napolione D, Siminovich-Blok B. Acupuncture and multiple sclerosis: a review of the evidence. Evidence-based complement. Altern Med. 2014;2014:1–9.
99. Guo P, Gao F, Zhao T, Sun W, Wang B, Li Z. Positive effects of extracorporeal shock wave therapy on spasticity in poststroke patients: a meta-analysis. J Stroke Cerebrovasc Dis. 2017;26(11):2470–6.
100. Wang T, Du L, Shan L, Dong H, Feng J, Kiessling MC, et al. A prospective case-control study of radial extracorporeal shock wave therapy for spastic plantar flexor muscles in very young children with cerebral palsy. Medicine (Baltimore). 2016;95(19):e3649.
101. Park D-S, Kwon DR, Park G-Y, Lee MY. Therapeutic effect of extracorporeal shock wave therapy according to treatment session on gastrocnemius muscle spasticity in children with spastic cerebral palsy: a pilot study. Ann Rehabil Med. 2015;39(6):914–21.
102. Mirea A, Onose G, Padure L, Rosulescu E. Extracorporeal shockwave therapy (ESWT) benefits in spastic children with cerebral palsy (CP). J Med Life. 2014;7 Spec No. 3:127–32.

Correction to: Treatment of Focal Muscle Stiffness with Hyaluronidase Injections

Preeti Raghavan, Alexandra Gordon, Ryan Roemmich, and Antonio Stecco

Correction to:
P. Raghavan (ed.), *Spasticity and Muscle Stiffness*,
https://doi.org/10.1007/978-3-030-96900-4_13

This book was inadvertently published with incorrect affiliation of Alexandra Gordon in Chapter 13 and in the contributors list. The initially published version has now been corrected as follows:

Albert Einstein College of Medicine, Bronx, NY, USA

The updated original version of this chapter can be found at https://doi.org/10.1007/978-3-030-96900-4_13

P. Raghavan (ed.), *Spasticity and Muscle Stiffness*,
https://doi.org/10.1007/978-3-030-96900-4_15

Index

P. Raghavan (ed.), *Spasticity and Muscle Stiffness*,
https://doi.org/10.1007/978-3-030-96900-4

MIX
Papier aus verantwortungsvollen Quellen
Paper from responsible sources
FSC® C105338

If you have any concerns about our products,
you can contact us on
ProductSafety@springernature.com

In case Publisher is established outside the EU,
the EU authorized representative is:
Springer Nature Customer Service Center GmbH
Europaplatz 3, 69115 Heidelberg, Germany

Printed by Libri Plureos GmbH
in Hamburg, Germany